How To
Look Great
& Feel Sexy!

Revitalize Your Energy in 9 Days

By Nick Delgado M.S., Ph.D.

Published by: Dr. Nick Delgado
25422 Trabuco Road #105-141
Lake Forest, CA 92630 U.S.A.
800-631-0232
E-mail: NickDelgado@msn.com

All rights reserved. No part of this book may be reproduced or transmitted in any form or by any means, electronic or mechanical, including photocopying, recording or by any information storage and retrieval system without written permission from the author, except for the inclusion of brief quotations in a review.

Copyright 1997 and 1992
by Nick Delgado
First Printing 1992
second Printing 1997 revised

ISBN 1-879084-04-X $31.95

Table of Contents

ABOUT THE AUTHOR

More than 20 years ago, Nick Delgado was 50 lbs. overweight, had high blood pressure and was considered clinically obese. In his search for a solution to his own health problems, he discovered that the best approach was a unique nutrition and exercise program. Following this approach he lost 50 lbs. of unwanted fat and reduced his blood pressure and cholesterol to safe levels permanently. Nick was awarded a full State and University scholastic scholarship to the University of Southern California, where he received a B.A. in Psychology in 1977. He completed six months of Master's work in Physical Therapy at USC's Rancho Los Amigos Hospital in 1977. He went to Loma Linda University in 1982, where he was accepted into their Health Science program as a Masters and Doctoral candidate. Nick worked with the Nathan Pritikin Longevity Center in Santa Monica, California as Director of the Pritikin Better Health Program presenting education conferences and scientific studies from 1979-1981. Since then, Nick has professionally conducted 3,200 seminars, workshops and conventions from 1979-1997. Topics have included stress and weight reduction, nutrition, exercise, prevention of disease, quality health and happiness.

Nick Delgado, founder and Director of Healthy Studios, Inc. now offers a mobile screening program for companies of any size where you will learn revealing facts about how to improve your health and he makes guest appearances regularly on radio and television programs.

Nick's goal is to establish health education programs nationally and internationally and in the process help everyone become as healthy and happy as they can be.

FOREWARD

Good health is our birthright. We should live our years actively, in lean, light bodies, with abundant energy, flexibility and muscular strength throughout our life span. Along with sensible exercise and emotional happiness, proper diet is essential in creating a state of vibrant health. Fortunately, much progress has been made towards knowing what constitutes ideal nutritional choices - a most excellent presentation of that knowledge is in your hands, right now. In "*How to Look Great & Feel Sexy*", Dr. Delgado has assembled the best medical and nutritional opinion, plus the fruits of his own vast experience in nutritional counseling, to create a superb, common-sense guide to optimal nutrition through healthful (and delicious!) food choices.

The guidelines presented in this book are based upon sound nutritional science and clinical experience, and reflect the growing awareness that an evolution past our current, high fat, low fiber, animal-based diet is essential if we are to create optimum health. Numerous medical studies now show that common maladies that plague our society - heart disease, high blood pressure, obesity, adult-onset diabetes, gout and other forms of inflammatory joint disease, and other degenerative conditions - are commonly prevented and often improved or actually cured by eating in the dietary style described in the pages to follow.

The human body has absolutely no requirement for the flesh of animals, nor for the milk of cows - and actually functions superbly without these cholesterol-laden, artery-clogging substances. All the protein, vitamins and other nutrients required for human health are abundantly found in the delicious grains, legumes, fruits, vegetables, seeds and other bountiful plants given to us by the Earth - the foundation of **The Delgado Health Plan**.

In "*How to Look Great & Feel Sexy*", Nick Delgado presents sound and practical advice for implementing healthful eating into a busy daily life. Far from a "diet of deprivation," the wonderful ethnic and other cuisines from which these foods are prepared provide a constant parade of taste delights, that are easy to make and satisfying to enjoy. "*How to Look Great & Feel Sexy*" and the life-affirming dining style it presents, is a gateway to glowing health, and great eating. I recommend it most highly.

Michael Klaper, M.D.

i

This book represents the "state-of-the-art" in dietary management of health preservation and disease avoidance (and reversal). Dr. Delgado has taken the principles of diet and exercise fostered by his predecessors and adapted them into a daily living program that is easy, practical and toothsome! This program was formulated with the busy person in mind. Unlike many other books on nutrition, recommendations for food additives, and other artificial remedies, is kept to a minimum. In addition, no guarantees are made for this program - other than optimal nutritional health.

I heartily recommend this book to anyone who is truly serious about preserving health and longevity!

Joseph T. Broderick, MD
Diplomate, American Board
of Internal Medicine

A WEIGHT LOSS AND HEALTH PLAN WITH GREAT TASTE

The second section of the book has tasty recipes that are zero cholesterol, low fat, low salt, low sugar and ideally balanced in protein. The utilization of the book can help you reduce the risk of health problems like high cholesterol, hypertension, adult onset diabetes, hardening of the arteries, some types of cancer of the breast and colon, certain forms of arthritis and digestive disorders. **The Delgado Program** is a natural approach using nutrition and exercise, without any drugs and free of surgery.

If you want fast weight loss, then select the recipes labeled as such, these are highest in water content and lowest in food density, such as soups, salads, fruits, and vegetable dishes. As you approach your ideal weight, you will need to start eating foods that are lower in water content and higher in food density, such as grains, pastas, rice, breads, beans and sweet potatoes.

All of the recipes in this book are low in fat, sugar and salt. These foods are high in fiber, vitamins and minerals. Your whole family can benefit from following this nutritional balance plan.

We have purposely designed our recipes without any meat, dairy products or oil for six primary reasons.

1. Meat, chicken, fish, turkey and dairy products contain cholesterol which clogs arteries. Any food that has legs, wings, a tail or that could wiggle or move has cholesterol in it.
2. Dairy products are the leading cause of food allergies.
3. Meat, dairy products and oils are devoid of fiber, which leads to digestive disease.
4. Meat, dairy products and oils are more concentrated in pesticides, chemicals and hormones than any other food group.
5. Meat, dairy products and oils are higher in fats than all other foods. Excess fats are associated with obesity, cancer, high blood pressure, diabetes and arthritis.
6. Meat and dairy products are too high in protein, which is the major cause of osteoporosis and kidney damage.

The recipe section of this book contains virtually no meat or dairy products. You can avoid meat and dairy products for the reasons listed above, and you will feel the greatest you ever have. If you add meat or dairy products to any of these recipes, it should only be on a limited basis, and certainly not for every meal. A safe level of use would be less than two or three times a week.

As you eat less fat and more natural foods, you will notice a need to eat a larger volume of food, along with additional in-between snacks. This is because complex carbohydrates digest at a faster rate than fatty foods. This is a good sign that you're following the plan correctly. Dr. Delgado conceived this rejuvenating, and amazingly successful program that has helped literally thousands of people.

Nick Delgado also offers cassette tapes, CD-ROMs, books and video tapes on health and nutrition for additional support. Please see the end of the book for further detail.

For more information, requests or brochure, call **Healthy Studios** at **800-631-0232**; NickDelgado@msn.com (E-Mail)

COLLEN GRAJEDA, "I lost 42 pounds in four months and I have maintained my new ideal weight for eight years. I lost all the excess fat from my hips and thighs. This is the only program that works for me because it is a way of eating good for life, and not a fad liquid diet. It's easy to follow the Delgado Plan for a lifetime."

JOAN POLLACK, "Most expertly presented program on health and nutrition I have ever attended. Dr. Delgado, teacher and founder of Healthy Studios, teaches and inspires one to study and practice good nutrition. His recipes in this book are terrific! Everyone should have this book for a lifetime of reference and use."

BOB WEILAND, "The Delgado Plan helped me reduce my weight of 242 pounds down to 130 pounds, a loss of 112 pounds in only nine months. My cholesterol dropped from over 300 mg. to 130 mg. Your plan helped me to have the energy to complete the walk across America - 2,994 miles - on my hands (Bob is a double amputee) in 3 ½ years, ending in a meeting with President Ronald Reagan, July 7, 1986."

WALT HERD, "I have a great feeling of excitement and accomplishment since starting the program. I started your program right after the results of my blood test came in. The results revealed a cholesterol level of 242, exactly 100 points higher than it should be for my age. This frightened me into action because my father had just had a seven-way - yes, 7-way bypass operation and in no way was I interested in being in that position in my future. So, in earnest I followed your program and in seven weeks my cholesterol was reduced to 144. AND I FEEL GREAT ABOUT IT!"

RICHARD DOLGENOW, "I lost 40 pounds. I have lost six inches in the waist, going from 38 to 32; dropped my cholesterol from 205 to 130. Not one day goes by without someone coming up to me, to tell me how good I look and asked me how I did it. I had stomach problems, headaches, hurt all over my body and felt very low about myself. In just a few months, many good things have happened to me. Many new friends. I feel like 18 and people say I look like 35 and I will be 50 in January. The only thing that I regret is that I do not have a before picture. I really did not believe this program would work. With all the odds, people at first poking fun at me, people pushing the wrong type of foods at me, and making me feel like a fool, I held with the program and won. Thank You."

HAROLD E. KIMZEY, "Now in my early 60's, I was 60 to 70 pounds overweight and a borderline diabetic. I had high blood pressure, high triglycerides and suffered from irregularity of my bowels. In the short time that I've been with the Delgado Program, I've found that my blood pressure is returning to normal, my triglycerides are coming down, I am no longer diabetic, I have regular bowel movements and I've lost 20 pounds. Also, my energy level has increased and I'm aware of a keener sense of wellbeing. With a record like that, it's difficult to say just what I like about Delgado best. I am on a diet that is working and I'm NEVER hungry. The food that I eat is good (and quite normal) and I can have it in quantity. Who can beat that?"

1

Fountain of Youth
by Nick Delgado, Ph.D.

Director, **Healthy Studios**
25422 Trabuco Road, #105-141
Lake Forest CA 92630
800-631-0232

Anti-aging, preserving our youth and reverse aging is a hot topic because it affects all of us. The people most interested in looking and feeling younger represent a growing segment of "Baby Boomers" past the age of 35. Visit a retirement home or convalescent hospital and you will see the ravages of aging in our senior citizens. By the year 2030 we will have 52 million Americans past the age of 70.

Some people age more rapidly than others, because of a breakdown in our body's aging clock. Our organs age, shrink in size and produce fewer hormones. This reduction in available hormones leads to a slow deterioration of all of our vital body systems. The declines in the Immune system, Reproductive, Neurological, Metabolic and Circulatory systems, cause us to look and feel old.

I have spent over twenty years studying aging, nutrition, exercise physiology and reviewing medical research. I reviewed over 250,000 reports and lectured with Nathan Pritikin of the Pritikin Longevity Center. I conducted tests on over 10,000 participants at Mastery University events with Tony Robbins. I believe that you can remain physically and emotionally strong with advanced age.

We have all heard about the need to consume healthy foods and supplements. We know about the benefits of exercise. My experience as a seminar speaker, TV and radio talk show host shows me that only about 10% of the people follow a good lifestyle plan. Some people are confused and they make the excuse they do not have the time or money necessary to do independent research to know which is the best program for them. How can we help the other 90% that are in need of help and how can we improve the performance of the 10% interested in outstanding results? People want a simplified and practical program that I call the "Fountain of Youth".

The "Fountain of Youth" involves understanding the aging process. There are eight critical hormones that decrease as we grow older causing us to age rapidly. Reversing the clock is a matter of simply restoring these eight hormones to your youthful levels. I have seen numerous examples of people looking and feeling ten to twenty years younger within only ninety days.

The first critical hormone which controls several other important hormones is called **DHEA**-dehydroepiandrosterone (De-hydro-epi-an-DROS-ter-own). DHEA is a hormone that can be transformed into almost any other hormone as the body needs it. DHEA is concentrated in the brain six times more than in any other tissue or organ. Humans produce the largest amount of DHEA as compared to other primates or other animals. Every tissue of the human body has enzymes necessary for the metabolism of DHEA. DHEA is produced in the adrenals, ovaries, testicles and brain.

Dr. Cranton M.D. has been carefully monitoring patients on small amounts of DHEA for over five years. He gave the example of a forty one year old man who had low levels for his age. After a few months on DHEA, his blood levels of DHEA were restored to youthful levels. He noticed his energy level was markedly higher. His skin was thicker and moister, and he was sleeping six and a half hours a night instead of eight and waking rested. He felt six or seven years younger, his sex drive increased significantly, and he said, "When you're on DHEA, it feels as if every cell in your body is just humming."

A female patient with Asthma experienced astonishing results, she said, "Within an hour after taking my first capsule of DHEA, I suddenly found I could breathe again. That month my periods, which had been irregular, went back to normal-I was on my old regular twenty-seven day cycle-and my headaches disappeared. My depression lifted within the first few days. Two months after I started DHEA I joined a dance class. It had always been a childhood dream to dance. I feel like a teenager, as if I were renewing myself."

Dr. Yen reported in the Journal of Clinical Endocrinology and Metabolism 1994 giving men and women age 40 to 70 years old, DHEA (50 mg taken orally) at bedtime for 6 months. In two weeks the blood levels of DHEA were restored to youthful levels (double blind, placebo cross-over study). There was a remarkable increase in perceived physical and psychological well-being in 67% of the men and 84% of the women. The participants said they slept better, had more energy, handled stress better, with no side effects. DHEA helps maintain the immune system, providing a protein sparing effect while improving glucose levels.

DHEA decreases abnormal platelet aggregation and LDL ("bad") cholesterol levels. This reduces the risk of heart attacks and stroke. DHEA enhances the immune system and the thymus gland, reduces the rate of infection, Epstein Barr, Lupus, herpes and cancer. DHEA reduces the stress hormone cortisol and helps offset caffeine and the catabolic effects of exercise. DHEA increases serotonin naturally, which decreases food consumption and helps speed weight loss.

People taking higher amounts of DHEA (1,500 mg per day) for 28 days have reduced body fat by as much as 31% with an equal gain in muscle mass, and no loss of weight. DHEA helps to burn excess calories instead of storing glycogen. Obese people tend to have higher insulin levels. DHEA helps to lower insulin levels by pushing glucose into your cells to be burned. DHEA helps reduce appetite by creating a feeling of "fullness".

DHEA has many of the benefits of estrogen, with little or no side effects. It helps women with vaginal atrophy to stimulate the cellular growth of the vaginal wall, increased vaginal secretion, thus restoring the vagina to its youthful condition. Studies on female cancer patients that had ovaries removed reported little or no change in sex drive. The ovaries produce estrogen and testosterone. However, after removal of the Adrenal glands, the site of DHEA production, four out five women experienced a total loss of sexual desire and responsiveness. A combination of DHEA and Free Testosterone are the most important hormones for sexual interest and desire in women.

DHEA produces the pheromones that emit our scent through the skin. Pheromones act on our brain to receive the scent of the opposite sex. It may influence our choice of mate, if we become pregnant, and the bonding with our babies. DHEA is produced by the fetus two hundred to eight hundred times higher than the levels of progesterone, testosterone, and estrogen.

This tremendous amount of DHEA present during youth has intrigued longevity researchers. DHEA drops to near zero in all people at death. Will we prolong life an additional ten or twenty years if we take supplements of DHEA to maintain youthful levels? Studies show that an increase in blood levels of DHEA sulfate is associated with a 36% less mortality rate from any cause.

DHEA precursors do not convert very well into DHEA, so I prefer to use the actual DHEA grade.

DHEA declines from heavy alcohol drinking, birth control pills, stress, hypothyroidism, lack of exercise and obesity. More is not necessarily better in the case of hormone replacement. High dosages of DHEA (1,600 mg a day) can cause acne, unwanted hair growth, irritability, headaches, and rapid heart beat. If you are having any side effects, reduce the dosage gradually down to lower intakes. Have your DHEA levels checked by saliva tests to monitor your progress and maintain ideal levels.

Stay within the safe guidelines for anti-aging of 25 mg a night for women and 25 mg morning and night for men. Some people need up to 100 mg of DHEA a day to reach ideal levels. The goal is to bring DHEA sulfate and Free DHEA combined up to youthful levels of a person aged 20 to 25. Blood tests for serum DHEA goal is 300-400 mg/dl for women and 450-600 mg/dl for men. Ideal levels for DHEA (Free unbound) is 700-1200 ng/dl for men and 450-800 ng/dl for women. Saliva DHEA for men is 10.9-16.9 Nmol/L or 200-300 pg/ml and for women 7.2-8.5 Nmol/L or 125-170 pg/ml. DHEA is available as capsules, tablets, liquid sublingual under the tongue or transdermal cream applied to the skin.

The next critical hormone that slows aging is **testosterone**. Free & total testosterone are found naturally circulating in the bloodstream of baby boys creating the male testes and penis. Small amounts of testosterone produced in women's ovaries and adrenals provide energy, libido and a feeling of well being. Young teenagers and adult men have large increases in free testosterone followed by a gradual decrease after age 30. Free testosterone becomes bound and unusable as we age by Sex Hormone Binding Globulin (SHBG).

A 73 year old Doctor said, "I take testosterone because I want to feel the same way I did when I was in my prime. I want to have the same sexuality that I did when I was young. I want to maintain my muscle strength. I want to feel vital. Testosterone makes it all possible."

Research during W.W.II on testosterone showed the powerful effect on the immune system. A physician transplanted testes from a dying soldier into the abdomen of a soldier suffering from gangrene caused by a gunshot wound. The soldier would have died, but the gangrene was cured following the transplant of the testes. In 1934 a scientist isolated the testosterone make up and received the Nobel Prize. Discoveries in 1951 reported that testosterone improves nitrogen balance, increases muscle mass and repairs damaged bones and ligaments.

In the 1960's it was discovered that testosterone lowers cholesterol, improves abnormal EKG's of cardiac patients, helps claudication (clogged leg arteries) and angina pectoris (chest pain) -clogged heart arteries. Free testosterone maintained at youthful levels protects men against atherosclerosis - hardening of the arteries. Testosterone also improves diabetic retinopathy, helping eye sight, lowers insulin requirements and enhances glucose tolerance of diabetic patients.

Testosterone decreases body fat, improves waist-to-hip ratio of fat and enhances lean body mass. It has a protective effect against auto immune diseases such as lupus and rheumatoid arthritis. Studies show that men with high testosterone levels live longer, healthier lives and maintain sexual potency. Men over 50 years old with low testosterone levels, in a double blind, placebo-controlled study, were given either replacement testosterone for 90 days or a placebo. They found the hormone renewed strength, improved balance and increased libido. Restoring testosterone increased red blood cell count, lowered LDL ("bad") cholesterol and enhanced feelings of well-being.

In July 1996 New England Journal of Medicine researchers discovered that testosterone significantly enhanced muscle size and reduced body fat even in men who do not exercise or go on a diet. Three groups of male weight lifters did the same exercise or no exercise. The men were given testosterone or placebo every week for ten weeks. The men given testosterone had much more muscle whether or not they exercised.

The American Journal of Physiology reported in men age 67 after only 4 weeks with the addition of testosterone an increase in leg muscle strength and restored muscle size. In another study at the University of Washington, men past the age of 60 who were given testosterone for three months lost fat and gained muscle without going on a diet!

Crossover studies where the placebo group was given testosterone, and the group given testosterone was taken off, men reported being more aggressive and energetic at work. The men with normalized testosterone levels found that their relationships improved with their wives because of better sexual performance, initiation of sexual intercourse and increased ability to maintain an erection.

In older men, ages 31 to 80, high levels of Sex Hormone Binding Globulin reduced free testosterone in 74% of the men complaining of sexual dysfunction. Nearly 80% of the men had a reduction in libido (interest in sex), difficulty in getting or maintaining an erection, rarely had early morning erections and 92% experienced a reduction in sexual satisfaction.

In addition, these men with low free testosterone levels reported fatigue, depression, irritability, aches, pains and stiffness. A significant drop in free testosterone can occur as early as age 40. At age 60, 18% of men are impotent and at age 80, 75% are impotent. Once a man becomes impotent he loses his drive for life, has impaired erections, his muscles become thinner, he becomes depressed and mental acuity fades.

All healthy males get erections, mostly during the REM dream stage of sleep every night without exception. These erections are not stimulated or associated with the content of dreams. The penis of a medically fit man erects more than 100 times a night! Erections occur in cycles lasting about 30 minutes, although the penis is not fully erect the entire time.

If a man wakes up in the middle of the night with an erection this is a normal healthy sign. If he gets an erection early in the morning, he can rest assured that his penis is in good working order. If he is not having good erections during sex, any difficulty is probably psychological. That is assuming random erections occur. You can do a simple test using postage stamps to test for erections. Take a roll of postage stamps and wrap it around the flaccid penis before sleep. If the perforations between the stamps tear by morning, then the man had an erection during the night. If no erection, then the problem is organic and physical.

The following three tests can determine what type of organic problem exists.

1. Vascular disorders are the most common causes of penile erection dysfunction. High cholesterol levels will clog arteries that bring blood to the penis or by leaks in the venous system that result when the blood in the shaft of the penis drains out prematurely. A doctor can use one simple injection of vasoactive drugs (Papaverine or Prostaglandin-E) to determine whether the arterial system is intact. The drug produces an immediate erection in healthy men regardless of the mental factor. The penis either gets hard or it does not. If it does not, then you need to clean the arteries. Change to a cholesterol free vegetarian diet, take soluble fibers, reduce alcohol, stop smoking, especially before sex, increase free testosterone to reduce atherosclerosis and see a doctor for treatment.
2. The test for neurological problems is performed by inserting a gloved-finger one inch into the man's anus, to feel the sphincter muscle and with the other hand gently squeezing the tip of the penis. If the nerves to the penis are working properly, squeezing the tip of the penis will cause the anal sphincter to contract firmly against the finger.

3. Hormonal disorders are the third common cause of erection failure. Diabetes, overactive or under-active thyroid and low growth hormone levels can cause erection failure. Lack of testosterone can also cause erection failure. These hormone disorders can be tested by saliva or blood. Restoring hormone levels to normal levels can solve these erection problems.

The herbs Avena Sativa (Green Oats), Nettles and Saw Palmetto can restore free testosterone to the youthful range for men and women. One gram per day of the B-Vitamin niacin also reportedly helps lower Sex Hormone Binding Globulin and releases the free testosterone. Another supplement, Testron SX, and the mineral zinc, has been reported to increase natural testosterone production. Testron SX also helps keep DHT (dihydrotestosterone) in a free state, non binding. In most people, the natural herbs and vitamins restore youthful levels. In some people, replacement therapy with gel or transdermal testosterone may be necessary. This can improve the quality of life for adults.

Salivary testosterone levels ideal for men is 200 to 400 pmol/L. Men with saliva levels under 120 pmol/L can benefit from supplements. Free testosterone blood levels for men should be 19 to 40 pg/ml. Men with low levels of 1 to 9 pg/ml will benefit from supplement therapy. Ideal **blood** levels for total testosterone for men is 500 to 1200 ng/dl (nanograms per deciliter). Men with low levels of less than 400 ng/dl bearing watching and under 250 ng/dl need treatment. If you restore these low testosterone levels to what they should be you may feel like you were 25 years old again! By the age of 30 free testosterone levels start to drop gradually with age. Have your level checked with a simple saliva test.

Ideal range for women **salivary** testosterone is 80 to 155 pmol/L. **Blood** tests for free testosterone during ovulation, age 20 to 29 is .9 to 3.9 ng/ml, and total testosterone levels of 16 to 100 ng/dl. This is the time when women are most fertile. Past the age of 50, post menopausal women have their lowest blood levels of free testosterone at .3 to 2.7 pg/ml. Past the age of 40, menopausal women's total testosterone levels can drop to zero to 64 ng/dl.

It is best to stay in the youthful range, not too low or too high. Excessive levels of testosterone in women can occur from ovarian or adrenal disorders or excessive dosages of supplements leading to acne, increased body hair growth, deepening of the voice or balding.

The combination of bound and free testosterone is total testosterone. Doctors mistakenly usually only check total testosterone. Yet it is the free testosterone that is the only biologically active part from a health and sexual point of view. Even if an adult has total testosterone levels above normal, but has below-normal free testosterone, your sex drive will probably be sluggish and nonexistent. Think of free testosterone as the only active part with high impact on your health.

Saliva tests for free testosterone and DHEA can be provided by contacting us at Healthy Studios, 800-631-0232. We can provide you a test kit that you send back with a fee to have your level of free testosterone and DHEA checked. Saliva tests are easy to collect and mail to the laboratory without involving clinic staff, no biohazard, no mess, no blood, very convenient and economical.

Saliva tests are accurate with over a 90% correlation to blood tests results. Saliva tests can measure the effects of supplements better than blood, because spinning blood separates out cells that may have 75% of the hormones. Your supplements for testosterone or DHEA may be working, but blood tests may not pick up the improvements as well as Saliva tests. Saliva tests pick up the full tissue levels for hormones. We can measure other important hormones in saliva including melatonin, estradiol, progesterone and cortisol.

Testosterone, estrogen, progesterone and melatonin are cyclic, going up and down throughout the day, night and month. Saliva tests for free testosterone are performed with three samples taken morning, afternoon and late night. A man's testosterone level is highest in the morning. The levels change every 15 minutes. Testosterone can vary by 100 ng (serum) or more with variations from day to day by as much as 50%. By taking a series of samples we can accurately track the average range and a doctor can determine if you need replacement therapy.

DHEA sulfate is very stable with very little change in levels from day to day. A single saliva test for DHEA can tell us if your levels are below ideal. We need to take supplements of DHEA to prevent the decline associated with aging. The addition of DHEA can convert into the necessary testosterone as the body needs. The DHEA and herbs like Avena Sativa may completely restore the free and total testosterone to normal levels in most of the cases. However, if it doesn't normalize your testosterone levels then see your doctor for a prescription of testosterone patch or gel to solve the problem.

Surprisingly it takes very small amounts of testosterone to physically maintain an erection and enjoy sex. The problem is that a man low in testosterone may simply not care enough to pursue it. Once testosterone levels are replenished a man will find that he has recaptured a healthy interest in sex. Men have went from zero libido to a vigorous sex life within ten days.

The saying, "if you don't use it you lose it" applies with testosterone. Frequency of sex increases testosterone in both male and females after sex. Salivary testosterone concentrations were measured in a study of four couples on a total of eleven evenings before and after sexual intercourse and eleven evenings when there was no intercourse. Testosterone increased in men and women when there was intercourse and decreased when there was none. Your relationship plays a meaningful role in immunity, health and longevity.

Women during menopause who have tried hormone replacement with estrogen and progesterone are starting to be given a small amount of testosterone which replenishes energy, libido and feeling good again. Remember, women need testosterone to be healthy maintain strong bones and proper balance.

Testosterone is the ultimate aphrodisiac. Testosterone along with DHEA is responsible for the sex drive of both men and women; stimulating our desire for sexual activity and orgasm. It is testosterone, not estrogen that causes the heightened erotic sensitivity of the clitoris, breasts, and nipples. Testosterone encourages a woman to go after a man. She becomes more sexual, more responsive and more assertive. It does not influence the frequency of intercourse. Testosterone improves self-confidence and serves as an antidepressant in women.

Testosterone is regulated by **LHRH**-(Luteinizing Hormone Releasing Hormone), the director of testosterone. **PEA**-(phenylethylamine) is the hormone that releases when you see someone you're interested in causing attraction to the opposite sex. DHEA contributes to the sex drive in both men and women, increasing your libido by sensitizing your erogenous zones to touch and promoting positive sexual scents called **pheromones**. **Dopamine** increases our receptivity to pleasure. High **serotonin** levels reduce our interest in sex and inhibits orgasm in both sexes. Low serotonin levels caused by diet pills can increase aggression and excessive sexual aberrations.

Estrogen is a warm, receptive, willing, passive and seductive hormone. Progesterone and prolactin are nurturer hormones, reducing sex drive. Oxytocin increases during touch creating bonding and a feeling of love. Vasopressin is a peptide like hormone that bonds and enhances parenting feelings.

Another critical hormone that decreases with age is progesterone. The use of natural progesterone from wild yam is a better choice in place of synthetic progesterone like Progestins or Provera. Many women feel remarkable better using the natural cream or transdermal form of natural progesterone. Natural progesterone increases bone density preventing osteoporosis.

For years doctors have known about the need to replace estrogen in women after menopause. However, synthetic hormones caused many women to stop their prescription because of side effects. By using natural Es Gen Cream, Pro Estron™ plant supplements, Estraderm skin patch, Estrace tablets, and vaginal cream you can avoid the usual side affects of synthetic hormones. Synthetic estrogen know as Premarin can cause irritability, fluid retention, and breast tenderness. You gain all the benefits using natural estrogen such as reduced hot flashes, night sweats, better memory, alertness, and reduced aging of the skin. Natural hormones may also reduce the incidence of Alzheimer's disease, heart disease, and colon cancer.

More and more doctors are starting to ignore advertisements to use synthetic hormones by pharmaceutical companies and they are allowing their patients the safer alternative of hormones derived from plants, wild yams or soy products.

Another anti aging hormone to monitor includes thyroid. If your thyroid level is low try taking supplements of desiccated thyroid. This is a natural form providing T3 and T4 that is more like that which the thyroid gland produces. People will feel better on it. Also be sure to use kelp for the iodine necessary for thyroid metabolism.

Thyroid & Thyroid Stimulating Hormone TSH benefits include:
- Improved sex drive, energy, less fatigue, move faster, stronger
- Less colds, viruses, respiratory ailments, better breathing
- Warm hands & feet, stronger heart pump action
- Less muscle cramps, reduced low back pain, stiff joints, arthritis
- Prevent bruising, less dry skin & leathery skin, avoid brittle nails, hair loss
- Ideal thyroid levels help mental acuity, improve memory, less emotional crying, upset
- Reduce Atherosclerosis, less headaches

Pregnenolone is another important hormone that is key to keeping our brains functioning at peak capacity. It is a potent memory enhancer that improves concentration, fights mental fatigue, depression and reduces arthritis. Pregnenolone is produced from cholesterol. DHEA, testosterone, and estrogen are also made from cholesterol. Low cholesterol levels will not interfere with the maintenance of proper normal levels. However, as we age the ability to convert cholesterol to proper hormonal levels is a problem. Take supplements providing 50 mg per day to replace what you need to restore your levels. Pregnenolone adult blood levels should range between 50 to 350 ug/ml.

A startling experiment on anti-aging demonstrated the power of **melatonin**, the actual hormone that controls the aging clock. The scientists transplanted the pineal gland from old mice into the young mice. They took the pineal gland from the young mice and transplanted it into the old mice. Melatonin is released in smaller quantities from the pineal gland as we age. The transformation was incredible! The older mice looked younger, with rejuvenated bodies. They were more active with a 30% extension in life span. The young mice with the old pineal gland aged rapidly and died 30% sooner than normal. The aging clock had finally unlocked the mysterious mechanism that determines not only how we age but why we age.

The pineal gland in humans also sends out a message through melatonin to preserve the organs and the body in a healthy state. As we age, we must replace the dwindling melatonin to continue to preserve youth. It's best to take very small amounts of melatonin of one half mg to five mg a night sublingual, dissolved under the tongue before you go to sleep. Increase gradually, so that you awaken in the morning alert and rested. If you awaken groggy, reduce the dosage back down by one half milligram increments. Melatonin acts like a natural sleeping pill, enhancing REM dream sleep. Melatonin reduces jet lag, and resets the biological clock.

In a marriage, day people and night people can learn to match their schedule using melatonin. The person that tends to stay up late can take Melatonin at the time their spouse wants to go to sleep.

Melatonin has other benefits. It is a free radical scavenger serving as an antioxidant inside the cells. It lowers cholesterol, heart disease, and cataracts. It may help Parkinson's disease, Alzheimer's and asthma and keep you young, vigorous and sexually rejuvenated.

Another hormone that declines with age is **Human Growth Hormone** (HGH). In senior citizens the use of homopathic **Insulin Like Growth Factor** (IGF-1) can turn the clock back because the function of HGH is restored.

At this time, studies by Dr. Yen suggest that we may replace some of the drop in Human Growth Hormone with DHEA. There was a 10% increase in Insulin Like Growth Factor (IGF-1) levels and a 19% decline in Binding Protein (IGFBP-1) creating a 50% ratio improvement. This was the benefit of taking 50 mg of DHEA nightly for six months.

William Regelson M.D., age 71, has been taking 50 mg of DHEA everyday and one-tenth of a milligram of melatonin every night for eleven years. "I feel the difference. We need to treat aging as a disease, not just an irreversible condition." Dr. Regelson is a researcher at the Medical College of Virginia in Richmond.

Dr. Cranton M.D., told the story of a man age 72 years old who felt as if his life was winding down. He had no energy, reduced muscle tone, and he was falling asleep while driving. After eight months of hormone replacement he no longer needs as much sleep and he does not fall asleep while driving. The muscles in his legs and arms are strong and hardening. Now he runs up the steps in his house "as if I were twenty years younger. I thought my life was almost over, but now I'm planning to go on to one hundred ."

Now that you have learned about the latest research on anti-aging and hormone replacement let's not forget the important principals of healthy eating. People who want to look and feel great will do the following. I encourage the use of whole food concentrates, antioxidant's vitamin A, E, C, B complex and whole food origins for minerals. Eat as much raw food as possible in the form of vegetables, fruit, sprouted seeds, sprouted beans and sprouted grains. I use a Vita-mix whole foods machine to blend whole vegetables and fruit, retaining the fiber and all the vitamins, minerals and organic pure water. Use gluten and soy replacements for meat and rice milk for dairy product substitutes. Frequently nibble small meals, whenever you feel empty or hungry.

Exercise and activity has also been proven to reverse and slow aging. By following the Fountain of Youth hormone replacement program you will have more energy to be able to workout with weights and do aerobics at least three times a week. Be physical and active. Enjoy holding, hugs, kisses and intimacy. Physical activity and intimacy will also increase your natural hormone production.

What can you expect from the Fountain of Youth program? After only nine days most people will notice an improvement in energy levels, mental abilities, sleep habits, and sexual energy. After 90 days the fat on your body will begin to melt away using only natural approaches to enhance your body's proper metabolic levels. Your new Fountain of Youth habits will allow you to look and feel years younger. Your family and friends will notice the transformation and ask you what you have done.

What will you be like five or ten years from now if you do not even try the program? Can you afford to wait until it is almost too late? Can you see yourself looking and feeling better than you have in years? How will the Fountain of Youth plan help your career, relationships and feeling of well-being?

You do have a choice. You could choose to do nothing and continue to do what you have been doing. Will you be happy with the rate at which you are aging? Is it worth the risk of illness, pain of degeneration and loss of function? You could try the Fountain of Youth program for just 90 days. If you follow the plan as I have explained it you will get tremendous results. The older you are the more dramatic the results will be, and the closer you are to age 30 the better you will preserve yourself.

How to Look Great & Feel Sexy

2

Feed Your Hunger - The Easy Solution

Do you want to eat delicious foods (Italian, Mexican, Chinese and American), enjoy frequent meals without hunger, increase your energy and look fit for a lifetime? To have constant energy and achieve your ideal weight, eat low fat foods just before you get hungry.

Anticipation of hunger is one of the keys to the success of **The Delgado Program**. It is very important you learn to eat more frequently. We tell our patients to eat just before they get hungry. Be sensitive to that earlier signal of weakness your body sends you about thirty minutes before hunger. It could be a feeling of slight weakness, distraction or an empty feeling in the stomach. On other diets, you're told to fight the natural urge of hunger. Then, finally you're so hungry you lose control and give in to the greasy temptations of our fast-paced environment.

Haven't you ever gone to the supermarket on an empty stomach and noticed how many fattening foods you bought? You know you should eat before going to the market. However, most dieters make a terrible mistake going to a restaurant or relatives house to eat when they're starved. Why not eat (fruits, vegetables or soups) before you go to a restaurant, a friends' or relatives' house for a meal? In this way you will be in control to avoid temptations and make better food choices.

Why do you think fast food restaurants are so successful? Have you noticed how liquor stores and markets have two thirds of the cash register area filled with candy and snacks? We have discovered your only protection from this powerful temptation, to control temptation, is simply to anticipate your hunger. You must eat low calorie, high fiber foods the moment you feel a slight drop in energy or have an empty feeling in the stomach. When you're trying to lose weight, you have to eat a lot more fruits (three to eight pieces a day) and a lot more vegetables - up to four pounds worth (raw, cooked, steamed, microwaved or in soups). Vegetables and fruits are high in water content, so you won't have to drink eight glasses of water a day. Two to four glasses would be sufficient depending on how much you exercise. Many overweight people fear overeating. On **The Delgado Plan**, a compulsive eater can "overeat" fruits, vegetables, soups and salads and still lose weight. For example, if you consumed four pounds of vegetables and fruit in a day, you would have taken in an average of only 550 calories. There would have been no room left for the fattening foods like meat, cheese, milk, eggs and oils.

An experiment was conducted requiring the participants to eat ten potatoes a day. They could eat anything else, as long as they ate the ten potatoes first (potatoes have only 69 calories each x 10 = 690 calories). The participants all lost fat weight during the three month experiment. There was little room for any other food! Of course, **The Delgado Plan** encourages you to eat a variety of natural foods, not just potatoes. **The Delgado Plan** will work best if you don't smother your vegetables with fatty, oily dressings and cheese.

Veggies and fruits are so low in calories that they are actually digested within 15 to 45 minutes (the initial absorption of most of the glucose). This means the next meal should be every 15 to 30 minutes to get sufficient glucose and rarely longer than 90 minutes in between. You must learn to eat the moment you feel empty, weak, or slightly hungry. That is the signal from your body that your glucose level has begun to drop. The signal to eat will vary by how much and what kind of food you ate at your previous meal or snack. The constant presence of glucose will allow your body to burn fat consistently.

The Krebs cycle is a complex biochemical energy-producing process during which your body must have glucose to burn fat. Glucose is very important to the production of energy. If you don't eat complex carbohydrates to get the precise amount of glucose needed your body will actually break down amino acid (body protein from muscle and organs as a last resort) into glucose to get the necessary amount. Your body cannot convert fat into glucose quick enough to meet the body's needs. This is why foods high in complex carbohydrates are called "protein sparing foods". We spare the protein of the body by getting the glucose fuel we need from the food, allowing the protein to be used for its special purpose.

Complex carbohydrates should be eaten frequently to protect the body's stores of protein. Don't get the mistaken idea you need protein from meat and cheese when you feel weak (a common misconception). You are only in need of slightly more calories from complex carbohydrates with a greater food density, like grains. The lighter fruits and vegetables simply need to be eaten more often. Eating enough grains, breads, cereal and pastas will give you additional calories, strength and the necessary protein your body requires.

The Delgado Plan allows our bodies to continue to use mostly glucose, along with a constant attack focused on fat in the blood and the storage of fat in the cells.

The quickest way to burn fat is to eat vegetables and fruits approximately every thirty minutes. The frequency between nibbles depends on how you feel, how much activity you're involved with and how big you are. For example, a big, muscular man who is also overweight and doing heavy labor, will need a higher volume of low fat foods than a small lady, who is slightly overweight, working at a desk. The big man will need more food in his stomach to feel good and get through his workday without undue weakness or fatigue. The smaller woman will feel good eating smaller, less frequent meals. It may not be practical to eat as often as every fifteen to thirty minutes during certain times of the day. If this is the case, then eat more bread, cereals, grains or beans that can sustain you for one to two hours before your next meal.

For example, before a seminar, athletic event or a prolonged business meeting I eat a bowl of cereal or two vegetable sandwiches, or one or two bean burritos (without cheese). After the two hours, I return to eating vegetables and fruit for the rest of the day.

Your comfort zone of eating also must be considered. There may be times when you notice it's hard to eat enough fruits and vegetables to feel satisfied. You may start to feel too hungry, weak or bothered by having to eat so often. At that point you should eat grains, breads, pastas, cereals or beans. This will reduce the number of meals you have to eat for convenience sake and will provide a feeling of strength and satisfaction.

Be sure the food you eat has a rich nutritional value. Make calories count! Your body needs fiber, vitamins, minerals, glucose, fat, protein and water. Which food do you think is going to supply these nutritional needs? Liquid diet drinks, which are loaded with sugar, fructose, dairy whey, synthetic chemicals and processed protein? Certainly weight loss is best accomplished eating nature's balanced food supply of fruits, vegetables, grains and legumes that are rich in vitamins, minerals and fiber.

We've become a desperate society bent on self abuse and denial. People divert their attention from the need to eat properly by blaming the psychological aspects associated with overeating. Feelings of guilt arise from the resulting appearance of obesity caused by eating fatty foods. This vicious cycle of wanting to punish yourself through starvation for the "sin" of overeating can be broken by simply choosing to eat low fat, high fiber foods.

Follow the guidelines for **The Delgado Program**. Forget the out-dated "four food groups" and starvation diets. Reward yourself, don't punish yourself. You will be surprised at how great tasting fruits, vegetables and grains can be and what a wonderful reward it will be for you to nibble each hour or two. All people enjoy eating and **The Delgado Program** will satisfy that powerful urge of hunger. The weight loss you experience will astonish you.

Large servings of potatoes, fruits, vegetables and soups are satisfying foods that fill your stomach's four cup capacity. Compare this to very small servings of fatty foods that concentrate twice as many calories into your stomach. Your stomach sends signals to your brain when it's empty. Your stomach cannot tell the difference in calories; it can only report to the brain when it's empty. By eating frequent meals, eight or more nibblings per day, you will not have as much of a desire for sweets or fatty foods. You will gradually recondition yourself into this new way of eating on **The Delgado Plan** and become lean and fit for life.

The body panics when food isn't provided regularly and often "saves" calories by storing them as fat. Studies on food intake have shown you will lose weight more easily if you spread 1500 calories over eight or more meals per day, as compared to only three meals or less. Fewer calories are stored as fat when you nibble all day as compared to eating the same food consumed three times per day. Fasting, skipping meals or eating only one meal a day puts your body into a panic, increasing the output of certain hormones that encourage fat storage (adipocyte enzyme activity). You can control your body by eating when your stomach feels slightly empty, and you feel weak or hungry. Don't ever wait to eat until you're starved.

In the Oct. 5, 1989, New England Journal of Medicine, David Jenkins, M.D., and associates proved the superiority of the Delgado Way of frequent nibbling. People were given seventeen snacks a day, as compared to gorging on three meals per day on the same food. Several metabolic advantages were shown: The "frequent nibblers" experienced a significant reduction in cholesterol by as much as 10%, a 15% reduction in the "bad" LDL cholesterol, 30% less serum insulin output and 20% less output of C-peptide and cortisol in the urine. They also found the most effective diet in controlling lipids was the high carbohydrate, high fiber, low fat diet with 70% carbohydrate, 15% protein and 15% fat. In two weeks, the Delgado type of program lowered cholesterol down to an average of 189 mg. People eating three meals a day from the four food groups averaged a level of 244. This fattening Weight Watchers type diet is 33% fat, 15% protein and only 52% carbohydrate.

Increased meal frequency, with low fat, high fiber foods can reduce the rate of obesity in children and in adults. Stop discouraging your children from eating between meals and telling them it will spoil their dinner. We encourage you and your children to eat between meals. We want to stop the bad habit of eating three big meals per day and start eating lighter, more frequent meals. It won't work to eat candy, potato chips and soda pop between meals. Have bowls of cold fruit and veggies cut up in the refrigerator for the family. Each member of the family also should carry a food sack that we call the Delgado Cool Tote - (see next section) to work or school and nibble between breaks. The whole family can stay healthy, fit and trim.

How to Look Great & Feel Sexy

3

The Delgado Cool Tote

Most people who are unable to maintain high energy or lose weight rely on fatty foods, without fiber. Great health begins with selecting high energy, low fat foods. This idea will save you money and time as you lose weight and improve your health in the process. Almost every person following **The Delgado Health Plan** who has tried this easy technique described in this chapter has reported fantastic results within weeks. Are you interested? Consider the following:

When you go to work or leave your home for more than a few hours, there is a tendency to eat whatever is available - candy, doughnuts, fast burgers and fries. As protection from fats and sugars, I would like to tell you about the Delgado Cool Tote.

Every busy person will benefit from this simple idea if used daily. Let me explain how this works. Get yourself an insulated bag with blue ice (Delgado Cool Tote) designed to carry food. Then, once every three days (twice a week) go to the biggest produce market in your area, and buy a selection of your favorite veggies fruits and breads. Take the Delgado Cool Tote with you wherever you go (especially to work and keep it under your desk). You can nibble on low fat foods when you feel weak, empty or hungry.

The Delgado Cool Tote idea allows and encourages frequent snacks between meals. Frequent eating from the Cool Tote to overcome hunger, overeating and binging may sound like a contradiction; however, it is actually an easy solution. In a recent poll, it was shown most people snack on extremely high fat foods (ice cream, potato chips, doughnuts, candy and sodas) between or after meals. Our approach - eating tasty, low fat foods all day long - will protect you from giving in to eating the wrong foods.

I have been training and educating busy people to follow a low fat, nutritional program since 1978. I found many ways to help people to comply with and follow the program, but none as effective or long lasting as the Delgado Cool Tote. For three years I helped thousands of people to follow the plan, while I only told a handful of people about my special Cool Tote idea.

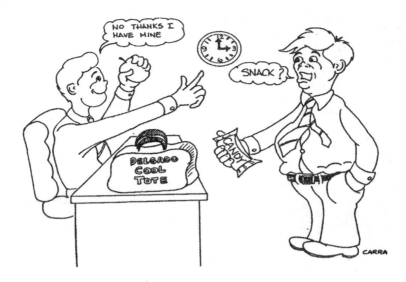

It was in early 1979 that I hired Bea (Delgado) Campbell (my mother), as a health educator. She spent countless hours with me learning the ideas, teaching students and working with me to help participants follow the program. By the end of 1979, I hired several health educators. I noticed they always followed the program better than anyone else, because they were required to prepare the foods for our food demonstration classes for as many as forty to one hundred people. The educators had to make five-course meals complete with soups, salads, whole grain breads, main dish casseroles and desserts at least four times a week. They were encouraged to eat the unopened, unused leftovers. They followed the low fat diet perfectly because it was the only food they had in their refrigerator and kitchen. I also noticed the educators began carrying their foods with them in ice chests or sacks, as I had been doing for years, to guarantee the right food was eaten at all times.

The Delgado Cool Tote should contain your favorite types of fruits, vegetables and breads you enjoy eating. The average food sack filled with fruits and vegetables weighs about ten to fifteen pounds. If you want to lose weight, purchase those foods that are low in calories.

Buy vegetables that are easy to carry: a basket of cherry tomatoes, yellow or red bell peppers, etc. Eat the peppers raw and you will be surprised how refreshing and crisp they taste.

Red bell peppers are four times higher in Vitamin C than oranges, and green peppers are twice as high. White corn and yellow corn in the husk can be peeled and surprisingly, tastes mildly sweet when eaten raw. Take along one or two carrots and a small stalk of celery.

I also get vegetables in a jar like new potatoes (which are small, bite-size, and already cooked), green string beans and green peas. I take a spoon with me, pour off the juice and just eat the peas, potatoes or string beans right from the jar. Chinese snow peas are delicious eaten raw so take enough to last a few days.

You can microwave vegetables in the morning. Pour salsa, low- sodium Worcestershire Sauce or mustard on them, take a fork in your tote and eat them on the way to work. Many of our participants put cooked potatoes - red rose or white - in a baggy to be eaten during the day from their Cool Tote. It's best to remove the skin from the potato. The green substance under the skin called solanine has been known to cause liver problems when consumed in excess. You can microwave your veggies at work if you prefer. However, many busy people have to eat on the go and save themselves time by taking a bite of potato or fruit at a stop light on the way to and from work.

You should purchase enough vegetables and fruit to last about three days. Some fruits take two to three days to ripen. Leave unripened fruit at home in a paper bag to ripen. When they are ready to eat, take them with you in your Cool Tote. A ready supply of fruit for your Cool Tote can help reduce the number of visits you need to make to the market.

Your Cool Tote would be complete if you make sure there is a variety of fresh fruit. Favorite selections for your tote can include Rainer cherries (yellow), or bing cherries, grapes, pears, plums, peaches and bananas. Bananas can be eaten daily on our weight loss plan because they have less than 2% fat and are relatively low in calories per volume. Eat fresh apples, nectarines, blueberries, blackberries and raspberries. Frozen berries can be placed in a lid-tight container and eaten as they thaw during the day. The best way to design your Cool Tote contents would be to carry a variety of each fruit, and snack from whichever item your heart desires at the moment.

People who are accustomed to starvation diets, calorie restriction and skipping meals will be afraid to try this. However, you will find yourself several pounds lighter in six months without any deprivation, weakness or danger associated with those old ways of dieting.

The Delgado Plan will work for compulsive eaters, busy people and all for whom diet plans have failed. Your food bill probably will drop dramatically, since you will reduce your expenditures on prepared foods. Also, you may find yourself routinely skipping restaurant stops. Most of my busy participants (Delgado seminar graduates and patients) go to restaurants for variety or for special occasions. As you reduce the frequent restaurant trips, you can save literally hundreds of dollars. On those occasions when you do go to a restaurant, be sure to nibble from your Delgado Cool Tote in the car on your way to the restaurant. By doing so, you will find yourself ordering less or no fatty foods from the menu.

If you're in the car for long periods or going to be in warm weather, you should invest in the Delgado Cool Tote, which is available by mail order. The tote also comes with a blue ice packet to keep your fruits and veggies cold. You should freeze the ice packet every night and put it back in your tote every morning. If you travel and you don't have access to a refrigerator-freezer, just put ice in a plastic ziplock bag with the blue ice. Place the bag upright in the tote and at the end of the day, drain the water and add new ice cubes. We cover the ice bag with one or two paper towels to absorb the small amount of moisture from the condensed water. At night when you get home from work, put the veggies and fruit into the refrigerator crisper. Leave them in the bag so you can just put them in your Cool Tote without delay. You must plan to carry your Cool Tote with you every day. Don't forget to assemble your foods in time for work the next day. The Delgado Cool Tote provides an easier, safer method of food transport.

It will be necessary to keep your Cool Tote with you, at your work station. If you are unable to keep your tote near you, then take a banana, apple or some bread to nibble. If your food is left in the refrigerator, you may not get the chance to snack when your body signals hunger. You may get distracted by your busy work schedule, and when you finally do eat, you'll be ravenous. You'll eat that doughnut, chocolate, cheese or potato chips that add fat. Just pinch yourself on your hips or waist! RIGHT?!

Nibble every thirty minutes to an hour if you're eating fruits and veggies to lose weight. When eating more grains, breads, beans and casserole dishes, you'll find you only need to eat every two hours. Remember, grains and beans will sustain you longer since they are lower in water content than fruits and vegetables and are more concentrated in food substance. We encourage you to have a whole grain brown rice bread in your Cool Tote and eat at least two slices a day. You also need the high fiber, vitamins and minerals that grains provide for long-term good health.

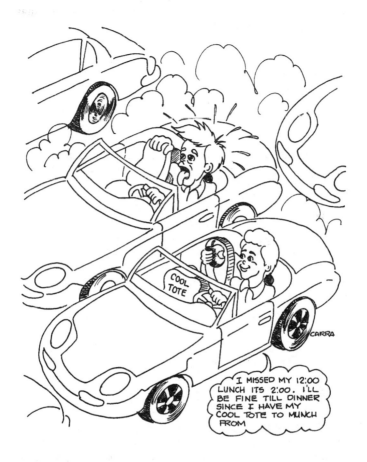

Eat from your Cool Tote right up to the time you're going to eat at a restaurant or go home for lunch or dinner. You will be able to maintain control and select foods properly at these traditional set meal times. You may find you won't need to stop for lunch or dinner and many days you'll just eat straight from your tote. Consider the time it will save. Time that can be allocated for a family walk, swim or outings to the park, beach or movies (take your Cool Tote!). You can read to your children, or take turns exercising on mini-trampolines and stationary bikes while you watch TV. Besides the suggested snacking, we encourage you to have family meals together. Your family will benefit as they enjoy improved health and fitness on **The Delgado Plan**.

How to Look Great & Feel Sexy

4

Ten Rules
For Fast Fat Loss

In the United States today, obesity effects more than 70 million Americans, and taken as a whole, we carry around 2.3 billion pounds excess body fat! To achieve Optimum Weight Control, we must choose a water rich high-carbohydrate, low fat, high-fiber diet combined with a consistent exercise program. Let's first discuss our diet as compared to those of other countries.

In our country, only 22% of our diet is composed of complex carbohydrates (unprocessed whole grains, beans, fruits and vegetables) and as a result, over 32% of our people are obese. In countries such as Uruguay and Venezuela where they eat a diet higher (53-60%) in fiber and starchy complex carbohydrates, only 20% of the people are overweight. Yet when you examine countries where the diet is composed of over 70-80% complex carbohydrates, obesity is almost nonexistent.

THE FIRST RULE for weight loss is simple: The more complex carbohydrates (potatoes, fruits, vegetables, salads, spaghetti squash, brown rice, etc.) you eat, the more likely you'll have an ideal body weight.

THE SECOND RULE is to eat large amounts of soups because they are filling and satisfying. Make very thick, flavorful vegetable soups and you will lose fat weight quickly, without being hungry.

THE THIRD RULE would be to keep several containers of chopped vegetables in your refrigerator. These vegetables can be used to make large salads and casseroles. When you begin using a large serving bowl in place of a small, standard size bowl, you will be eating your way to a more slender body!

THE FOURTH RULE is to eat more fruit, because fruit (like vegetables) is high in water content and high in fiber, both of which have almost no calories. Even watermelon is a good weight loss food (along with apples, pears, nectarines, oranges, etc.) You will lose fat if you snack on fruit and vegetables constantly, day and night, with meals or between meals. If you have a sweet tooth and you have trouble resisting fatty candy bars, then you can eat fruit like cherries, blueberries, grapes and watermelon in place of those sweets. You will still get those cravings for candy; however, if you have a ready supply of fruit to eat at all times, then you can successfully resist temptations.

THE FIFTH RULE of weight control is by reducing fat you reduce calories. Every gram of fat has 9 calories. Yet every gram of carbohydrate or protein provides just 4 calories. Remember, fats have 2 1/4 times more calories, which is why they're called "fats" and why they are so "fattening". Read labels on the foods you buy to be sure you're eating less than 45 grams of fat per day. On a 2,000 calorie diet this works out to be 20% fat; on a 1,000 calorie weight loss diet, you should eat less than 22 grams of fat daily. Generally, a food should contain less than four grams of fat per one cup serving. You must limit or avoid fats, oils, margarine, eggs, low fat and whole milk, cheese, peanut butter and fatty meats.

THE SIXTH RULE to weight control is to be sure to eat more foods high in fiber and low in food density. Your stomach can hold about four cups of food before a signal is sent to the brain that tells you that you're full. If you begin eating large amounts of complex carbohydrates that are naturally high in fiber, most of the food you eat will be low in food density and very low in calories. This is because fiber by definition is non-digestible. Because you can't digest fiber for calories, it just passes out of the body. So, if you ate four cups of food for breakfast (cooked oatmeal or cracked wheat with bran and fruit), four cups of food for lunch (salad bar of vegetables and fruit, sandwich of whole grain bread with veggies or beans inside), and four cups of dinner (salad bar, soup, fruit, potato, corn and Spanish brown rice), with light snacks of veggies and fruit between meals, your stomach capacity would be fully satisfied throughout the day. The best thing is even with all this tasty food, you would have only consumed about 900 to 1600 calories for the day! This would allow you to lose weight at a safe and healthful pace, free of hunger.

Always ask yourself these questions: Does this food contain fiber? Is it of plant origin? Is it unprocessed? For example, do cheese, steak, chicken, fish, milk, yogurt, eggs, hamburgers, mayonnaise or vegetable oil have fiber in them? The answer is no. Foods of animal origin have no fiber. They are totally digested and absorbed as calories. Foods like sugar and vegetable oil have lost their fiber through man-made processing. One of the worst examples of man's intervention into Mother Nature's food supply is corn oil. It takes over 14 ears of corn to make one tablespoon of oil! These concentrated foods are fattening because Westerners eat them every day.

Dr. Denis Burkitt was able to show the importance of eating foods high in fiber in his study of 23 young Irishmen. They were told to eat two pounds of potatoes (about 10 large potatoes) every day for three months. Since they ate their daily ration of potatoes, they were allowed to add as many other foods as they wanted. During the study, every man had lost weight. The 4-cup capacity of the stomach was filled after eating three or four of the large potatoes, and there wasn't much room for other high calorie foods. In fact, two pounds of potatoes have only 690 calories, and a cup of potatoes has just 115 calories. Yet one cup of french fries contains 450 calories! A cup of so-called "lean" hamburger labeled 21% fat would have over 750 calories. A cup of sugar has nearly 800 calories, while the original sugar beet, with its fiber intact, has only 54 calories. And while a cup of corn has only 137 calories, a cup of corn oil has a whopping 1,927 calories or 120 calories per tablespoon.

WEIGHT LOSS GUIDE
by Food Density, Fiber and Calories
(Number of calories per 8 oz. serving)

Low density, fibrous foods
UNLIMITED USE for weight loss
10 Lettuce
16 Cucumbers
20 Celery/Mushrooms
24 Cabbage/Bok Choy
28 Cauliflower/Squash (summer)
31 Turnip greens/Green beans
32 Mustard greens
33 Bell peppers (green)
36 Asparagus
40 Broccoli/Spinach
45 Tomatoes
46 Carrots
47 Bell peppers (red)
54 Brussels sprouts/Beets
64 Artichokes
70 Grapes/Peaches
70 Gazpacho soup
73 Apples
79 Apricots
81 Oranges/Pineapple
93 Squash (winter)
101 Pears
109 Peas (green)
118 Potatoes

Medium density, fibrous food
MEDIUM USE
125 Corn grits
132 Oatmeal
137 Corn
191 Bananas
195 Bread (whole)

High density, high fiber foods
MODERATE USE
224 Beans: lentil, pinto, kidney, etc.
232 Brown rice
291 Sweet potatoes

High density, low fiber foods	High density, no fiber foods
OCCASIONAL USE	RESTRICT/AVOID
(High calorie or cholesterol	(High fat or cholesterol)
88 Skim milk	159 Milk (whole)
117 Apple juice	222 Eggs
124 Yogurt (skim)/Egg whites	342 Ice cream
125 Cottage cheese (uncreamed)	345 Evaporated milk
145 Low fat milk	420 McDonald's Quarter Pounder
148 Shrimp	450 Cheddar cheese
170 Clams	750 Hamburger meat patty (21% fat)
188 Oysters	667 Chocolate
218 Fish, halibut	770 Sugar (white)
232 Chicken (no skin)	794 Maple syrup
234 Soybeans	821 Sugar (brown)
246 Turkey	1520 Peanut butter
250 Liteline cheese	1625 Butter
384 Avocados	1634 Margarine
430 Flank steak	1927 Corn oil
799 Cashews/Walnuts/Pecans/	
Sunflower seeds	

Beans, grains and cereals are a great source of fiber, however, these foods are high in food density and higher in calories. So eat grains, brown rice, whole wheat bread and beans in small portions (up to four cup servings of grains per day) after eating foods that are low in food density like fruits, veggies and soups. Also, to lose weight when you do eat grains, you should eat hot, cooked cereals (cracked wheat, oatmeal, 4-grain, etc.) or puffed cereals for breakfast, as opposed to flakes or granola cereals. Cooking cereal with water will cause 1/3 cup to enlarge to fill the whole bowl. Flakes and granola cereals have more calories because they are heavier and concentrated in food density. Puffed cereals are lighter in food density, which makes them a good choice for weight loss.

You may include wheat bran in your diet to speed food through your digestive tract so you can absorb fewer calories and lose weight faster.

THE SEVENTH RULE is to reduce sugar consumption and to substitute whole fruit (pineapple, strawberries, etc.) for sugar wherever possible. Sugar or fruit juice causes your body to release too much insulin, which can cause reactive hypoglycemia. This makes you extremely hungry, a condition to avoid when dieting! Also, insulin promotes additional fat storage throughout your body. Use apple butter or apple juice concentrate, but use them in small amounts to avoid reactions.

THE EIGHTH RULE would be to eat frequent meals or snacks whenever you're hungry - be sure NOT to skip meals. Body fat is burned most efficiently in the presence of carbohydrates and burning the fat properly is comparable to making a fire with the proper wood. Eating meals high in complex carbohydrates regularly also will "spare" body proteins, organs and muscles from being used as fuel. The body prefers to burn glucose from carbohydrates. So don't skip meals, or you will lose body proteins that can be converted to glucose more easily than body fat.

THE NINTH RULE is to exercise consistently and properly for maximum weight loss. Recent experiments have shown exercises involving the largest muscle groups (legs, hips and back), such as walking, jogging, dancing, using mini-trampolines, stairsteppers, treadmills and exercise bikes, will burn off more fat from the hard-to-lose areas like the stomach, thighs or hips, than will specific exercises like sit-ups and bending motions.

In one important experiment, 13 college men completed 5,004 sit-ups during a 27-day program, averaging about 187 sit-ups daily per person. Each man's fat content was measured both by fat biopsies and water immersion. As we suspected, there was no greater fat loss in the abdominal fat cells than in the fat storage in cells located throughout the body. This means spot reducing (sit-ups or arm exercises) will tone up specific muscles, but will not reduce fat cells in specific areas. So, the best way to burn fat is to do exercises using the largest muscle groups because more total calories will be burned up in a given amount of time.

To burn off the most fat from your stomach, hips or whichever part you're trying to reduce, you should walk, jog, dance, etc. continuously for at least 15 to 60 minutes a day. Although the stomach muscles are too small a group to get maximum fat burning, you should still do toning exercises for all specific muscle groups to keep firm. In addition, it's been found exercising about 30 minutes just before your evening meal will help to reduce your appetite by releasing glycogen (storage glucose). This will help you to burn more fat weight and maintain muscle tone. However, the best time to exercise for most people is in the morning. Studies have shown long term adherence to an exercise plan is better for morning exercisers as compared with evening exercisers.

DELGADO EXERCISE FOR FITNESS AND FAT LOSS
Aerobic walking with Heavy hands, stairstepper, jogging, stationary biking for long, slow distances: 15-60 minutes per day, 5-6 days a week. Light weight lifting for muscle toning: 20 minutes, 2 days a week.

THE TENTH RULE is to remain patient. Don't be discouraged with seemingly slow weight loss. If you had been on a high protein diet, your tissues would have been dehydrated. As you follow **The Delgado Health Plan**, your muscles will reabsorb vital fluid. Also your body will hold 4 to 10 lbs more bulk food in the intestines. You may believe you're gaining weight during the first month following the program. Actually, you'll be burning fat at the most rapid pace of any program yet developed. Stay on **The Delgado Plan** at least six months and you will appreciate how easily those inches of fat will shrink away, without being hungry. Calorie and portion restricted programs leave you hungry, but on **The Delgado Plan** you can eat tasty, low fat foods whenever you feel slightly empty or hungry. You will always feel good, month after month, which is strong motivation to stay on this plan for life.

Men tend to carry fat weight around the waist area. Women retain fat mostly in the hips, thighs and buttocks. This is a genetic problem that will take about six months to two years to resolve on the best possible program, **The Delgado Health Plan**. Fat can take months or years to get rid of, which is why you must establish this plan as a way of life. When you lose the fat, by changing your daily eating and exercise habits, you can keep it off for a lifetime. Listen to The Delgado "How to Look and Feel Great" cassette tapes daily for long term motivation, support and instructions. Feeding your mind with positive thoughts will help you to keep on track and achieve your weight loss goal.

TEN RULES FOR FAT LOSS SUMMARY
1. Eat more water rich complex carbohydrates.
2. Eat large bowls of soup several times per day.
3. Eat large servings of veggies for lunch, snacks and dinner - salad bar, soups or casseroles.
4. Eat whole fresh fruit (3-8 pieces per day).
5. Reduce fats to less than 22 grams per day.
6. Eat high fiber, low density foods.
7. Reduce sugar (simple carbohydrates).
8. Eat frequent meals whenever you are slightly hungry.
9. Exercise daily (15 to 60 minutes): do aerobics, walk, or jog, etc.
10. Be patient: expect great results in six months to two years.

Follow the ten rules listed above and you will attain your ideal weight. After you've achieved your perfect weight, you may increase your intake of grains, beans, sweet potatoes, breads, uncooked cereals, and reduce the use of vegetables, fruits and wheat bran.

SELECTION OF FOODS FOR FAT LOSS

EAT OR SNACK (EVERY 1/2 HOUR TO 2 HOURS) WHEN YOU FEEL WEAK, EMPTY OR MILDLY HUNGRY. IF YOU ARE NOT MILDLY HUNGRY OR WEAK, THERE IS NO NEED TO EAT AT THAT TIME. WAIT FOR YOUR BODY'S SIGNAL TO EAT. EAT UNTIL SATISFIED THE SOUPS, VEGGIES, FRUIT BELOW:

SOUPS: broths, vegetable, tomato (no milk).

VEGGIES: cucumbers, cauliflower, tomatoes, broccoli, cabbage, squash, snow peas, potatoes, carrots, mushrooms, bell peppers, bean sprouts, seed sprouts, grain sprouts, etc.; vegetable casserole, salads.

FRUIT: melon, oranges, grapes, apples, pears, berries, bananas, plums, cherries, nectarines, etc.

LOW DENSITY GRAINS: hot air popcorn, rice cakes, puffed cereal, cooked oat bran cereal.

DESSERT: sorbet, strawberry ice, frozen banana.

FIBER: psyllium husk, wheat bran, corn bran, oat bran.

SPICES: garlic, chili, pepper, dill, onion, cilantro, etc., non-fat salad dressing, mustard, catsup, vinegar.

HERB TEAS: chamomile, red bush, chinese, linden.

BEVERAGES: mineral water, lightly flavored fruit drink, 2-4 glasses water per day, tomato juice, carrot juice, grain drinks as a coffee replacement such as Postum.

RESTAURANT DINING - FILL UP ON SOUP & SALADS. ADD ONE PLATEFUL OF A MAIN DISH SELECTION LISTED BELOW:

AMERICAN: soup and salad bars, fruit, baked potato, hash browns (dry), Egg Beaters or egg whites (no cheese).

DELI: whole wheat sandwich w/lettuce, tomato, vinegar, pepper, bell peppers, onion, mustard, no oil.

CHINESE: (order no oil, no MSG, no egg) mixed vegetables, chop suey, broccoli, snow peas, vegetable soup, hot & sour soup (no pork), vegetable chow mein, moo-shu (no meat), steamed rice.

JAPANESE: (sushi-California roll - no fish eggs, cucumber roll, miso soup, cucumber salad, noodles.)

MEXICAN: steamed corn tortillas, lettuce, tomato, salsa, gazpacho soup, tortilla soup (no cheese), black bean soup, lentil soup, cocido (vegetable), tostada, burrito, veggie taco (no cheese), beans, rice, salsa.

ITALIAN: green salad, minestrone soup, steamed mushrooms, zucchini, cheeseless pizza (w/mushrooms, bell pepper, pineapple, tomato), pasta with "fat free" tomato sauce (no oil, no meat, no cheese), sourdough bread.

EAT SMALL PORTIONS,
LIMIT TO 2 TO 4 CUPS PER DAY:

GRAINS: cooked cereals (cracked wheat, oatmeal, 4-grain, etc.), cereal flakes, granolas, muesli, brown rice, millet, whole wheat pastas, wheat meat.

BREADS: whole wheat or corn tortillas, Essene or Manna sprouted bread, whole wheat pretzels, crackers (low fat), oat bran muffins (no yolk).

LEGUMES: beans (pinto, black, navy, lentil), black-eyed peas, tostada or burrito (no cheese), hummus, garbanzo.

VEGETABLES: yams, sweet potatoes.

DESSERTS: fruit pie (whole wheat crust, no sugar), whole wheat or oatmeal cookies (low fat, no sugar)

BEVERAGES: rice milk, fruit smoothies.

FOODS TO LIMIT OR AVOID(AS NOTED)
HIGH FAT OR HIGH SUGAR FOODS - LIMIT
TO 1-2 OUNCES PER DAY:

NUTS/SEEDS: almonds, cashews, pecans, nut butter, sunflower seeds, sesame seeds.
SNACKS: potato chips, corn chips, crackers.

MISC.: soybeans, soy cheese, tofu, avocado, olives, coconut, rice bran.

SWEETS: Rice Dream (non-dairy ice cream), raisins, dates, apple butter, pancake syrup, jams and jellies (unsweetened), angel food cake.

SAUCES/SPICES: A-1, Worcestershire (vegetable-based), barbeque sauce, Molly McButter or Butter Buds.

HIGH PROTEIN FOODS - LIMIT TO 1 OUNCE PER DAY OR AVOID:

DAIRY: low fat cheese (Lifetime, Liteline, Weight Watcher's), nonfat milk, nonfat yogurt.

LEAN FISH: halibut, sole, scallops, clams, sushi.

CRUSTACEA: shrimp, crab, lobster.

LEAN MEAT: chicken, turkey, range-fed beef, flank steak, Canadian bacon, fat-reduced ham, lamb.

HIGH SUGAR OR CAFFEINE - LIMIT TO 4 OUNCES (4 CUPS) PER WEEK OR AVOID:

BEVERAGES: soda pop, diet drinks, alcohol, coffee, tea.

SUGARS, SALT:
LIMIT TO 1/3 TSP. PER DAY OR AVOID:

SUGARS: sugar, fructose, chocolate syrup, sugar cereals, artificial sweeteners.

SPICES: salt, garlic salt, soy sauce, Accent (M.S.G.).

HIGH CHOLESTEROL OR HIGH FAT - AVOID:

EGGS: egg yolks, products with whole eggs added, caviar.

FATS: butter, margarine, lard, vegetable oil, olive oil, corn oil, canola oil, fish oil, cod oil, etc.; mayonnaise, nondairy creamers, oily or creamy dressings.

DAIRY: cheese (jack, mozzarella, cheddar, Swiss, etc.) cream, ice cream, yogurt, whole milk, powdered milk.

SWEETS: chocolate candy, cake, cookies.

MEAT: steak, ham, bacon, pork, sausage, salmon, organ meats, liver, hot dogs (beef, chicken or turkey franks), bologna, etc.

SAMPLE "FAST" FAT LOSS MEAL PLAN
DAY ONE

BREAKFAST: Bowl hot cereal (oatmeal, wheat, 4-grain or 7-grain with peaches, pears or prunes and 2 tbsp. wheat bran.

SNACK: Fruit and vegetables.

LUNCH: 1 large bowl veggie salad w/non-fat dressing, 2 fruits.

SNACK: Potato, herb tea.

DINNER: Chinese restaurant - veggies, chop suey, broccoli, mushrooms, cabbage, (NO MSG, NO OIL), add spicy szechuan.

DAY TWO

BREAKFAST: Oat bran cereal cooked in 1/2 apple juice & 1/2 water, 1/4 cantaloupe.

SNACK: Vegetable, water w/3 tbsp. psyllium husk.

LUNCH: Minestrone soup, 2 fruits, baked potato w/salsa.

SNACK: Green peas, tomato juice.

DINNER: Cheeseless pizza w/mushrooms, tomatoes, peppers.

DAY THREE

BREAKFAST: Potatoes (microwave - cover with glass bowl), mixed veggies, soup.

SNACK: Tomatoes, corn, peas.

LUNCH: Vegetable soup, salad, fruit.

SNACK: Banana, grapes, nectarine.

DINNER: Potato pancakes, veggies, soup, fruit, frozen banana ice cream (dairy free).

DAY FOUR

BREAKFAST: Whole grain muffins w/apple butter, fruit.

SNACK: 1 slice bread, tomatoes.

LUNCH: Veggie sandwich: cucumbers, cauliflower, tomato, artichoke hearts (packed in water), mustard, barbeque sauce.

SNACK: Fruit, carrot juice.

DINNER: Mixed veggies, casserole, soup, fruit, baked potato with ketchup or Molly McButter.

DAY FIVE

BREAKFAST: Puffed cereal with added two tablespoons wheat bran, use rice milk, water or juice, fruit.

SNACK: Fruit.

LUNCH: Veggie taco (soft corn tortillas, salsa, lettuce, sprouts, mushrooms, tomato, potato), cabbage soup.

SNACK: 1 bread roll, mineral water with lemon or cherry flavor.

DINNER: veggies, soup, fruit, Sorbet.

NOTE:
If you have to leave home to go to work, be sure to take your Delgado Cool Tote (filled with your favorite fruits, vegetables and bread) to nibble from during the day.
For good nutrition be sure to eat the following daily:
> Two different types of whole grains, at least 1 citrus fruit, 1 green vegetable, 1 yellow vegetable and a small serving of beans or peas in a soup or salad and a supplemental source of Vitamin B12 or foods like cereals fortified with B12.
> Repeat any breakfast, lunch or dinner you like. Keep it simple and convenient. Eat until you feel satisfied. Don't let yourself get weak or hungry by not eating.

How to Look Great & Feel Sexy

5

Protein Myths and Facts

In this chapter we will look at some myths surrounding protein. The most common myth is that egg proteins are a high quality nutritional source of protein. This has spread through the scientific community as well, and we'll help you dispel this myth. Do you still eat two or three eggs per week because you believe that egg proteins are a good source of nutrients? If so, you may develop several degenerative diseases later in life (if you haven't already developed them).

So why has this myth spread throughout our culture? Why do people believe eggs are good for us? Much of the fault lies with invalid rat studies.

In 1914 Osborne and Mendel did their first research studies attempting to determine which foods were the highest quality protein. They decided to use rats as subjects because rats have a short life cycle and are easy to monitor. They found when they gave rats animal-type proteins, such as eggs, meats, cheese, etc., they grew very large. In fact, when rats ate eggs they grew the largest. However, when the rats were fed potatoes, whole wheat, beans, peas or grain as their only food, the rats hardly grew at all.

Scientists thought there must be something nutritionally lacking in wheat, for example, because the essential amino acid, lysine, was too low in concentration to provide for proper growth in rats. (Am. J. Clin. Nutr., 27:1231, 1974). In fact, when they added lysine to the wheat in a diet for rats, the rats grew suddenly. This began the idea of needing complementary proteins or complete proteins. You may have heard of people trying to eat beans and rice at the same meal to be sure they receive adequate protein.

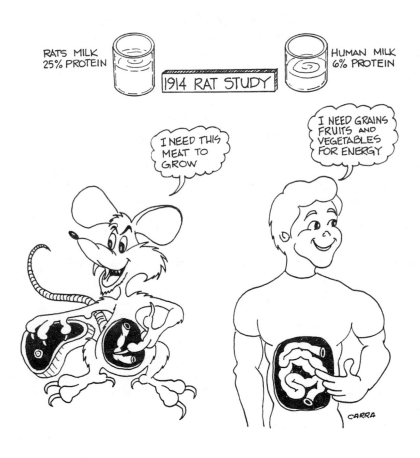

Let's understand what this theory is based on. It is based on the belief eggs are of superior quality, because of the rat studies. But rats are carnivorous. They have sharp teeth and claws, and they have a short digestive tract designed to get meat-type protein in and out before it rots. In contrast, humans have a long, convoluting digestive tract designed to handle whole grains, fresh fruits and vegetables. Our teeth are mostly molars for chewing fiber.

Rats grow to full size in nine weeks time. Humans take nearly 20 years to reach full size. Rats need a concentrated source of protein (rat's breast milk is over 25% protein). In a follow-up study rats were given human breast milk and hardly grew at all because human breast milk is low (under 6%) in protein.

If a nutritionist were to analyze human breast milk based on this information, we would all be led to believe human breast milk is a very poor source of food for infants. Yet, as we all know, it's one of the best sources of food we could supply our infants. When children are growing at their most rapid growth rate, nearly doubling in size, human breast milk allows for maximum growth.

Let's make a comparison to food. Brown rice is merely 6% protein. If you give rice or wheat to rats, they don't grow very well. By comparison, we find children respond very differently. Children given various vegetable proteins, grow just as well, calorie for calorie, compared to animal proteins. (Knapp, Am. J. Clin. Nutri. 26:586,, 1971).

One group of children at age 2-5 (a rapid growth rate period), were given only wheat proteins, which is 14 % protein. This group was compared with children given egg-type proteins (which is a combination of wheat with lysine to make up for the limiting amino acids). The first group grew just as well, if not better, than the egg protein group. (Ready, Am. J. Clin. Nutri. 24:1246, 1971).

The claim that animal protein is "superior" to vegetable protein is false. The truth is all natural foods of vegetable origin contain all the amino acids to satisfy human needs. The most recent findings suggest we do not have to combine beans with rice or other vegetables to get a complete protein. Frances Moore Lappe, author of *Diet for a Small Planet,* agrees in her 10th year revised edition human needs are easily met without combining vegetable proteins. In 1988, the American Dietetic Association position paper emphasized it is not necessary to combine protein foods at each meal. The human body makes amino acids that combine in the intestines with amino acids from foods to meet our nutritional needs. Adequate amounts of amino acids and protein will be obtained from a high complex carbohydrate diet supplying a variety of grains, legumes, seeds, vegetables and fruit.

Researcher Dr. C. Lee reported a study (Am. J. Clin. Nutr. 26:702, 1971) in which a group of college-aged students were given two different types of diet, adding support to this contention. One group was given only cheap, starchy white rice, which consisted of just 6% protein. The other group was given chicken and rice. They compared how much nitrogen and protein was absorbed into the body and how much was excreted. Again, everyone was surprised to find the group eating the rice alone had absorbed 20% more nitrogen (or protein) than the group eating the chicken and rice!

There is something special about the vegetable proteins: they seem to have been designed more efficiently for our bodies. We absorb them better than animal-type protein foods. When Dr. Kempner at Duke University gave people protein intakes as low as 22 grams per day (a 94% complex carbohydrate diet from rice and fruit), the result was a protein-sparing effect. The carbohydrates eaten were used for energy, protecting the protein so it could be used for other essential use.

According to Contemporary Nutrition (Volume 5, 1980), a group of men, weighing 154 lbs each, were given a protein-free diet, and the protein lost from the body was measured. They excreted about 24 grams of protein per day. So we know we need to replace at least 20 to 24 grams a day to meet a person's needs.

It's been established approximately 40 grams of protein would meet anyone's needs. If you make certain you get enough calories and carbohydrates it will surpass a person's requirements. Eating grains, beans, peas, fruits and vegetables provides over 60 grams of quality protein a day.

According to the National Academy of Science (1980), even a pregnant woman needs only 4 more grams of protein per day than a non-pregnant woman, which would be just 44 grams total. This would satisfy the total known needs of a 9 month fetus.

Another myth is that fish is a brain food. Although the brain does require essential nutrients, it's been found the primary source of food energy to the brain is glucose, which comes from complex carbohydrates. If you do not have enough glucose supplied to the brain you'd become very hypoglycemic. You might even black out because the brain is in need of the nutrients supplied by glucose. But, it's not really protein that gives us glucose, because protein does not convert nearly so readily into glucose as do the complex carbohydrates.

World-class athletes, including bodybuilders, have recently changed their views on protein. For years they have been telling us they needed large amounts of protein. Chris Dickerson, Mr. Olympia and winner of eleven other pro bodybuilding titles (he's won more bodybuilding titles than Arnold Schwarzenegger), has recently stated, "I used to follow a low-carbohydrate diet, which worked well enough for me to win Mr. U.S.A., Mr. America and two Mr. Universe titles; but since I moved back to California in early 1979 to train for the pro shows I've followed a low fat diet since the body prefers to use carbohydrates for its energy needs. I feel more energy in my workouts when I'm on a low fat diet than when I was on a low carbohydrate regime."

Carbohydrates are your preferred source of energy. It's the high carbohydrate, low fat diet that is the best kind of diet even for a bodybuilder. Chris doesn't add extra protein foods to his diet. He has found he gets the protein from the whole wheat, beans, peas, fruits and vegetables in his diet.

Mr. Universe, Tom Platz, wrote in "Muscle and Fitness" (Oct. 1984), "If you're going to build an 'out of this world' physique, you need to experiment constantly. Therefore, I increased my consumption of complex carbohydrate foods and immediately noted an upsurge in my strength and size levels. My energy was increased and my blood sugar level seemed to stabilize. Today, I follow a high-carb, medium protein and low fat diet . . ."

Natural Mr. Universe heavyweight bodybuilder Skip LaCour is training for competition, using **The Delgado Health Plan**. Skip is inspiring the world of bodybuilders to take drug-free training to the next level. Skip carries a Delgado Cool Tote so he can eat every one or two hours. He uses high quality supplements including DHEA, purified colloidal minerals and multivitamins. He also consumes raw sprouts, vegetables and fruits.

Mr. Olympia 1983, Samir Bannout, uses a high-carb (70%), moderate protein, low fat (10-20%) diet. So, many top bodybuilders are switching to a Delgado-type plan. Tennis stars like Martina Navrotilova and Jimmy Connors also use a high complex carbohydrate, low fat, adequate protein diet. The world record in the "Ironman" Triathalon (112-mile bicycle, 26-mile marathon, 2.4 mile swim) was set by Dave Scott, who also follows this low fat approach.

On a strict vegetarian or "vegan" diet (which includes no eggs or dairy products) there would be more than enough protein for muscle growth and maintenance, if an athlete ate enough foods to maintain his weight. I have followed a "vegan" diet, weight lifting, and running program since 1978. I get all the protein I need from raw sprouts, vegetables, fruit, tubers and grains.

Athletes perspire heavily and lose nitrogen in their sweat. While losing a smaller amount of nitrogen in their urine. Only during muscle building are small amounts of extra protein needed. This amounts to merely 25 grams (less than one oz) of protein, which is met by an increased intake of food to meet the caloric needs of the body.

The "zone diet" is higher in protein and fat with less carbohydrates. Zone dieters have lipid studies with results higher in serum LDL cholesterol. The excessive protein and fat is toxic to the human body over long periods of time.

A gorilla is almost pure vegetarian! They eat tubers, grains, vegetables and fruits and they are one of the most powerful, muscular animals on earth. They don't need to eat meat to be strong.

In elementary nutrition textbooks across the country, there is a great misunderstanding about what our protein needs are. In a textbook by Helen Guthrie, there is a chapter about protein requirements. It has a picture of a big rat and a little rat and the caption reads, "For human requirements." The book states, "Rats will gain more weight on an egg diet than on a whole wheat diet" suggesting there is a correlation between weight gain in rats and tissue protein synthesis. If you read the chapter on protein there are no studies indicating what the protein absorption is when humans eat various foods. The only studies they support that give false credence to the assumption humans need eggs are rat studies! Why do they leave out the human studies?

We found out who sponsors the production of textbooks on nutrition: huge budgets are provided by the Dairy Council and meat industry. They have found it is worthwhile to spend millions of dollars to teach our doctors and dietitians nutrition - based on those old rat studies! Further, they choose to include certain studies they want seen and leave out those they don't. It's a strong statement to make, but this has contributed to the worst epidemic of degenerative diseases seen in this country's history!

At universities pamphlets are provided by the Dairy Council promoting the benefits of eggs, milk and meat proteins. We asked the professors why the Dairy Council is providing so much of this information. They responded by saying the literature is provided free and they can pass it out to their students so our future nutritionists, dietitians and doctors can learn "good nutrition."

What if you still decide you need more protein? Should you eat more chicken and fish and get as much protein as you can because you're getting older?

We have to disagree strongly with that idea. Our protein requirements are best met by whole natural foods. If you choose to add excess protein to your diet, the result will be devastating, starting with dehydration - a rapid loss of fluids.

Test this for yourself. It won't hurt you to eat a high protein diet for one day. Eat large amounts of chicken, fish, add some egg whites to your meal all day long. See what happens to you - you'll be very thirsty, very quickly. In a couple of hours you'll be surprised at the amount of water you'll need to drink. This happens because your body is building up excess waste products - urea, ammonia and uric acid from the protein that must be diluted by your vital tissue fluid. After several years on a high-protein diet you can develop severe gout, kidney stones, liver disorders and osteoporosis (a loss of minerals, calcium, magnesium and zinc from your bones).

X-rays of bones show us people who eat large amounts of meat, eggs, cheese and milk protein develop holes in their bones as they get older. By comparison, people who eat less protein and more complex carbohydrate foods have greater density and strength in their bones.

Now try another experiment. Two days later switch over to potatoes, fresh fruits, brown rice, whole wheat bread, spaghetti and other carbohydrate foods. Eat these for two days and watch how drastically your requirements for water are reduced! You'll also notice you'll start to feel better.

It is true we need protein for muscles, tissue repair, hormones, antibodies, enzymes and hemoglobin to transport oxygen and clotting ability. Protein is essential to life. Yet we get enough quality protein from whole natural foods that meet our caloric needs, for example:

FOOD GRAMS OF PROTEIN

1 cup of split peas	16
1 cup navy or kidney beans	15
1/4 cup almonds	6.5
1 cup oatmeal	6
1 whole wheat pita bread	6
1 cup corn	5
2 oranges	2.5

All vegetables contain protein. Don't be misled by people who tell you these foods are a poor quality protein source.

You also may want to include small amounts of low fat animal products (and B-12 supplements) to your regular diet. You don't need animal protein, but some people enjoy the taste variety. These can be used as a condiment in stews, casseroles, etc. However, an excellent replacement for meat in any recipe would be "wheat meat" or "seitan." Wheat meat is available in some health food stores packaged in a jar, or in the refrigerated section with barbecue sauce called "Wibs". You also could make your own using the recipe in my book under "Vevestake". Try it, you'll like it.

Protein deficiencies (kwashiorkor) are due to starvation. A diet of whole, complex carbohydrates contains all the protein you'll ever need, as long as you get sufficient calories. Once you reach your ideal weight you will need to eat fewer fruits and vegetables and more grains, legumes, peas, nuts and seeds in sufficient quantities to maintain your weight.

The Delgado Health Plan is a proven concept. Within several months you'll feel better than you ever have. This is an opportunity you will benefit from for the rest of your life. Start today.

PROTEIN QUESTION AND ANSWERS
Q. Is it possible to be protein deficient?
A. Protein deficiency generally occurs only due to a lack of calories. It's not the lack of protein in the diet; it's the lack of proper whole foods to meet your needs.

Q. Will I find the best source of quality protein by eating grains, vegetables and fruit?
A. Yes, according to recent studies on humans, your best protein sources are from these foods. Protein is not as efficiently absorbed when it comes from animal sources. This is based on very thorough research with humans instead of rats.

Q. Name some of the best protein sources for humans.
A. The best sources of protein would include whole sprouts, brown rice, grains, whole wheat bread, beans, peas, potatoes, along with a variety of vegetables and fruits. **The Delgado Health Plan** would give you at least 40 to 70 grams of protein a day, which is more than sufficient. There is no need to include meat, eggs or dairy products for protein needs, unless you're a rat, dog or cat!

Q. Name foods and approaches that would build muscle and gain weight.
A. The best approaches would include the high complex carbohydrate diet with sweet potatoes and whole grains to give you enough calories to build muscle. You would want to begin exercising, especially with weight lifting. That will help to build lean tissue.

Q. Is it always necessary to combine vegetables and protein, like rice and beans, at the same meal to obtain a complete protein?

A. No, it's not necessary. The foods supply all the amino acids in each vegetable and grain. Those people who say there are amino acids missing in certain foods are not correct in that assumption. The nutritional analysis of foods shows us the amino acids are present; they're just in different balances and patterns. They don't have to be in the same pattern as eggs, for example. Eggs were not a good comparison base.

Q. Will I have to worry about getting enough protein during weight loss?

A. When you are losing weight you are getting a supply of calories from your body's storage of fat. At the same time, if you eat the high complex carbohydrate vegetables, fruits and smaller amounts of grains, you'll have glucose present to spare your body proteins. Inside the starchy complex carbohydrates there will be sufficient protein to meet your needs. Once you reach your ideal body weight, however, you'll need to maintain a steady calorie intake, possibly adding more grains, beans, yams and pastas to meet your needs.

Q. Are there any people that have special needs to ensure they get enough protein, and how can this be accomplished without adding protein to the diet?

A. Growing children, pregnant women, athletes, and people at or below their ideal body weight will need slightly more protein. This protein need can be easily met by eating less vegetables, soups, and fruits, while being sure to eat more whole grain breads, cold cereals, rice, pasta, beans and yams

How to Look Great & Feel Sexy

6

Exercise For Busy People

Set a goal to exercise twice a day, a minimum of 15 to 30 minutes every morning and again in the evening. If you miss a session, you will at least have gotten in one exercise period a day. Studies show those people who exercise in the morning are more likely to continue exercising one year later, as compared with those who try to exercise in the afternoon or evening.

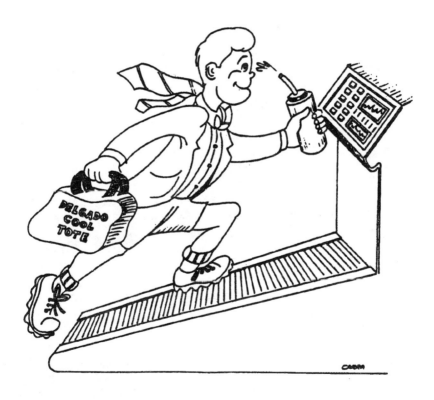

I always drink two or three glasses of water and I eat a few grapes, an apple, banana or orange just before I start exercising. You must be well hydrated, otherwise you will become fatigued quickly. In addition, I bring water and some fruit with me to the gym during my workout in case I get thirsty. If you drink fluids before, during and after your exercise, you will find your performance and energy improving dramatically.

Do an exercise that is simple and aerobic in nature. It should employ the largest muscle groups of the body (legs or back). You may want to exercise to an aerobic video tape. You can use a mini trampoline, stationary bike, Nordic track, treadmill or stairstepper. Try out each of these exercises and acquire the necessary equipment to begin your program today.

I have found the motorized treadmill to be one of the best overall fat burning and conditioning exercises available. You can purchase a good treadmill with variable speed control for under $500. If your home has adequate space, place the treadmill in front of the television or stereo. If you are overweight, you should exercise at a walking speed of between two and four miles per hour. It is important that you can talk during your exercise without becoming completely out of breath. Slow your pace down until you find the most comfortable rate. It has been shown walking one mile will burn nearly as much fat as running one mile.

The key to optimum conditioning is long, slow distances as opposed to short, intense workouts. Exercising at your "target heart rate" according to so-called fitness guidelines may be causing you to exercise beyond or below your capabilities. Certain fitness experts may have led you to believe exercise was of no value unless you worked out hard and intense, at a certain target heart rate (220 - age X 65 to 85%). For most people, a target heart rate of 65-85 % will be too intense, and lead to avoidance of your daily sessions. For long term success, a slower, consistent pace will give you the best results. For example, a target of 50-65% for a 40 year old would equal 90-117 beats per minute, sustained during exercise. However, if you can carry on a conversation during your exercise, and go a long, slow distance (LSD), then you don't have to monitor your pulse rate.

A stairstepper is another great indoor exercise that is a better conditioner than a stationary bike or mini trampoline. You will find you can read a book as you step in place on the foot pads. This will help you to lose track of time so that you will exercise for a longer period. However, if you find the stairstepper too hard and intense, and it leaves you "huffing and puffing", then stay with the more gentle bicycle or trampoline exercise session.

A daily walking program of fifteen minutes to one hour a day will burn fat all over your body. If you have a desire to rid yourself of a fat midsection, don't waste time with sit-ups and spot reducing schemes. Lying on a floor and moving your legs is not as effective as moving your whole body upright and supporting your whole weight and walking. Though riding a bike will help those who can't walk, due to knee or ankle problems, it's still not as effective as walking. Here again, don't expect one walk to shed 20 lbs for you. Daily walks, either alone or in addition to other forms of exercise, will have a cumulative effect, and will greatly improve your body's fat-burning capabilities.

Exercise will strengthen your muscles so that your body will burn fat more efficiently. Mitochondria, the power house of the cells, will increase in number, which will improve your body's ability to burn fat. People who are overweight burn fat less efficiently. By following **The Delgado Plan** of daily exercise and frequent low fat meals, the process of fat-burning can be accomplished easily.

Daily aerobic exercise will help your body's fat cells to release more fat into the bloodstream sooner to be burned by your muscles. This will allow your body to burn more storage fat during and after exercise, instead of burning mostly glucose. Fit people who exercise daily become "fat burners." Unfit people, who are unaccustomed to daily exercise start out burning mainly glucose and not much fat. Your body has two fuel tanks to choose from, one filled with glucose and one filled with fat (unlike your car that has only one fuel tank of gas.) Eventually, after several months of rhythmic, distance exercise your body will select fat as its preferred fuel. This happens because glucose and storage glycogen is used up so quickly that your body will conserve glucose and become conditioned to burn fat. If you follow our low fat diet, there will be almost no fat in your bloodstream, so your body will focus on burning released storage fat from your fat cells as you exercise.

How to Look Great & Feel Sexy

7

How To Look Great
By Shrinking
Your Fat Cells

The **Delgado Diet and Exercise Plan** is designed so that you can stay on it for a lifetime. Women can develop and maintain that new attractive figure, a leaner body with a firm abdomen, curvaceous hips and a radiant face with the cheeks of a model. Men will have a muscular, firm, better proportioned appearance. You will get compliments from men and women who remember your past struggles with starvation and food restriction diets. Failure, pain, hunger and weakness can all be turned into success, pain free satisfaction and energy on **The Delgado Plan**.

Women need fat, but in the right places - distributed evenly over the body for a smooth, soft look. For example, a 130 lb., 5'4" ideally proportioned woman, participating in daily exercise classes and capable of running a 26-mile marathon may have 15% body fat. Therefore, 15 to 20% body fat would be a lean, athletic, well shaped woman. The breakdown of fat distribution may be as follows: 2 - 4 lbs for breasts, 4 lbs of fat in the intestinal area, 4 - 5 lbs under the skin and 5 lbs of fat on the back of each thigh. There is also a need in both men and women for about 15 - 30 lbs of essential body fat in the organs and for insulation.

Men look their best when the body fat level is between 5-17%. In 1978, when I was overweight, Dr. Bob Girandola of U.S.C. measured my body fat. He used the water immersion method and my body fat level measured over 25%. He told me I was classified as obese! However, after less than 5 months on my low fat, high carbohydrate diet, and with exercise, my weight had reduced from over 200 lbs to 159 lbs Dr. Girandola repeated the test on body fat 4 months after the first test and was amazed that I had reduced to under 9%.

Selecting the right foods for your caloric needs is an effective way to reduce body fat and look years younger. Excess fat leaves a puffy, grotesque look (fatty stomach, hips and face) that makes people look years older.

One study has shown that when subjects were given extra fat added to a low calorie diet, 33% of the fat went right to the fat storage cells. It was discovered by using radioactive tracers placed on the fat in the diet, that the fat was stored instead of being used for fuel. The body is not capable of burning more than a certain amount of fat from the diet. The excess will simply be absorbed and stored by the billions of fat cells of the body. Fat storage cells (adipose tissue) act like billions of small sponges. Excess fat from your diet is absorbed by these fat cells daily, even if you are consuming fewer calories.

Your body receives most of its needed fuel for energy (over 80%) from carbohydrates that break down into glucose. Fat is a secondary fuel that can only be used at a constant slow rate. If you remove carbohydrates from a low calorie diet, your body will continue to burn the same constant rate of fat; however, the rest of your caloric needs will come from glucose stored in your liver and muscles. This stored glucose amounts to less than 12 hours of fuel. After 12 hours of avoiding carbohydrate foods, your entire body storage of glucose will be depleted. When this happens, your body then will quickly begin breaking down your muscle proteins into glucose for fuel, instead of burning more fat. This is why the best diet for you should be very low in fat and high in complex carbohydrates, not just low in calories. Your body can only release more fat from the cells than it stores if there is less fat in your diet and more complex carbohydrates.

Fat provides 9 calories per gram, whereas carbohydrate and protein have only 4 calories per gram. This means fat is twice as fattening as any other nutrient.

We all have different capacities to retain or lose fat. Every day that you eat low fat foods and exercise fifteen to sixty minutes, you will be establishing a pattern of success. Month after month you will see your results improving as your fat cells shrink. The actual number of fat cells we have is influenced by three critical periods of time during our lives.

The first comes before birth, during the last three months of pregnancy. If your mother was led to believe good nutrition meant eating more eggs, cheese, milk, butter and meat, then the excessive amount of fat and calories would have stimulated an increase in the number of fat cells in the fetus. If your mother had followed a Delgado type of nutritional plan with whole grains, cereals, rice, bread, pastas, beans, peas, fruits and vegetables without added fat, you may have developed fewer fat cells.

The next critical period of fat cell development occurs during the first year of life. If your mother gave you high fat (bottle) formulas and introduced fat and sugar-laden foods, then the fat cells would have increased beyond the expected number. Fat cells could double or triple during the first year after birth. However, if you were breast fed, then your body would have produced fewer fat cells.

In the final, critical period, which is during childhood and youth, the fat cells grow both in size and number. This is followed by another significant increase because of hormonal changes (puberty for teenage girls) and a fatty diet.

However, if you did develop a large number of fat cells, for any of the above reasons, there is no need to be discouraged. **The Delgado Program** will slim down the size of your fat cells.

It may take several months or even a full year or two to get to your goal of ideal body weight. However, if you consider that this plan will enable you to achieve a fat free body permanently, it's worth the wait, isn't it?

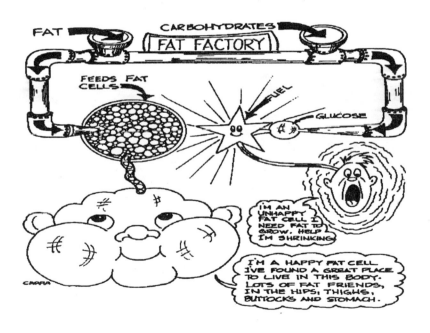

How to Look Great & Feel Sexy

8

Fat Loss Goals

Successful participants on **The Delgado Plan** who lose fat weight permanently, reduce at a consistent rate of 1/4–2 lbs of fat loss per week for women and 1 to 3 lbs for men. Even very fit athletes with high metabolic rates and muscular bodies that are efficient at burning fat would never burn more than 5 lbs of fat in a week. In most cases, weight loss more than 3 lbs a week would be mainly water, body protein and emptying of food from the digestive tract.

If the weight loss is over 3 lbs per week, you will be losing mostly muscle and water which is deceptive. When you lose muscle you are losing your best friend in the fight against fat. Muscles burn fat faster than any other body tissue. When you lose muscle, your percentage of body fat may actually be increasing! You could lose as much as 8 lbs of muscle in a month and up to 12 lbs of water. Starvation, liquid diets, and portion control (restricting complex carbohydrates) cause you to lose mostly muscle and water, leaving you weak and gaunt-looking. Also, losing body protein (muscle, heart, organs) and water weight is dangerous and can be fatal. Most of the current diet fads promote rapid weight loss to entice you to follow their programs.

Don't be discouraged by slow weight loss - you're losing fat weight on **The Delgado Plan**. Losing fat weight at a 1–3 lb. rate per week is ideal. The following ideas will help you to understand expected fluctuations in weight. You're body is composed of over 80% water. If you drained and dehydrated all your body fluids - blood, etc., bone, protein and fat are all that would remain. Fat tissue contains a low percentage of water as compared to muscle that has an extremely high water content.

Your muscles are made up of over 60% water, whereas fat tissue contains less than 10% water. When you lose water on high protein, starvation diets like "Slim Fast" or "Herbal Life" drinks, you are losing a lot of muscle. The emptying of food from the digestive tract, loss of body muscle and water can be done by not eating food for two days, but what have you accomplished? Nothing but a temporary reduction on the weight scale with no change in your appearance and no loss of fat. You need to look at this fact seriously now and consider what is happening. You must reduce your fat intake daily by making the proper food selections or those fat cells in your hips, thighs and stomach will become bigger.

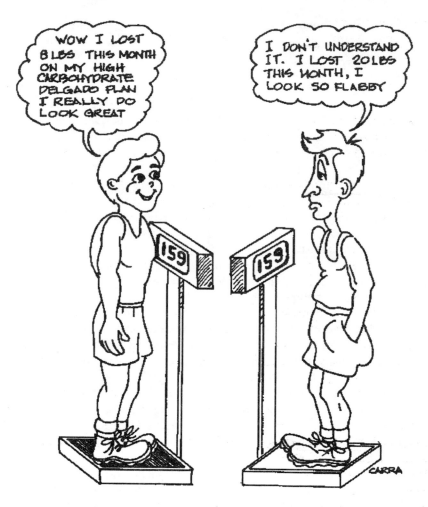

The Delgado Plan increases the complex carbohydrates to over 70% and less than 5% of simple sugar carbohydrates. The average American eats less than 25% complex carbohydrates and as much as 25% simple sugar carbohydrates. Our program also reduces the American diet from over 43% fat down to under 15%.

The shift in calories will work as follows:

	American Diet	Delgado Plan
Complex Carbohydrates	22 %	70 % or more
Simple Carbohydrates	20 %	5 % or less
Fat	43 %	15 % or less
Protein	15 %	10% to 15 %
	100 %	100 %

This change toward a higher complex carbohydrate food plan will cause some immediate shifts in body water levels accounting for a temporary gain in water weight. However, the great news is you will notice rapid fat reduction. You'll look in the mirror and see bulges of fat getting smaller. Your percentage of fat by body composition testing will show marked drops at the 6 month and 12 month point after starting **The Delgado Plan**. It will be easy for you to stay on the plan for the necessary 12 months or more to get rid of excess body fat.

However, be prepared for major changes in body water levels in the first week to three months. You may even gain weight while you lose body fat. If you gain weight, don't let it discourage you for these reasons:

1. An increase in carbohydrates allows nearly 60% more glycogen (stored carbohydrate) in your muscles and liver. Glycogen absorbs three grams of additional water for each additional gram of glycogen. Your muscles will absorb this needed vital water, but this weight gain will be far offset by the amount of fat lost in the next thirty days.
2. Exercise in the first two weeks will cause a significant expansion in blood volume by as much as 30%. This increase in body fluid will make you weigh more on the weight scale, despite appreciable fat loss. Remember, our goal here is fat loss to get rid of those unsightly bulges, not just a deceptive and temporary water loss.
3. High fiber complex carbohydrate foods provide needed bulk to the stools. Your intestinal tract holds up to 10 lbs worth of food which can add to your weight. This satisfied, full feeling may be a new experience for you if you're accustomed to starvation and liquid diets or limited portion control plans that always leave you feeling empty. Stepping on the weight scale in the first month may be discouraging but, 12 months after starting the program you will appreciate how sensible and easy it is to eat high fiber, low fat foods.
4. Menstrual cycles can cause several pounds of fluid retention. This is one reason women should only weigh themselves from month to month and not be worried about weekly changes in weight.

5. **The Delgado Plan** can help you reduce your dependency on medications such as diuretics or Beta Blockers that will cause a significant regaining of vital body water. This is another temporary change that your body will adjust to in a matter of weeks. (Be sure to have your dosages of medications monitored by a physician willing to help you reduce your dependency on chemicals).

9

Pesticides Exposure - Highest in Meat, Fish, Dairy

If you want to lose weight you must eat a large amount of fruits, vegetables, salads and vegetable soups, smaller amounts of grains and beans, and little or no meat and dairy products. The concern of pesticides is not overlooked here in regard to eating more fruits and veggies, but let us remind you that eating closer to the origin of the food chain - fruits, vegetables, grains, beans and peas - is much safer than eating high on the chain (animal products) because of biomagnification.

Biomagnification is the increased concentration of chemicals, pesticides and toxins that results when animals eat grains and vegetables exposed to pesticides, which concentrate 1,000 times in the animal's fat. When you eat the animal, the pesticides and heavy metals like mercury or lead can concentrate in your body not just double, but 1,000 X 1,000 or one million times! The concentration of these potentially deadly chemicals increases the higher you eat on the food chain. Meat, fish and dairy products expose you to the highest concentration of these deadly chemicals. Grains, fruits and vegetables are comparatively safe.

Small fish and plankton consumed by larger fish like tuna or swordfish, and eventually eaten by humans, have potentially high concentrations of chemicals that are dose related. The higher the dosage, the more dangerous the chemicals become as they concentrate in your body to lethal levels that may induce cancer or liver failure. Meat, chicken and fish have 10 times more pesticides than plant foods: fruits, vegetables or grains.

Drinking the milk of animals (cow or goat) is equally dangerous because of the buildup of harmful substances that end up in the secretions (milk) of the animal. Dairy products (milk, cheese, sour cream and eggs) have 5-1/2 times more toxic pesticides than do plant foods. A woman who eats low or at the origin of the food chain (fruits, vegetables and grains) will be eating lower - fat foods with fewer chemicals, and in turn with fewer chemicals for her baby. According to the New England Journal of Medicine, March 26, 1981, only 2% of mothers' milk from women eating only grains, beans, fruits and vegetables (no meat) was found to contain significant levels of DDT and other toxic chemicals. By contrast, 100% of mothers eating meat and dairy products produced breast milk with significant levels of DDT, pesticides and toxic chemicals.

Health-conscious people prefer to buy organic fruits and vegetables. Purchasing organic, seedless red and green grapes, potatoes, apples or carrots is worth the extra 10 to 60 cents a pound to avoid chemicals and pesticides. The average person eats at least 4 lbs of food a day, so for a mere $1.40 extra a day we will be supporting those farmers who care about future generations. This may force other farmers to begin farming pesticide free.

If you do buy non-organic fruits and vegetables, like cabbage or lettuce, then take a moment to peel the outer leaves. Rinse broccoli, cauliflower, nectarines, pears or grapes in water. You may want to soak them briefly with a dash of liquid soap or use one of the vegetable cleaner solutions currently available at health food stores. Peeling non-organic apples may be necessary, since the wax seals the pesticides onto the apples. It's far better to eat the fruits, vegetables and breads as they are, as compared to the fast foods and deadlier T.V. dinners. Less than 7% of the pesticides we consume come from grains, fruits and vegetables. However, 55 % of the pesticides come from meats and 33% come from dairy products.

10

Avoid the Mistakes
of the Other Programs
Use the Delgado Six

Phen-Fen is a combination of obesity drugs such as Phentermine and Fenfluramine or Reduxdexfenfluramine. People taking these weight loss drugs have suffered from over 47 serious side effects. Doctors monitor patients and prescribe these drugs for short term weight loss in place of lifestyle modification. Follow-up studies done show almost all the people eventually regained the lost weight and more. Suppression of appetite apparently occurs because Fenfluramine causes brain damage by destroying brain cells that produce seratonin. Seratonin is a neurotransmitter that regulates appetite, and it gives you a sense of feeling good. Phentermine acts like an amphetamine to stimulate metabolism. Redux (dexfenfluramine) reduces peoples' craving for carbohydrates. People have died from pulmonary hypertension taking this weight loss drug. There is no way ahead of time to know who will die and who will live, when taking this drug, like in a deadly game of Russian Roulette.

Another misleading diet is called the "zone". The "zone diet" is based on the Glycemic Index and insulin response to various foods. In the original studies, people were fed typical high fat American foods (fat desensitizes insulin). They measured high insulin levels after fasting one day and eating single carbohydrate rich foods. When Dr. Anderson, at the Kentucky Medical Center, later tried to duplicate the study using low fat foods, he came up with completely different results. Insulin levels were normal when complex carbohydrate foods were measured (after eating lowfat foods for one week) and fasting one day. The "Zone Diet" book based all their information on an original false premise. They even claimed lowfat, cholesterol-free diets would raise serum cholesterol levels. My studies of twenty years proves the exact opposite. "Zone dieters" have much higher cholesterol levels and plaques in their arteries over time compared to those eating whole natural complex carbohydrate foods. Vegans eat a diet highest in complex carbohydrates with the lowest cholesterol levels and the cleanest arteries based on world wide studies. The only part of the "zone diet" that makes sense is eating more vegetables and less bread or cereal. I do not agree that adding more fat or protein to your diet is safe. If you want to reduce body fat, eat less fat, protein and dense carbohydrates.

To lose weight, stay fit and have energy, you need to stop adding fat to your diet now, today! The four food groups and the pyramid food group (a slight improvement, but too many servings of protein are encouraged) are this country's worst diet mistake - it forces you to select food from fattening categories such as meat (beef, pork, chicken, fish) and dairy products (cheese, milk, yogurt, butter, etc.). Two of the four food groups are extremely concentrated in fat. That is partly why the American diet gets nearly 50% of its calories from fat. Grains, vegetables and fruits are the only acceptable foods from the basic four. Diets by Weight Watchers, Nutri-System, Jenny Craig, Diet Centers and the like are forcing you to follow the old "four food groups." You are led to believe that you cannot have a "balanced diet" without keeping meat and dairy products in your diet.

The four food groups got started many years ago to simplify the public need for food during war time. The basic food groups have led many people to consume products to which they are allergic, like milk and other dairy products. Also, people with an excessive capacity to retain fat are struggling to overcome the inherent disadvantages of consuming meats and dairy products. Meats and dairy products are totally without fiber, deficient in complex carbohydrates and low in water content. Chicken, fish, red meat, yogurt, cheese, milk and butter are generally higher in sodium, fat, calories and cholesterol than complex carbohydrates, starches, fruits, vegetables, beans and peas. Cheese, milk, eggs, meat and oils are concentrated in food density. Put simply, every bite of food from meat or dairy products is so concentrated in calories that it goes right to your fat storage. This concentrated source of calories can't possibly be used by sedentary people.

You are being misled by sales and marketing gimmicks that trick you into buying high fat, high sugar and salty products with taste-tempting pictures and healthful sounding names like Weight Watchers. The name Weight Watchers automatically means low fat, light foods to most people, which is not always true when you look at the labels of their frozen foods. The only redeeming value of these weight control programs is you are asked to eat fresh fruits, vegetables and whole grains besides the frozen foods. It's these fresh, whole natural foods that keeps the dieters intake of fat and cholesterol in check in spite of the fat and cholesterol-laden packaged foods.

Weight Watchers	Compared to	Swanson's
So. Fried Chicken Patty		Fried Chicken
		(white portions)
FAT:	16 grams	16 grams
% of fat:	53%	41%
Serving Size:	6.5 ounces	6.5 ounces

So called diet foods like Weight Watchers and Lean Cuisine are as high or sometimes higher in fat by percentage of calories than the regular food brands. The average frozen food line of Weight Watchers contains 37% fat (11 grams of fat, 290 calories, 60 mg of cholesterol and 800 mg of sodium.) Lean Cuisine averages 9 grams of fat, 260 calories, 60 mg of cholesterol, and 930 mg of sodium. The reason they may have fewer calories is that they give small portions or they use non-nutrient fillers and thickeners. The unsuspecting, uninformed public blindly trusts the name Weight Watchers, NutriSystems and Jenny Craig.

For example, here is the entire ingredient list from the Salisbury Steak Champignon, Jenny Craig's best selling prepared "diet" frozen dinner:

Cooked **beef**, water, cooked potatoes, carrots, green beans, onions, **cheddar cheese**, bread crumbs, **eggs**, mushrooms, **white wine**, **margarine**, **vegetable oil**, demi glace (wheat flour, starch, **lactose**, dehydrated onions, **salt**, tomato starch, hydrolyzed plant protein, **vegetable oil**, yeast extract, **beef extract**, **sugar**, caramel, corn starch, **wine powder**, spices), modified food starch, tomato paste, **nonfat dry milk**, **salt**, flour, natural flavorings, **beef flavor** (**salt**, **corn syrup solids**, **beef fat**, hydrolyzed plant protein, celery, and other spices, onion powder, starch, **beef extract**, caramel color, garlic powder, spice extractives of pepper, **disodium** inosinate, **disodium** guanylate), Worcestershire sauce, spices, **chicken flavor** (**corn syrup solids**, **salt**, **chicken fat**, **all vegetable shortening** [**soybean**, **cottonseed oil**, onion powder, starch, **disodium** inosinate, **disodium** guanylate, spice extractives of celery and turmeric), garlic, parsley, xantham gum, annato color, **artificial color** (contains FD & C Yellow #5.)

Now that you've read this list of ingredients from their label, does this look like a food that would be good for your health? Your cholesterol level? Or for weight loss? It's no wonder why you have to eat such small portions of these frozen "diet" dinners. We challenge you to read the labels of other "diet" system programs. They derive most of their profit from selling packaged foods.

The name on a label can say anything because it's considered part of the title. So beware of misleading words on food products like "pure virgin" olive oil, "natural" sugar and "unrefined" flour. Remember to look on the back or the bottom of the container and read the nutrition information under "ingredients." The ingredient list is strictly controlled by the Food and Drug Administration (FDA). The listing must be accurate, be in a particular sequence and leave nothing out. Always look for oils, butter, margarine, sugar, fructose and salt and if any of these fattening ingredients are listed first on the label, you know the food is concentrated in calories.

As you read labels, also look at the total grams of fat and if there are more than four grams of fat per serving don't buy it. If the food product has less than 4 grams of fat, then it's generally okay to buy. This simple rule of buying food products with zero, one, two or three grams of fat per serving will help to keep your average fat intake per day to less than 20 grams of fat and under 20% of your total calories from fat.

The average American man or woman consumes over 125 grams of fat per day adding up to a whopping 43% fat diet. Multiply the number of grams of fat by 9 and then divide that number by the total calories listed on the label to determine the percentage of fat. For example, Promise margarine, approved by the American Heart Association has 10 grams of fat and 90 calories per tablespoon (10 grams X 9 calories/gram = 90/90 = 100% fat!). Promise margarine, Heart Smart and "I Can't Believe it's not Butter" have the most amount of fat of any foods on Earth! Read the labels. The first time you go to a market armed with this information you will be shocked at the amount of fat in slickly packaged foods. 2% low fat milk has 32% fat with it's five grams of fat per 140 calories in 1 cup. It should be called high fat milk, and whole milk with its 50% fat and 9 grams of fat should be called greasy milk. Figurines, the diet bar, has 5 grams of fat per serving, exceeding 45% fat. This should be called a "fat" bar, not a diet bar.

Now, let's review the latest liquid drink craze - "Slim Fast." The following is a comparison of a 1200 calorie-per-day intake:

THE DELGADO PLAN	VS	LIQUID SLIM FAST DIET
(one day example)		
4 pieces of fruit (banana, peach, pear, nectarine)		3 liquid Slimfast
1 large potato, w/salsa		3 oz water packed tuna
2 slices of bread, w/apple butter		1 tsp diet mayonnaise
2 bowls of soup		lettuce, tomato
2 large salads, w/oil-free dressing		bread, 1 slice
1 cup of brown rice, or pasta		1 diet coke
1 bowl of sorbet ice cream		
High fiber, low fat, no cholesterol		High protein, sugar and cholesterol

The Slim-Fast directions recommend you use their product three times a day for breakfast, lunch and as a snack, which adds up to as much as 600 calories. For dinner eat a specified meal, such as the one above. The ingredients of the Slim-Fast are whey powder, sucrose, nonfat dry milk, dextrose, calcium caseinate, purified cellulose, soy protein, bran fiber, fructose, natural and artificial flavors, malto-dextrins, carrageenan, lecithin, DL Methionine, aspartame, vitamins and minerals. This product contains four forms of sugars. It is also concentrated in dairy product from whey, nonfat milk and calcium caseinate.

Slim-Fast also contains several harmful ingredients that may elevate triglycerides and cause allergic reactions. These products are only for quick weight loss, but do not help to change your bad eating habits.

In 1990, 20 million Americans spent over one billion dollars on liquid weight loss products and liquid fasting programs. Well known celebrities advertise and endorse these fads, but they rarely keep the weight off. As an example, you may have heard of Oprah Winfrey's attempts to reduce her weight. As you recall a number of years ago she lost 67 lbs thanks to a 400-calorie-a-day liquid protein plan. At that time, she vowed to never be fat again. Unfortunately, she regained all of the weight she lost initially, plus a few pounds more! The problem with these fad diets is that they do not retrain your eating habits. After you lose weight on these plans, inevitably you will gain it back. After regaining the weight that she had lost, Oprah was educated in and incorporated into her lifestyle a diet modification, and exercise program which has helped her to accomplish a maintained level of weight reduction.

Why not introduce these dieters to **The Delgado Health Plan** to get the best weight loss, save money, and improve total health? You will be successful in losing weight if you follow **The Delgado Plan,** which encourages you to change your eating habits for a lifetime.

Become knowledgeable and don't be afraid to eat more of the whole natural foods on **The Delgado Plan**. Your friends might lose weight faster initially on their Weight Watcher's or starvation liquid diets, but you will pass them up in a few months and never be fat again, unlike your friends who will always struggle until they also learn **The Delgado Plan**.

You will lose fat weight effectively if you eat less than 20 grams of fat per day and never more than 40 grams. Your total percentage of calories from fat should be under 20%. This is the **Delgado 20-20 rule:** less than 20 grams of fat, under 20% fat to lose fat and keep it off. Your calorie intake will be under 2000, with an average of between 1000 and 1700 calories per day. To keep under 1700 calories per day just be sure to eat generous helpings of soups, fruits, vegetables, potatoes and complex carbohydrates without added fats and sugars. Eat more of the fiber and balanced foods that nature has provided.

Here are the **DELGADO SIX FOOD GROUPS:**

1. Green vegetables
2. Yellow/orange vegetables
3. Tuber-root vegetables (potatoes, beets, etc.)
4. Citrus and non-citrus fruits
5. Grains (two or more types per day) plus a Vitamin *B12 fortified cereal
6. Beans and peas (green, Chinese, split, black-eyed, chick) *or B-12 supplements preferably in combination with a B complex.

Note: include a weekly serving of sea vegetables (kelp, kombu, wakame, nori) and nuts and seeds for additional trace minerals.

Low fat meats, chicken, fish, turkey, flank steak and nonfat dairy products should only be used as a condiment and never as a main dish (you may choose not to use any meat or dairy product). You should say, "We're having potato pasta casserole," instead of saying, "We're having chicken tonight with a side dish of vegetables."

A 1989 survey by the California Department of Health of 1000 consumers discovered that over 25 % of those questioned ate no fruits or vegetables on any given day. Nearly two-thirds of Californians don't eat enough fruits and vegetables. Mass media advertising has led to reliance on fast food burgers, frozen dinners and fatty dairy products. The information in this book will show you how to improve your diet dramatically and gain control over hunger and improper food selections.

11

How to Increase
Your Energy

One of the key reasons people participate in **The Delgado Health Plan** is to increase their energy levels. The complex carbohydrates are your best source of energy. Fat provides you with less quality energy. Protein would be the least acceptable energy source and cause the most fatigue. To have more energy, therefore, eat potatoes, vegetables, fruit and whole grains that are high in complex carbohydrates.

Plan ahead, carry food with you in a sack lunch, ice chest or a Delgado Cool Tote as I carry with me. This will maintain even glucose levels, giving you a high energy level. The moment you begin to feel weak, an empty stomach or hungry, go ahead and eat lightly. Frequent small meals of complex carbohydrates will be digested into glucose at a slow, consistent rate. Big, heavy meals tend to lead to a build-up of fat in the blood known as triglycerides.

Triglycerides are the way fats are carried in the blood and are stored in your fat cells. Pinch the fat on your body and you are pinching triglycerides. To experience high energy, you must maintain low fat levels in your blood. Strive to keep your triglyceride levels under 100 mg and total lipids ideally under 500 at all times during the day, especially after eating.

Fasting for blood tests have misled people and physicians into ignoring poor dietary habits. By eating frequent, small meals that are low in fat, you can maintain low fat levels in your blood all day and night. This will allow for excellent circulation. The red blood cells will flow freely to carry the maximum amount of oxygen to your brain and all the cells of your body. One fatty meal can cause the blood to become sticky, resulting in clumping of the red blood cells for over 9 hours. If less oxygen reaches the brain, you will become sleepy and tired. This is probably why so many people drink coffee (caffeine is a drug stimulant) to try to stay awake and alert. However, by maintaining low fat triglycerides and total lipids you will experience an incredible increase in energy as more oxygen reaches your brain.

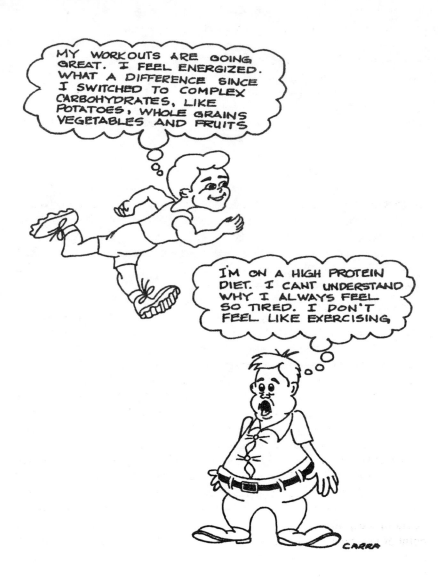

How to Look Great & Feel Sexy

The following steps are necessary to reduce fat in your blood:

1. Avoid all oils: polyunsaturates like corn oil, safflower oil, etc., monounsaturates like canola oil, olive oil, etc., and saturated fats found in butter, cheese, red meat, etc.
2. Avoid excessive use of sugar, alcohol, fruit juice or dried fruit. Sugars convert into fats if used beyond your caloric needs. Sugars are devoid of fiber so they rush into your bloodstream too quickly and turn into fats.
3. Maintain your ideal weight - obesity can cause high fat levels in the blood. In order to have more energy, you must achieve your ideal body weight. If you are currently overweight, choosing all the recommended foods and exercising daily, you may not begin to experience high energy levels until you reach your ideal body weight. If you are carrying 10 to 40 extra pounds on your body and that extra weight is in the form of fat that can enter your bloodstream at any time and slow you down, just as if you had eaten fat. You can reach your ideal body weight by following the recommendations we offer in this book.
4. Exercise daily to maintain good circulation and low fat levels. Daily exercise will begin to fire up your system to give you more energy. If you do the minimum of 15 minutes a day, that is fine. But why not plan to do 15 minutes in the morning and 15 minutes more at night? By exercising in the morning, you will burn fats that have accumulated during the night while you were sleeping and inactive. Since your triglycerides will be lower, you will have more energy throughout the day. Then at the end of the day, when there is a tendency to have a slight elevation of triglycerides, exercising again for 15 minutes will reduce the fatty levels in your bloodstream. If you want to maintain high energy levels all day long, avoid excessive or intensive exercise. Long, slow distance exercises (walking, swimming, light weights) are better than fast, overly demanding runs and heavy weight training sessions. If you are an athlete or you are accustomed to intense workouts, anticipate a need for several additional hours of sleep to allow your body to recover each day. Training to the point of muscular failure on every exercise is terribly taxing to your energy levels. Start your exercise plan slow, be consistent and you will look forward to each day with excitement and vigor. If you find yourself avoiding exercise sessions, you probably have been training too hard.
5. Reduce stress by focusing on the good things in people and in life. If adrenaline builds up, it can increase blood fats for several hours.

Have your triglycerides, cholesterol and total lipids checked every three weeks until you can maintain ideal levels on a regular basis. After consecutive low readings, you can check your levels every three months to be sure you're still on the right track.

Make sure you get enough sleep each night. Most of our participants notice they require much less sleep as they eat better and exercise. You should feel rested and good in the morning without needing coffee, tea or cokes all day. A thirty minute nap during the day may be beneficial for people who work long hours (12 to 16 hours a day.)

Your physiology, posture, stance and walk are also important to feel energetic. If you slump and slouch you will feel tired. Try sitting up straight and erect and you will notice an immediate improvement. Tony Robbins taught me the importance of frequent exercise, breathing, massage and "peak state" sessions to maintain high energy.

Some people suffer from "chronic fatigue syndrome", which can be caused by a number of different conditions. See a doctor to check your thyroid, blood counts, B-12 and iron for anemia, possible viral conditions like Epstein-Barr, mono, etc., allergies and other metabolic diseases like cancer. **The Delgado Plan** can serve as a cornerstone to enhance treatment and in many cases provide full recovery from various energy robbing diseases.

The final key to high energy is to fill your mind with good news, good thoughts, read positive books, listen to motivational tapes, attend church sermons and success seminars.

12

The Ideal Diet & Exercise for Peak Performance and High Energy

Wouldn't you like to perform at your absolute best always?

Athletes, sales people, children, housewives, and senior citizens can reach their peak potential and enjoy life more fully be eating more raw, sprouted, uncooked food, exercise, and hormones . The Peak performance plan requires a degree of discipline, commonly found in high achievers. Many people choose the immediate gratification of eating sweets and fats (short term goals of taste). Successful people have experienced the sweet rewards of security and happiness that comes with ideal health.

Successful people choose more healthful food selections and exercise to reach their long term goals. They will bypass the temporary pleasure of sweets and select the foods necessary for performance at peak levels. Feeling good and looking great is a powerful motivation for health conscious people, isn't it?

People who value health, will exercise their bodies and minds daily to be as sharp as possible. Commit to 30 minutes of daily exercise and one hour of reading a night. You might make the excuse that "you don't have the time to exercise or to read" when in reality you do. Studies show that watching television dominates most free time. Yes, that means the three to eight hours of television that most people watch every day can be allocated to more productive pursuits. If you must watch television, then exercise aerobically on a reclined bike, stairmaster, or treadmill while you watch. Better yet, consider reading while you exercise. You can be a wonderful role model for your children.

Here is the first key dietary principle to follow for peak performance:

- Consume foods rich in complex carbohydrates in the raw state. Raw foods, such as fruit vegetables, sprouted grains, sprouted legumes, and sprouted seeds are rich in digestive enzymes. The moment you heat the food by any method (lightly steaming, microwave oven, or stove) you destroy all the digestive enzymes in the food.

- Enjoy more fruits of various types for breakfast, lunch, dinner, and snacks. Fruits provide the purest source of fresh organic water, minerals, vitamins, fiber, and enzymes.

- For a rich supply of enzymes, organic vitamins, and minerals, add to your lunch, dinner, or late meals a big bowl of raw vegetables with fat-free dressing. Have sprouted sesame seeds, sprouted sunflower seeds, sprouted garbanzo beans, sprouted peas, sprouted bean mix, tomatoes, raw celery, carrots, broccoli, etc. We need a constant supply of fresh foods to get enough enzymes. Enzymes are essential to all of life's processes.

If you deplete your enzyme supply you may weaken your immune system (increasing the risk of disease) and create malfunctions of other bodily systems such as your nervous system, respiratory, musculature, and skeletal systems. This can shorten your life span by as much as twenty years, according to Dr. Edward Howell.

There are three ways to deplete our bodies supply of natural enzymes. One way to deplete our enzyme supply is by eating processed sugars, fats, and proteins. Sugars, fats, and proteins completely lack enzymes. They require excessive amounts of enzymes from the pancreas, stomach, and liver to complete digestion.

The second way to deplete our supply of enzymes is to eat too many cooked foods. The mildest form of heating food (over 118 degrees F) destroys all enzymes in the food. Lightly steamed, stir-fired, microwave or stove cooked destroy enzymes. A temperature that would be uncomfortable to the skin on your hand will destroy enzymes. Pasteurization is carried out at 145 degrees F. Water boils at 212 degrees F. Most cooking is carried out at 300 degrees F. or hotter!

The last way to deplete our enzymes is by consuming raw seeds, or raw nuts that have not been sprouted. Raw food that has not been sprouted contain enzyme inhibitors. Avoid enzyme inhibitors in raw foods (raw seeds, raw nuts, raw grains, or raw legumes), because they destroy your bodies limited supply of enzymes. Chickens and rats fed raw soybeans not sprouted or cooked become sickened and fail to grow. If you do eat any of these foods, be sure to sprout them. Sprouting the raw seed gets rid of enzyme inhibitors. Remember, legumes (beans) and grains are actually seeds before they are sprouted. Another way to get rid of enzyme inhibitors in seeds is to cook the seeds. This is the only condition that we should cook any food.

Nature provides enzyme inhibitors in seeds, nuts, grains, and legumes to prevent premature growth until being planted in a proper place. Seeds' thousands of years old found in pyramids, still contain enzyme inhibitors. These enzyme inhibitors serve a vital role in preserving the plant species. Seeds that are extremely old, will sprout and grow within twenty-four hours after being planted in moist soil. The water soaks into the seeds, nuts, legumes, or grains and completely deactivates the enzyme inhibitors within twenty-four hours.

After three days, the sprouts are now little plants fully concentrated in beneficial enzymes. These digestive enzymes inside vegetables, fruits, sprouted wheat berries, or bean sprouts help our bodies during digestion. Without these plant enzymes, our bodies must draw on our own limited supply of enzymes to digest the food. Also, our body will convert some metabolic enzymes to be used as digestive enzymes. Eating cooked food can dangerously deplete our vital metabolic enzymes.

We have over 1,300 types of enzymes used in every bodily process. We have enzymes in every cell of our body; in our lungs, arteries, brain, and muscles to produce rapid chemical reactions so we can breathe, move, and even, think! The ability to think requires several chemical reactions initiated by enzymes. The only difference between life and death of a cell, tissue, or system is the presents of enzymes. Enzymes provide the actual God given spark of life, the vital living force within each of us. Enzymes are biologically active proteins that we are born with. We have a finite, limited supply of enzymes and when we run out or become too low in enzymes we become ill or die.

The same process of life or death occurs in all other animals and plants. The genetic clock is present in all animals, influenced by hormone levels, enzymes, and a coded gene for life and death. Death occurs after the gene sends a hormone signal to stop enzyme activity. To extend life to our full genetic capability, we must preserve and protect our enzymes.

Every time we eat junk food, cooked, processed, without enzymes, we deplete more of our storage of enzymes. The normal process of digestion uses up some of our digestive enzymes (lipase, protease, and amylase) in the mouth, stomach, and intestines. We rapidly deplete our storage of enzymes by eating highly processed sugars and fats. Still, the average American consumes over 130 pounds of sugar per year from soda pop, candy, and packaged foods. We consume more than 100 pounds of excess fat, and concentrated protein from cheese, meat, and oils.

It is no wonder that our body, designed to live over 120 years of life, barely makes it through 70 or 80 years of life. Animals fed cooked meat, seeds not sprouted, and processed foods (fatty or sugary) die prematurely. The same species of animal in captivity fed raw meat, or raw organic vegetables, and sprouts live a much longer life.

When I refer too organic, I am not talking about pesticide free (foods free of pesticides and additives are important for a different reason- to avoid toxins). Organic food is enhanced by living organisms such as plants and microorganisms. Living food converts all the vitamins, minerals, and nutrients into organic substances. Organic minerals, vitamins, and water are superior to inorganic sources. Organic water in fruits and vegetables contain organic minerals chemically improved by living organisms.

Plain tap or bottled water has an inferior source of minerals in the inorganic form. The only time you should consume additional bottled water, is just before an exercise session. Ideally, most of your water supply should come from whole fruits and vegetables, because it is organic water containing organic minerals. Organic, colloidal minerals are better because they are smaller and have an electrical charge. Inorganic minerals are too large to be used by the human body.

Most people take supplements of inorganic iron, sodium, or potassium from rock or nonliving substances produced by chemical reactions or man-made extraction's. Synthetic, man-made vitamin C, Ascorbic Acid, lacks the beneficial properties of organic vitamin C bioflavinoids found in living, natural foods. The Ascorbic Acid is simply the outercoating surrounding the essential bioflavinoids.

The organic sodium and potassium in celery are beneficial to our bodies enhancing enzyme activity and detoxification. Yet the sodium and potassium we get in table salt are potentially toxic to our bodies, blood pressure, heart rate, and enzyme activities. The organic iron in beet juice, green vegetables, and apples (there is more iron in the tart apple varieties like Granny Smith as compared to sweet red delicious) enhances red blood cell development. Yet the inorganic iron (ferrous sulfate) in supplement pills destroys hemoglobin and is potentially toxic to the liver (inorganic iron overload from pans or pills can cause death).

The best supplement line we recommend comes from whole plant foods with capsules of concentrated raw vegetables, carrots, broccoli, grains and fruits. Capsules prepared without being heated are best. This preserves the enzymes, vitamins and minerals.

Raw vegetable juices and whole fruit juices can provide organic water, fiber, vitamins, minerals, and enzymes. Most centrifugal force blenders create too much heat that can destroy some enzymes. You can add ice cubes during blending to the new Vitamix blender to keep the food cool and preserve enzymes. The vitamix blender has a special motor that actually blends and retains all the fiber. Regular juicers discard all the essential fiber.

My favorite recipe includes sprouted sesame seeds, sprouted sunflower seeds, sprouted flaxseed, sprouted beans, sprouted grains with two carrots, one vine ripe tomato, one apple, blueberries, strawberries, and a banana. If it comes out too thick, I add rice milk or water to thin it out so I can drink the live blend of food. I keep fresh sprouts growing daily in four jars I rinse with water twice daily. The sprouts are ready in three to four days. The strong taste of sprouts is made palatable by the fresh fruit and carrots I add to this recipe. This makes about 44 ounces of blended thick juice for my family and me every morning. I notice I am not hungry for hours after drinking this wonderful life preserving drink.

If you choose to eat cooked food, you should eat mostly whole, natural vegetarian food. The best grains to use in the cooked form would include: rice, rice pasta, rice cereals, rice milk (Amazake, Rice Dream) etc. Rice grains are best since they are the least allergic producing grain for most people.

Other good grains low in allergy properties would include kamut, spelt, or corn grains. These grains are less allergic producing then gluten containing grains so try them and monitor how you feel. Spelt, spelt bread, spelt pasta, spelt cereal (an ancient wheat free of gluten) are available in the health food store. Corn, corn flakes, corn tortillas are also good choices for an allergy free plan.

Cooking any of the above grains into bread will cause a complete loss of enzymes in the food, but it will get rid of the enzyme inhibitors. It is best to consume grains of any type after being sprouted. Fermenting of grains or soybeans is another way to get a rich source of enzymes. Amazake rice milk with rice koji is in a fermented form, providing a good source of enzymes. Fermented, predigested foods such as tofu (select the lowfat version), miso, and tempeh are free of enzyme inhibitors, and are rich in good enzymes (if uncooked).

Add digestive enzymes from a plant source supplement sprinkled from the capsule into your food whenever you eat cooked foods. This will decrease the losses of you're limited supply of enzymes. Get an enzyme supplement that contains amylase (digests starch), protease (digest's protein), and lipase (digests fat). Open the capsule and sprinkle it on the cooked foods you eat. Sprinkling enzymes onto the food will allow the digestive process to begin immediately in the mouth and stomach. The addition of these supplements will help to preserve your enzymes. Be sure to select the capsules without bile. Bile is foul tasting. You should swallow and not break open capsules with bile.

Have you ever had constant, terrifying nightmares? I remember only too vividly, waking up in the middle of the night, drenched in sweat, as I struggled to get away from some ominous fate. Looking back on those episodes, I now know that came from eating too much meat (concentrated in fat and cooked protein) and dairy products (high in fat and pasteurized cooked protein). All of which can deplete enzyme levels and vitamin B complex.

A healthy individual should experience dream recall. If you cannot recall "good" dreams, and you only remember nightmares (You wake fearful, worried, upset, death thoughts), you may be deficient in Vitamin B6. A good source of B6 is brown rice, bananas, corn, and carrot juice. Take a supplement of B6 of 100 to 600 milligrams per day until dream recall begins to occur, then taper off the dosage down to 2 to 25 mg per day. According to Carl C. Pteiffer, Ph.D., MD, in his book _Nutrition and Mental Illness_, a health practitioner may have you use a maximum of 2,000 mgs. per day until you experience dream recall. If you awaken every two hours during the night with vivid dreams, and remember up to four dreams in the morning you are getting too much B6. If B6 produces numbness of fingers or toes, shift to pyridoxal phosphate at 200 mg dosage of B6.

For good mental health avoid being contaminated with copper from birth control pills, drinking water from copper pipes, or any supplement with added copper. Use other forms of birth control such as condoms. Use filtered water, and get most of your water from fruits and vegetables. When I'm thirsty, the first thing I eat is a juicy tomato, or grapes.

What if you have been exposed to any of the above sources of concentrated copper? Check with a doctor to have your copper levels in the urine, blood plasma and hair measured. Also ask your doctor to check your urine, blood, and hair for zinc levels. If copper is found to be elevated and zinc low, take the antidote of zinc gluconate, 15 mg to 30 mg a day. Also you should consume more tropical fruits like mangos and pineapples for a source of manganese. Zinc can cause an imbalance in manganese, this is why you need to add manganese when taking zinc supplements. Manganese gluconate of 10 to 50 mg a day will prevent any problems.

How to Look Great & Feel Sexy

Some conditions that have been helped by treating high copper levels, with added zinc and manganese include:

- Paranoia, fearful feelings, feelings of persecution, loss of contact with reality, disperceptions, schizophrenia (a misleading diagnosis or label), depression, compulsions, hallucinations, Autism, impotence, anemia, and nervous exhaustion.

Additional tests your doctor might run include blood and urine histamines levels. Also, check the blood for vitamin B6. You should have your cholesterol level done as part of a lipid panel, a chemistry panel with liver and kidney enzyme levels, and CBC with blood morphology.

Circulation to your brain will also effect performance and your energy level. Have a carotid artery ultrasound (ask the doctor or technician to identify for you even the smallest of cholesterol atherosclerotic plaques). Ask your doctor to refer you for a noninvasive, Ultra Fast CT Scan of the heart. The doctors were amazed to find how clean my arteries were without any calcification or cholesterol! When I was asked how I did it? I responded. "read my books as a reference source *Fatigue to Vitality, How to Look Great & Feel* Sexy, learn and incorporate the health plans and philosophies into your lifestyle and utilize the recipes that are included in my book, *How to Look Great & Feel Sexy*." Finally, have your bone density checked for osteoporosis with a duel density photon scan. My bones are in great shape, even without using dairy products for 20 years! Read my books for the secret. How are your bones of the spine and hips? A simple scan is available at certain hospitals without a prescription, call us for suggestions.

For peak performance and good mental health, avoid all dairy products and use rice milk, or Westsoy lite.

Avoid wheat products, barley, rye, and oats as much as possible and use the rice or the suggested grains listed above. Please see, *"Mastering the Powers of Your Inner Health"* for details. Gluten is a protein in wheat, barley, rye, and oats and it is very difficult to digest for many people. This may be because the digestive enzymes cannot digest the gluten. The undigested gluten protein leaves an accumulation of toxic material in the intestines. This irritates the lining of the intestinal wall, causing constant indigestion and malabsorption of all nutrients. It is also possible that endorphins found in gluten compete with our body's endorphins (vital brain chemicals involved in mood).

Whatever the reason, weeks and months may be required before a marked improvement appears after wheat, rye, barley, oats, milk, cheese, and yogurt are removed from the diet. Reintroduction of these grains and dairy products into the diet usually produces a relapse in days, or even hours! This is why it is important to maintain a strict adherence to the diet and to be aware of the exact ingredients of many foods. For more information, read my book "*Mastering the Powers of Your Inner Health*".

The results will be tremendous. Your brain will function best with ideal blood glucose levels (the brain can only use glucose for fuel). To prevent hypoglycemia (low blood sugar), eat frequent small meals of fresh fruits, vegetables, sprouted peas, and rice based products. Carry a cool tote and frozen blue ice, filled with fruits and vegetables, with you always. Take fresh food with you to the office and on the road. Nibble the moment you are hungry. Eat every few hours, or every twenty minutes if need be. Anticipate your hunger and eat if you feel weak or empty. The results will be tremendous within a short period of time.

Our studies show that the average person with an elevated cholesterol level can reduce it by as much as 30% by dietary changes alone. You can reduce and control triglycerides (fat in the blood) by as much as 40% within nine days (with added exercise). Improved circulation will do wonders for your performance, sense of well being, and energy levels.

To have high energy, exercise aerobically for about 30 minutes to an hour every day. You can sustain a pace based on your pulse rate with the formula 20 minus your age x .60 = your target pulse rate to maintain during each session. Also monitor your respiration rate during exercise. You should be able to carry on a conversation during exercise and not get out of breath. If you are out of breath, huffing and puffing then slow down. Your respiration rate is the best way to tell if you are in aerobic exercise.

Some people will do just fine with a brisk walk, slow walk, or jogging. Other exercise we recommend includes a treadmill, stairmaster, recline bike, and cross country skiing. Also, weight training at least four times a week for 30 to 45 minutes at high intensity will keep all your muscles fit and in shape. Start with aerobics for 30 minutes and then finish with some weight training.

Busy people may have time for only one session a day. Yet, as we age, muscles tone and strength can be improved if you perform two or three exercise sessions a day. Each exercise session should take less than 30 to 45 minutes. You will be amazed at your rapid progress. Allow for sufficient rest and recovery (about two hours) between exercise sessions. Rest restores enzyme reserves. Excessive exercise without rest may deplete too much of your enzyme stores.

I apply my own principles to my fitness routine by consistently lifting weights at least once or twice a day. I do "fun" aerobics at least four times a week such as dancing, or playing with my children. Aerobics that provides additional benefits such as time with family or social nights out are activities that I look forward to. Because I enjoy the exercise I do, I look forward to doing it on a daily basis. Doing business meetings, family activities, and social events can create challenges. And I am proud to say that even in the busiest of schedules I have been able to continue to improve my fitness level. Age is not something to fear, it is an issue that requires the most advanced program and planning.

I modified my diet using the Juice blend recipe in the morning to include additional sprouts, fruits and vegetables above my normally high raw foods intake. After only six months, I noticed increases in energy, less body fat and gain's of lean body muscle mass. This brought me to ideal levels as if I were twenty years younger. I have placed first and second in the best body contest "Mr. Mastery" at the Anthony Robbins event in La Jolla, California 1992 and Cancun, Mexico 1993. I live each day feeling and looking in the peak of health. How about you? Are you ready to experience a whole feeling of wellness?

Read my books, listen to the audio tapes, view the video tapes, come to our seminars (ask for an updated schedule), or make an appointment for our mobile wellness screening or individual and group counseling.

   HEALTHY STUDIOS ®

Reverse Aging Seminars & Testing T.V. Show Production

Call today for a special discount on all of our products 800-631-0232

How to Look Great & Feel Sexy

13

Eating at Home
Or Restaurant

At home you can prepare meals centered around several high complex carbohydrate dishes, with vegetables, salads, soups and fruit ice creams for dessert.

Microwave cooking is great for busy people. Look for pre-packaged, microwave-ready fresh vegetables that include squash, potatoes, broccoli, snow peas and carrots. Try potato pancakes (Manischewitz) that can be poured directly from the package into a Pyrex bowl. Mix with filtered or bottled water and cook for three minutes in the microwave. Eat them like you would mashed potatoes. Potato pancakes have a spicy, onion flavor and taste great without being fried. The sodium content is high (1400 mg per serving) so if you're on a sodium restricted diet, then limit the use of these pancakes to twice a week. Almost every big grocery store I've been to has these pancakes in the Jewish food section next to Matzo balls.

Frozen vegetables without oils, butter, sauces or salt are convenient and easy to prepare for busy people who want to lose weight fast. Brussel sprouts, broccoli, cauliflower, lima beans or green peas are favorites with a three minute average cooking time. Blend with a dash of mustard, salsa and Worcestershire Sauce or you may want to try all three condiments in different corners of the vegetable container. We suggest you try a variety of mustards: Dijon, garlic, or jalapeno. Try catsup from the health food store or diet section of the market without added sugar. Use chili salsas: red, green or mixed, or blends like Pace, Ortega, Rosarita and La Victoria (mild, medium or hot) on potatoes or vegetables. They're great! Barbeque sauce without sugar can be obtained at specialty stores, health food stores and at other supermarket locations.

Weight control can begin with breakfast, because that is how most people start out the day. If you want to drop fat weight fast, you might begin your morning with just fruit, vegetables or a soup. The ideal type of cereal for weight loss is a hot cooked cereal, because when you cook the grain (cracked wheat, old-fashioned rolled oats, 4-grain cereal, etc.), the cereal absorbs much of the water that fills up the bowl and reduces the density of food concentration.

The best hot cooked cereal for weight loss is oat bran cereal, since bran, by its very nature, is mostly non-digestible. Most of it passes through your system undigested. As a result, you feel full and satisfied while only absorbing a fraction of the 110 calories for one serving.

Maybe you would like to try puffed rice, wheat or kashi. Since puffed cereals are light and filled with air, the food density will provide fewer calories.

I encourage people to use water or diluted juice with cereals instead of milk to reduce food calorie concentration further and to lessen the potential of food allergy reaction caused by milk (bloating, diarrhea, skin or lung conditions). Milk is a leading cause of food allergies in people throughout the world. You might like Rice Dream Vanilla milk from the health food store. It's sweet and thick, and if you dilute it with water, it tastes very much like nonfat milk without causing allergic reactions. You may want to try cold bottled or filtered water mixed with a small amount of fruit juice (apple, berry, etc.).

It's okay to mix in your favorite fruit with cereal. Some researchers have confused the occasional reaction of indigestion to be caused by the combination of fruits and cereal starches. I have found certain instances of indigestion can be observed after the consumption of fruit and cereal because people usually use milk in their cereal. Despite whether fruit is added or not, even the small amount of milk added to cereal may cause an upset stomach, bloating, gas, etc. and that the response of indigestion, is an allergic response to added milk, and not caused by the combination of fruit and starch. In tests, when people who had been experiencing symptoms of indigestion, were given the replacement of rice or soy milk, instead of dairy milk, 98% of those who had been experiencing indigestion were alleviated of symptoms.

You will find that cereal and fruit with water or juice is actually tasty. I know the thought of water or rice milk in cereal may seem strange, but if you'll just try it, I believe, like most people, that you'll grow to prefer it. If you or your children want to maintain or gain weight, you should be serving high-density grain cereals. Mueslix, granola (without oil), Nutri-Grain, Nutty Rice and other whole grain cereals can be eaten with cold water, juice or rice milk. Growing children need to eat more cereals that provide more calories. My children have for some time enjoyed their old fashioned rolled oats (raw, uncooked) mixed with Nutri-Grain rice nuggets and water. Try vanilla, "No Sugar" Strawberry or Blueberry syrup, or a jam preserve without sugar for added flavor.

At restaurants you can order puffed rice and water with fruit. One of my favorites is Egg Beaters scrambled with mushrooms, tomatoes, bell pepper and chili salsa into an omelet. If they don't offer Egg Beaters, which is low in fat and cholesterol, you can simply order egg whites scrambled without the yolks. I always have one or two orders of dry hash browns (cooked without oil). At a restaurant I'll use the catsup, A-1 sauce or salsa. At home I'll use catsup without added sugar or salt that I purchase from the health food store.

Muffins can be a good choice for a simple meal or snack if they are low in fat. Try an oat bran muffin (made without egg yolk or milk) from specialty stores or homemade from our recipe book.

For lunch or dinner, you might have some microwaveable mixed veggies: potatoes, squash, broccoli or carrots that come in a plastic container. Microwave the veggies for four minutes and use low-sodium Worcestershire Sauce, mustard or salsa. You might even enjoy a hearty vegetable soup that was left over from the weekend pot of soup. You can use a canned soup such as minestrone or Cous Cous cup of soup without oil. Pritikin soup is acceptable; it's just not tasty enough and needs to be spiced up with Mrs. Dash's Spicy Seasoning. If you're trying to lose weight, you need to use soups every day. If not for breakfast, at least have soups for lunch and/or dinner. We have great soup recipes like black bean, gazpacho, minestrone and potato (without milk).

When eating out, it's true some soups have more sodium than you would normally use (less than 200 mg of sodium per serving is ideal and not more than 500 mg is acceptable). However, the vegetable soups are usually so low in fat they make a great filling meal for faster weight loss. If the soup is made with meat (chicken, pork or beef), you should spoon out as much of the meat as possible or when ordering, ask the waitress for less or no meat in your soup. Meat is dense in calories, fat and protein and is without any fiber, so it should only be used as flavoring in food and not as a main dish. Chicken and fish also should be limited to less than a few ounces a week because they have as much cholesterol as red meat! Even if you remove the skin, cholesterol is permeated equally throughout the lean flesh of the chicken or fish.

I love to stop in for a tureen of vegetable soup at Marie Calender's. Sizzler's, the Soup Exchange and Soup Plantation also have good soups. At a Thai restaurant, I order Yum Won Sen (spicy salad) and Tom Yum Pak spicy lemon grass soup, which is my absolute favorite. I ask them to substitute broccoli for the large amount of chicken they traditionally use. At Mexican restaurants, I order tortilla soup without cheese or chicken, albondigas soup without meatballs, black bean soup without sour cream or gazpacho soup (a cold traditional Spanish soup made with tomatoes, onions and vegetables).

Eat large amounts of salad for rapid weight loss. My favorite salad ingredients include palm hearts, capers, artichoke hearts packed in water, portebellos mushrooms, vine ripe tomatoes, grape leaves, cabbage, kim chee, hummus, salad olives, Greek olives, lemon grass and Thai fat free dressing. Restaurants offer salad bars with great selections and be sure to use a low-calorie or nonfat Italian dressing, vinegar or lemon juice. You may even want to try salsa or minestrone soup over your salad! The type of salad dressing that you use on your salads can profoundly influence your goal of weight loss or increased energy. What if you made the mistake of using bleu cheese, thousand island or ranch dressing? This adds as much as 30 to 40 grams of fat, (per three tablespoons of salad dressing) which is as much fat as a typical hamburger!

DINING OUT
Dining out in restaurants takes a bit of finagling and compromise. If you order right off the menu without a special request, you can be sure of getting a high fat, cholesterol, salt or sugar meal. To get what you want, you have to ask for what you want!

Dressings and sauces, except tomato sauce, are rich in fat, cholesterol and salt and are easily omitted from most dishes. Whenever possible, ask for your pastas and vegetables to be prepared without butter, margarine or oil. If you have zucchini, mushrooms, carrots or other veggies fried in batter, simply eat the vegetable, avoiding the fried batter.

ITALIAN
Call ahead to ask if they will cook without oil or salt. More restaurants are offering this option.

SALAD: Order a salad with no meat or anchovies. You can have a small amount of Italian dressing (vinegar or lemon juice would be better) and one or two black olives. The peppers and other vegetables are good choices, too.

SOUP: Minestrone is a good choice; most have only small amounts of oil, if any. If you see too much oil, avoid it.

PIZZA: Order your pizza without cheese and a selection of vegetable toppings. Request extra sauce so the crust doesn't become dry, sprinkle on a little Rice Dream Parmesan. Some pizza parlors offer a whole wheat crust that is preferable.

PASTA: They probably will not have whole wheat pasta, but any pasta, except egg pasta, is okay.

BREAD: Breadsticks or Italian bread are safe. Avoid garlic bread.

VEGETABLES: All vegetables are fine when served without butter, margarine or oil. Try a steamed artichoke or a baked potato with meatless tomato sauce.

FRUIT: A fruit salad or fresh fruit is good for dessert.

CHINESE, JAPANESE OR THAI
When you order, request no oil, eggs, M.S.G., sugar, or soy sauce.

VEGETABLES: Ask them to stir fry your vegetables in chicken or fish stock. They can add cornstarch to thicken and ginger and garlic to flavor. Hot mustard is good to use at the table. Try to select soups and vegetables with broccoli added instead of meat. However, you can have approximately 3 oz. of chicken or fish with your vegetables two or three times per week. Avoid beef, pork and duck. Order chop suey or chow mein with very little oil. For taste variety, try the spicy, hot Szechuan sauces on broccoli, eggplant or other vegetables.

RICE: Choose plain steamed rice instead of fried rice. It is browned by frying in soy sauce or oil. Avoid hors d'oeuvres because they are high in fat and cholesterol.

MEXICAN
Call ahead in the morning to order beans without lard; they may oblige you.

SOUP: Gazpacho, a cold vegetable soup, is good to start the meal. Also, albondigas soup without meatballs or tortilla soup without the cheese.

SALAD: Try a dinner salad with fresh lemon and salsa.

CORN TORTILLAS: Request 1/2 dozen soft and steamed to dip in the salsa. Avoid fried chips. (If they are crispy, they are fried).

ENTREE: Try enchiladas stuffed with rice and no cheese. Try a tostada - ask for a steamed corn tortilla bottom instead of fried. Top with plain beans, shredded lettuce, onion, salsa and just a dab of guacamole.

FAJITA VEGETABLES: Stir fried without oil, beans cooked in water, corn tortillas.

BURRITOS: Without cheese, add hot sauce to taste.

FRENCH

APPETIZERS: Vegetables in a light vinaigrette, vegetable relish, French bread.

SALADS: Salads of fresh or steamed vegetables, Salad Nicoise without oil or egg yolk may be a safe choice.

ENTREE: Ratatouille (cooked vegetables), a simple vegetable soufflé made with egg whites (without the butter), or a baked potato with chives are all tasty choices. Most restaurants will prepare a beautiful steamed vegetable plate to order even if it is not on the menu. Request no salt, butter, margarine, oil or sauces. If your cholesterol level is below 160, you may order broiled fish, chicken (or frog legs) once or twice a week.

AMERICAN

SALAD/SALAD BARS: Fresh vegetables are unlimited. Limit the marinated vegetables, as they may be salted. Request tasty vegetable soups, also try fruit salads. Avoid eggs, meat, excess chicken, turkey, cheese, oil or mayonnaise based salad dressings, and bacon bits. Try using vinegar or lemon juice with garlic and herbs, if available.

BREAD: Try for whole grain bread or rolls, but if they are not available, anything other than butter or egg bread will do.

ENTREE: Steamed vegetable plate can usually be ordered, even if it is not on the menu. Ask them to omit the butter, oil, margarine and sauces. A side order of baked potato (request chili salsa instead of butter) or the fresh vegetables of the day can be an excellent main course after the salad bar. You'll leave feeling full, knowing you haven't over stressed your body.

DESSERT: Try fresh fruit or fruit salad. Fruit sorbet is good, too. If you feel very decadent, split a rich dessert among several people - and take tiny bites.

BREAKFAST BONUSES:
- Ask for sugar and salt-free cereals such as oatmeal, Cream of Wheat, Shredded Wheat or Grape-Nuts.
- Try apple juice with water added instead of nonfat milk on cereal!
- Fresh fruit can generally be found at most coffee shops or breakfast houses. Order 1/2 grapefruit, orange sections, melon in season or sliced bananas.
- Always ask for dry toast or rolls, since most restaurants butter your toast for you. If you must, use jam for a spread on toast instead of butter.

LUNCH TIME SAVERS:
- Have hot soup, broth-based instead of creamed, as a main part of your lunch.
- Always order sandwiches on whole grain bread and hold the mayo.
- Look for eating places that offer minimally processed foods. Cafeterias and lunch counters have the advantage of showing you exactly what you are getting. The trick is to choose foods that are not swimming in fat, oil or sugar. Natural and vegetarian restaurants are good choices. They offer fresh vegetables and fruit salads, fruit and vegetable juices, whole grain breads, vegetable casseroles, etc. Beware of dishes laden with cheese, eggs or oil.
- Try creating your own vegetable sandwich with pita bread or crusty rolls filled with lettuce, tomatoes, pickles, beans, rice, pasta, cucumbers, carrots or cauliflower.
- Pick a fast food restaurant with a salad bar so you can fill up on raw vegetables. Otherwise order the simplest sandwich; leave off the fat-rich hamburger or chicken meat, instead request the bun, lettuce, tomatoes, pickles, mustard, catsup and hold the mayo; eat french fries on a limited basis (surprisingly fries may have less total fat than cheeseburgers or cheese tacos); order fruit juice instead of a milkshake (fast food restaurants probably will not have nonfat milk).
- Mashed potatoes (hold the gravy) with several ears of corn (hold the butter) can be a filling and healthy alternative to chicken.

RESTAURANT DINNER PREPARATIONS:
- Call the restaurant in advance for special requests. This courtesy will improve your chances of getting what you want. The worst that can happen is the restaurant will refuse. In that case, pick another restaurant.
- Eat something before you leave home and nibble from your Delgado Cool Tote in route to the restaurant. It will take the edge off your appetite so that fat laden temptations will not be as difficult to refuse.
- Think before entering. Have a good idea what you will order before you enter a restaurant - then stick to it. Try new dishes only if they fit your basic plan.
- Order a la carte to avoid unwanted courses and trimmings.
- Think in terms of low fat versus high fat choices for each course. For example, if appetizers are placed on the table, concentrate on celery and carrots instead of cheese, or for soup, choose hot consommé over cold vichyssoise.
- Order meatless dishes. Emphasize vegetables. Choose broiled or baked foods - not fried or french fried.
- Don't be afraid to split a meal with a friend.
- Skip dessert or have fresh fruit in season.

- Doggie bag your leftovers to enjoy the following day.

Remember, BE ASSERTIVE! Your integrity and strength of character will determine if the restaurant is going to serve you and your needs.

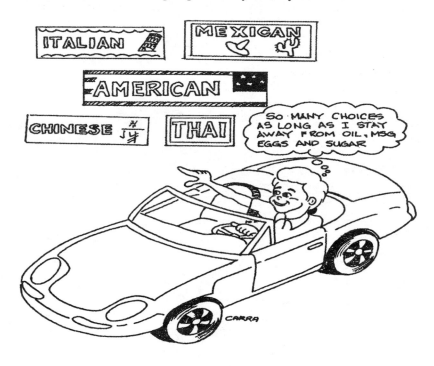

SAVING TIME IN THE KITCHEN
SECRETS OF THE PROFESSIONAL CHEF
You come home tired and face the task of preparing dinner for yourself and perhaps your family and friends. Maybe you have an evening engagement, and need to fix something in a hurry.

Certainly convenience foods were made for times like this. But we know what convenience foods contain - usually FAT, SALT AND SUGAR. So what do you do?

Don't give in to processed fast foods. Why not use the techniques of the professional chef, and prepare healthful convenience foods ahead of time to last you a week?

After all, many of us are professionals in our careers. Why shouldn't we apply the same organizational principles to our kitchens and to our health?

PREPARING FOODS FOR THE WEEK
HOW TO DO IT

You will need to set aside a block of time that you can be home, maybe Saturday afternoon, or Sunday, or even Monday evening. You'll probably want to allow a couple of hours. Then get set. The equipment you will need includes:

Large zip lock bags
A large stock or soup pan.
Individual or family-size plastic containers.
Sauce pans and utensils.
A food processor is optional.

First, you should wash, peel and cut several kinds of vegetables - the choice is yours. Fill a plastic container with some of them and set another batch aside for making soup.

If you own a microwave, you can prepare vegetables for freezing simply by cooking a dish full for one to two minutes. This "blanches" them, the same as if you had parboiled them.

Next, turn on the oven and throw in several russet potatoes, washed and scrubbed. While you're at it, cook a pot of rice, or a grain mixture. Portion it into Seal-a-Meal or Zip Lock bags and freeze, or store in the coldest part of the refrigerator.

Beans help control or reduce cholesterol levels, so now is the time to cook a pot of them. Use three to one proportions of water or chicken stock, add a bay leaf, onion and some garlic.

Make a basic soup or broth. The easiest way is to use Health Valley, Pritikin Unsalted Chicken Stock, or unsalted tomato juice, and add vegetables and herbs.

Here are some extras you might try that take about thirty minutes:
- Make some corn chips out of tortillas, or make wheat chips from chapatis (whole wheat Indian flour tortillas). Slice and place on a cookie sheet, bake at 350 degrees for 10 minutes or until crispy.

USES FOR PRE-COOKED FOODS
PREPARED VEGETABLES
Grab a handful of raw carrots, celery or broccoli for a quick snack. How often have you eaten some "forbidden" high calorie food, when you really wanted something light? Prepare some vegetables ahead of time, and you won't have any more excuses!

You also can take a plastic baggy of vegetables in your Delgado Cool Tote when you leave home and eat them for snacks.

Here are some vegetables you might like to prepare:

carrot sticks	jicama sticks
celery sticks	cauliflower-ettes
broccoli spears	cherry tomatoes
zucchini slices	green onions
red, green bell peppers	fresh baby green beans

Wash, peel and dry them thoroughly before storing them in containers. They should be good for two to three days.

SOME VEGETABLES THAT ARE GOOD
COOKED AND THEN EATEN COLD:
- artichokes with fresh lemon
- baked yam and sweet potato
- eggplant, cooked and pureed with garlic and basil

BAKED POTATOES CAN BE ENJOYED:
- sliced and diced in soups and casseroles
- grated and cooked in a nonstick pan, or oven-baked with onions as hash browns
- sliced and baked as french fries, or oven browned potatoes
- sliced and cooked with green onion and green chili salsa (Ortega or homemade) for Mexican-style potatoes
- red and white new potatoes can be cooked, chilled, diced and added to salads

SEITAN'S WHEAT MEAT CAN BE HEATED
AND USED IN APPROPRIATE
QUANTITIES:
- in sandwiches
- in soups
- as a crepe filling with stir-fried vegetables

BEANS CAN BE USED:
- pureed and served as a bean dip
- in Mexican dishes such as tostadas, chili's and enchiladas

BROWN RICE CAN BE USED IN:
- soups
- casseroles
- pilafs
- stir-fries
- desserts

You can make a pie crust by pressing rice into a pie shell and baking for fifteen minutes; then fill it with vegetable mixture or wheat meat for a delicious pie.

SAMPLE MENUS USING PRE-COOKED
FOODS PREPARED ONCE A WEEK
BREAKFASTS:
- Homemade granola with fruits
- Frozen whole wheat waffles or pancakes, with fruit berry topping
- Breakfast burritos
- Breakfast cookie bars

SNACKS:
- Crackers, bread or vegetable sticks with hummus
- A pouch of soup, heated in the microwave, or boiled in the bag
- Corn and wheat chips, bean dips and salsa dips

DINNERS:
- Wheat meat and vegetable stir-fry made fresh (it only takes fifteen minutes), frozen brown rice, reheated in the microwave, or boiled in the bag
- Banana-ginger freeze
- Spaghetti, served with marinara sauce, tossed green salad, minestrone - frozen, reheated in the pouch
- Tostadas, with low fat Rice Dream cheese (optional), pre-made bean dip, lettuce, tomatoes, salsa topping

EQUIPPING YOUR KITCHEN

Chances are, if you took a moment to review how your kitchen is set up, you'd wonder how you ever got dinner made. We put up with old pots and pans, cramped quarters and poorly designed preparation areas - conditions we wouldn't tolerate in our professional workspaces. If you take an hour or two to apply the same organizational abilities you use at work to your kitchen, food preparation may even be enjoyable!

THE WORK AREA

Make counter space available, with ample room for cutting. Have a permanent area set up for chopping and get rid of useless items and appliances not regularly used. Leave out the equipment you use most often. Knives should be next to the cutting area; spoons and spatulas close to the stove.

ALUMINUM

A growing body of medical evidence points to ingested aluminum involved in the process of Alzheimer's Disease. That means we should avoid:

- Covering foods directly with aluminum foil, especially acidic foods such as tomato sauce and citrus fruits
- Aluminum pots, pans, tea kettles
- Heating foods packaged in aluminum containers

RECOMMENDED COOKWARE:

- Silverstone - or other "non-stick" cookware
- Stainless steel with copper bottoms
- Porcelain
- Corningware
- Glass
- Iron skillets are excellent because they conduct heat well. But, they also add a significant amount of iron to your diet. Therefore, be careful not to use iron pots daily (iron overload can harm the liver), unless you're iron deficient as diagnosed by blood test.
- A chef's knife is indispensable. Make sure the blade is the right size for your hand. It should balance pleasingly. Nine-inch blades are about right for most women's hands. Stainless steel is easier to care for than carbon steel.

OTHER GREAT TIME SAVING TOOLS

- Microwave ovens
- Food processors with slicing and grating discs
- Salad spinners for drying lettuce, also doubles as a colander or drainer
- Pasta cooker

- "Gravy strainer" or "Soup strainer" - brand name for a clever container that separates fat from liquids
- Rice cooker
- Vegetable steamer
- Wok
- Crock pot

GUIDELINES FOR ADAPTING RECIPES

IF THE RECIPE CALLS FOR:	TRY INSTEAD:
whole eggs	egg substitutes, egg whites
whole milk	rice milk or soy milk
mayonnaise	non-dairy, low fat mayo
frying	baking, broiling, frying in non-stick pan, with minimum fat
salt	a blend of herbs and spices
ground beef	wheat meat or soy
oil for sautéing	chicken or vegetable broth
mustard	salt-free mustard
steak sauce	Mrs. Dash salt-free steak sauce
ketchup	basic recipe ketchup
baking soda, powder	low sodium baking soda, powder
graham cracker crumbs	low oil granola, ground Grape Nuts
sugar	less sugar, juice concentrates, low sugar jams, apple butter, vanilla, cinnamon, nutmeg, barley malt
cheese	low fat, low sodium Rice Dream cheese or Tofu Rella

Here is what to use instead of butter or oil in different cooking techniques:

SAUTÉING VEGETABLES: Use a little liquid - water, or vegetable or chicken broth, in the bottom of a skillet. Bring liquid to a boil, then add vegetables and stir until browned, allowing most of the liquid to evaporate. While sautéing, add extra liquid if vegetables look too dry.

You also can brown vegetables directly in a dry, non-stick skillet. Avoid using a high heat and watch the cooking process carefully to avoid scorching vegetables. This also can be applied to sautéing rice for a pilaf; or use a non-stick pan and oven-toast, watch carefully so the rice will not burn.

FRYING: On stove top, use non-stick skillet without fat to "fry" patties, potato pancakes, French toast, pancakes, etc. Use a non-stick baking sheet without fat to oven-"fry" breaded eggplant, potatoes, vegetables, etc. Some foods lend themselves well to either a skillet on the stove or a baking sheet for oven frying.

MARINADES: Replace oil or fat with compatible liquids: lemon juice, vinegar, vegetable broth or fat-free stock, tomato juice, fruit juice, rice milk, low salt soy sauce, cooking wines, etc.

BASTING: Use acceptable liquids such as those suggested under Marinades, as well as rendered juices from food being cooked.

SWEETENING TIPS: Fruits and fruit juices are most often required for sweetening. However, there are more subtle ways to sweeten foods. Cooking with carrots is one good way. They can give a sweet flavor to soups and entrees that normally call for a tablespoon or two of sugar, such as spaghetti sauce. If a little sugar is called for in a recipe, try adding a diced or chopped carrot. Or put in large whole carrot to simmer with the sauce, then remove it before serving. If you want to make the recipe even sweeter, add a swig of apple or pineapple juice. You can use carrots to sweeten a navy bean casserole, instead of the usual molasses and brown sugar. Cook the carrots and some apple juice in the bean liquid.

Naturally sweet vegetables like sweet potatoes, squash and yams make great pies and hot casseroles, and when chilled are gooey-sweet snacks. Sweet corn is another vegetable that lends a natural sweetness.

For some types of cooking and baking, to complement the sweetness you are trying to achieve, the flavor of vanilla will help. Use vanilla extract or whole vanilla beans. For chocolate, you can substitute carob powder, but beware of the carob bars sold in health food stores, which generally have sugar and fat additives comparable to a chocolate bar.

Also, use spices to best advantage. Certain spices, such as oregano or peppers, impart a slightly bitter quality, as opposed to sweet basil, for example. Spices such as coriander, cinnamon, nutmeg, allspice, curry, cardamom, ginger and mace tend to complement a sweet flavor. The omission of salt from recipes will also automatically sweeten a dish.

TO MAKE GRAVY FROM FAT-FREE STOCK: Remove all traces of fat from meat, fish or fowl stock by refrigerating or freezing the stock until fat is congealed. Remove fat with a large spoon and pour stock through several thickness of cheesecloth to remove remaining fat. You may want to freeze the de-fatted stock in pre-measured amounts or in ice cube trays.

Add to the fat-free stock desired seasoning and other liquids of choice, such as vegetable broth, rice milk or a dash of soy sauce. Then thicken according to the following methods:

THICKENING HINTS: For sauces, stews and many soups (cream-style and others), cornstarch or arrowroot can be used for thickening. Arrowroot clears completely, so it should be used where greater transparency is desirable. While it makes a delicate sauce, it does not reheat well. Cornstarch may leave a little cloudiness, but is preferable for some uses, such as thickening a white sauce, as it gives desirable color. (Arrowroot may be purchased at health or natural food stores).

To use cornstarch or arrowroot, follow these suggestions:

Make a thin paste of the cornstarch or arrowroot in a little cold liquid (water or other acceptable liquid). One level tablespoon of arrowroot will thicken one cup of liquid. Cornstarch has slightly more thickening capacity, so a little less will be needed to thicken the same amount of liquid.

Bring liquid to be thickened to a boil. If using cornstarch, simmer liquid gently as you slowly pour in the paste, stirring as you pour. With arrowroot, remove saucepan from heat as you do this step, then return to heat and again bring to a boil. Stir while liquid thickens.

Flours, such as wheat and potato, arc also good thickening agents and can be used instead of cornstarch or arrowroot for some recipes.

For some foods, a thickening agent such as those described is not required to get good results. For example, a spaghetti sauce is preferably thickened by reduction; that is, reducing it to the proper thickness. The sauce is slowly simmered, uncovered, until enough liquid evaporates to produce the desired consistency. This method also works well with soups. Another very handy way to thicken soups like split pea, minestrone, bean or vegetable is to puree a portion of it in the blender, and then return it to the soup pot. With this method, the blended soup vegetables act as a thickener.

INSTEAD OF 1 CUP ALL-PURPOSE WHITE FLOUR
1/2 cup barley flour
3/4 cup coarse whole wheat flour
3/4 cup barley flour
7/8 cup whole wheat pastry flour
3/4 cup buckwheat flour
3/4 cup coarse cornmeal
1 cup fine cornmeal
3/4-7/8 cup rice flour
1-1/3-1-1/2 cups rolled oatmeal
3/4-1 cup rye flour
1 cup rye meal
1 cup corn flour
3/4 cup 1- cup fine whole wheat flour
3/4 cup rolled oats plus 1/4 cup whole wheat flour
7/8 cup whole wheat flour plus 1/8 cup sunflower seed meal

INSTEAD OF AN EGG
1 tablespoon de-fatted soy or garbanzo flour
3 tablespoons potato flour or tapioca
1/2 cup cooked oatmeal
1 teaspoon Egg Replacer mixed with two tablespoons water (product is a mixture of refined flours and egg whites)

INSTEAD OF OIL
Butter, shortening or oil can be simply omitted in most recipes.

In baking, substitute applesauce or water for the oil used (usually no more than a quarter cup of applesauce per recipe; if more moisture is needed, replace the rest with water).

In cooking, the oils called for usually can be omitted, and an equal amount of vegetable stock or water is used instead.

For pie crusts, cookies and some desserts, cashews or almonds ground with a small amount of water help to hold the ingredients together.

ABOUT SWEETENERS
In general, the amount of sweetening called for in a recipe can easily be cut down. Start by cutting the amount in half. Use malt syrup or rice syrup as sweeteners instead of white or brown sugar. For a different flavor, use unsweetened apple juice concentrate as a sweetener, or ground up dates or raisins.

ABOUT LEAVENING
Use one teaspoon baking yeast dissolved in a quarter cup of warm water to which a half teaspoon of honey has been added. This works well in muffin recipes.

ABOUT NUTS
Nut or seed milk can be used in place of dairy milk in all recipes. It makes a good base for white sauces. Nuts can be ground up and used as a base for spreads or to hold crusts and cookies together. (Proportions: 1/4 cup nut meal to 1 cup water; mix in a blender or food processor).

HERBS, SPICES AND SEASONINGS
As you begin to cook without oils, fats, salt or sugar, you are likely to feel a little lost. These are, after all, the most common seasonings. However, you will soon find yourself more perceptive and appreciative of the unique flavors in foods. Herbs, spices and other appropriate seasonings can be used to vary and heighten flavor. Use twice the quantity a recipe calls for when substituting a fresh herb for a dry one.

PURCHASING HERBS AND SPICES
Fresh herbs - garlic, dill, basil, oregano, tarragon, parsley, cilantro, mint, ginger and chives - can often be found in the produce section of a grocery or health food store. You can buy potted herbs from a nursery and grow them at home in a window or your garden.

If you purchase dried herbs and spices in jars, you should read the label to make sure sugar and salt have not been added. If you are thinking of buying them in bulk at a health food store, buy small quantities: herbs and spices lose their flavor with age.

STORING HERBS AND SPICES
Fresh ginger and garlic can be peeled and stored in water or wine in the refrigerator. Fresh herbs can be stored in plastic bags or containers, in the refrigerator or freezer.

Dried herbs and spices should be stored in jars or containers with tight-fitting lids. It is essential that you keep them in a dry, cool place. If you store them near the heat of a stove they will quickly lose their flavor. Herbs and spices should be discarded when their flavor or aroma becomes weak.

Seasonings that add a licorice flavor:

fennel	star anise
anise	tarragon

Seasonings that add a salty flavor:
onion: fresh, flakes or powder
parsley: fresh or dried
garlic: fresh, granulated or powder
lemon/lime: juice or peel
celery: fresh, seed or powder
hot spices: cayenne, chili or Tabasco

Seasonings that add a sweet flavor:

vanilla extract	mace
mint	cloves
cinnamon	allspice
cardamom	nutmeg
ginger	

Seasonings used in ethnic dishes:
French:

tarragon	nutmeg

Italian:
oregano, basil, fennel, rosemary, garlic, parsley, marjoram

Mexican:
chili powder, chili pepper flakes, cumin, cilantro, oregano

Chinese:
ginger, star anise, fennel, curry, cayenne, cilantro, hot mustard, garlic

German & Scandinavian:
caraway, dill, cinnamon, cardamom, paprika, garlic, lemon

Indian:
cumin, curry, coriander, turmeric, fenugreek, garlic, saffron, cinnamon

MENU PLANNING

Quick, what's for dinner? Many people we know would say, "Well, I've got a chicken in the freezer," or "Don't we have some ground sirloin left?" or "Let's broil a couple of steaks!" Those of us who have been raised in the last fifty years are used to planning meals around animal protein. Our "side dishes" are the grains, fruits and vegetables that comprise the main calorie source of meals in much of the rest of the world. To develop healthier eating habits, then, we have to retrain ourselves to eat more like "primitive" man. This means basing our meals around complex carbohydrates, with the occasional meat, fish, or poultry we consume as the side dish!

This transition can be easier than you think! Thinking about the foods of your ethnic background is one way to get your imagination working. Eastern Europeans based their meals around buckwheat, potatoes and wheat. Oriental populations ate large amounts of rice. Africans lived on millet and tubers. South Americans grew yams and plantains. In Mexico and North America, corn, wild rice, squash and beans supplied the bulk of their nourishment. And where would Italy be without pasta?

In this section, we'll give you some pointers on menu planning and a week's menu for weight loss. Also included is brown-bagging advice. Bon Appetit!

EAT FIRST WITH YOUR EYES

Imagine sitting down to a dinner and seeing a white plate with a serving of mashed potatoes, cauliflower and basmati white rice in front of you. Perfectly nutritious, perhaps, but, how boring to the eye! Meals are much more appealing when planned to please all the senses. Season with aromatic herbs that tease the appetite with smell. Contrast colors like deep green broccoli, roasted red peppers, golden ears of corn and rich, purple kidney beans. This meal not only looks beautiful on a plate, but it also packs a powerhouse of good nutrition!

Contrast textures. Try serving crunchy, lightly cooked vegetables with smooth, creamy side dishes. Combine tastes, such as a spicy Indian Dal with a cool, minted vanilla Rice Dream topping, or a fiery Chili with sweet Texas Cornbread.

WHAT TO PACK IN A DELGADO COOL
TOTE, LUNCH BOX, OR PICNIC BASKET

* Sandwiches on whole wheat, rye or in whole wheat pita pockets with these fillings:

SPREADS/FILLINGS:
- Hummus
- Wheat meat or Nature burgers with barbecue sauce (no sugar)
- Sliced thin: cucumbers, carrots, tomatoes, zucchini, onions, red or green bell peppers, with no oil dressing

SALADS:
- Tabouli - Mid-Eastern Wheat Salad
- Potato Salad
- Rice Salad
- Fruit Salad
- 3-Bean Salad
  (Many of these salads can be stuffed inside a pita pocket)

ENTREES:
- Ratatouille
- Nick's Spicy Brown Rice
- Spaghetti
- Burritos

BREAKFAST FOODS:
- Homemade trail mix
- Banana Bread Pudding Square
- Whole wheat bagel
- Fruit salad
- Rice custard pudding
- Breakfast burrito
- Fruit juices
- Low-sodium V-8 or tomato juice
- Angeled eggs
- Oatmeal to make in a thermos (just add hot water and wait minutes, stir and serve)

WHEN YOU'RE THE GUEST
- If you can, let the host know in advance your dietary preferences, there is nothing worse than going to dinner and sheepishly telling your host you cannot eat the food.
- If you discover the food has been smothered with fat or salt, take a bite or two, and then rearrange the food on your plate.
- Eat some of your "legal" food at home before leaving so you are not at the mercy of your hunger and your host's fatty foods.

- Don't be the first guest to arrive. The time before dinner usually means high fat hors d'oeuvres and one too many cocktails! If you do arrive early, request sparkling water with juice.
- Concentrate on low fat appetizers, like raw vegetables, plain crackers or pretzels. Avoid salty and fatty snacks such as anchovies, caviar, cheese balls, sour cream dips, peanuts, etc. If an unwanted hors d'oeuvre is pressed on you, hold it in your cocktail napkin for awhile, then put it down and forget it!
- Circulate and find stimulating conversation. Concentrate on talking and listening instead of eating and drinking.
- Eat plenty of vegetables, a large portion of salad, rolls and other complex carbohydrates. Take only a small portion of the meat dish being served.
- Take fruit for dessert if there is a choice. If not, simply say you are stuffed and could not eat another bite - everything was just delicious! You can always have some fresh fruit, bread or vegetables from your Delgado Cool Tote in the car or you can eat when you get home if you are still hungry!

WHEN YOU'RE THE HOST

- Prepare the same low fat foods for your guests that you would normally eat. Explain to your guests why you eat the foods you do. Most everyone is enthusiastic about trying the foods even if they do not choose to live with the diet.
- Try gourmet recipes with the recommended substitutions. Dress up the meal for your friends with garnishes. Fix something fancy!
- Potluck dinners work well with a diverse crowd. Everyone can bring their favorites and you will have favorites too, and can stick with your diet without offending anyone.
- One important thing to remember: exposing your guests to your new way of eating may be the most valuable gift you could give them!

AIRLINE TRAVEL:

If business or pleasure finds you traveling on airplanes often, there is no need to worry about breaking your new good food habits. Special meals can be ordered in advance, when you make your reservations. The agent will present a list of different types of dietary plans - fruit plate, diabetic, low cholesterol, vegetarian and kosher. The best bet is usually a vegetable plate, or a low cholesterol meal or Hindu meal (dairy free vegetarian).

On the low cholesterol meal you'll still be given fats - margarine instead of butter, so avoid using these. Make sure the vegetarian meal is something comparable to pasta, or a baked potato with vegetables, as opposed to an egg and cheese disaster! This is called an "ova-lacto" vegetarian plate. DON'T ORDER IT! Just ask a few pertinent questions, the same as you would do in a restaurant. With a little patience, you'll fare well. My fellow passengers usually look on with envy as I enjoy a fresh meal instead of the standard T.V. dinner-type they sit viewing glumly!

The Delgado Cool Tote can be a lifesaver on a long flight. You can nibble on fresh fruit, bread and vegetables hour after hour. You will avoid weighing yourself down by passing up the salty peanuts, candy, buttery sauces and meats.

DELGADO TABLE
OF HEALTHIEST FOODS
EAT DAILY:
1. GREEN VEGETABLES: broccoli, mustard greens, kale, leafy lettuce, etc.
2. YELLOW VEGETABLES: carrots, squash, corn, sweet potatoes, pumpkin, etc.
3. HIGH WATER CONTENT/LOW CALORIE VEGETABLES: tomatoes, cucumbers, celery, cabbage, onions, cauliflower.
4. STARCH VEGETABLES: potatoes, jicama, yams, winter squash, parsnips, etc.
5. FRUIT: pineapple, strawberries, oranges, tangerines, apples, apricots, grapes, watermelon, cantaloupe, cherries, bananas, blueberries, pears, etc.
6. WHOLE GRAINS: brown rice, oatmeal, whole grain pastas, spaghetti, bread, millet, barley, nutty rice, corn or whole wheat grain tortillas, etc.
7. PEAS: split peas, green peas, yellow peas, black-eyed peas, chick peas, etc.
8. BEANS: pinto, kidney, navy, black, white, lentils, lima, green, mung, etc.
9. CHESTNUTS: (As many as desired)
10. BEVERAGES: Vegetable juice - tomato, carrot, V-8, red bush tea, linden, chamomile, Chinese herb; Caffix, Pero, Roastaroma grain drink; fresh water, Perrier water, Poland, low sodium club soda. (Daily as desired).
11. BRAN: Wheat bran - use 1-5 tbsp/day for weight loss and regularity. Psyllium husk, Colon Cleanse or Metamucil - use 2 to 3 tbsp per day to reduce cholesterol.

MODERATE USE FOODS
1. SOYBEANS: Tofu, soybean-meat substitutes - up to 6 oz per day.
2. NUTS/SEEDS: Walnuts, cashews, pecans, almonds, filberts, sunflower seeds, pumpkin seeds, coconuts, brazils, hazelnuts, almond butter, - up to 2 oz per day - 1/4 cup (a small handful of 24 nuts).
3. AVOCADOS: Guacamole - up to 1/4 whole. Black olives - 6 per day, Green olives - 6 per day.
4. FRUIT JUICE: Dried fruit, juice concentrate, canned, apple butter - up to 8 oz per day. If triglycerides are over 130 - up to 3 oz per day.

5. LEAN MEATS: Chicken, turkey, fish, cornish hens, flank steak; mollusks (clams, oysters, squid, snail, mussels, scallops) - up to 6 oz per week.
6. DAIRY: Nonfat milk, nonfat yogurt, evaporated skim milk, buttermilk (lowfat), low fat cottage cheese, hoop cheese, Liteline, Lifetime - fat reduced up to 1 oz per day due to milk allergies we recommend no more than 8 oz milk, 1 glass nonfat or 2 oz per day of yogurt. Instead, we suggest trying lite soy milk or rice milk.
7. SPICES/CONDIMENTS: Pepper, cayenne pepper, garlic, onion, oregano, "uncatsup" (low sugar, low salt), mustard, chili-salsa, No-Salt Vegit, vinegar.

FOODS TO LIMIT OR AVOID
AND RECOMMENDED REPLACEMENTS
1. CHOLESTEROL
LIMIT: Crustacean (shrimp, lobster, crab, crayfish, etc.) to 1 oz per week.
AVOID: Egg yolks, organ meats, (brains, liver kidney, heart)
REPLACEMENT: Egg whites in place of egg yolks, Egg Beaters for occasional use. Replace all foods (bakery, etc.) that have egg yolks with those that are egg free. Replace organ meats with Vitamin A Beta-carotene foods, i.e., carrots, yams or peppers. Use vegetarian based B-12 supplements. Eat iron-rich foods like wheat bran, garbanzo beans, lentils, etc.

2. FAT
LIMIT: Fats to 1 tsp per day.
AVOID: Vegetable oil-corn, olive, peanut, palm, safflower, polyunsaturated oil, linseed, coconut; margarine, lecithin, shortening; non-dairy creamer, salad dressing, whole milk, low fat milk, peanut butter.
REPLACEMENT: Use nonstick pans, Pam, chicken broth, no-oil Italian dressing. Butter- replace with butter flavor extract, butter buds, apple butter.

3. CHEESE
LIMIT: 1 oz per week low fat cheese
AVOID: Cheddar, Swiss, American, Blue, Colby, Jack, Parmesan, Mozzarella, Ricotta, Cream Cheese, String, etc.
REPLACEMENT: Rice Dream cheese, Liteline, Lifetime.

4. MEAT
AVOID: Sirloin, T-bone, club, hamburger, bacon, sausage, bologna, hot dogs, sardines, ham, duck, pork, lamb, veal.
REPLACEMENT: Seitan's wheat meat, with spices, tofu, tempeh etc.

5. SUGAR

AVOID: White, brown, turbinated, honey, fructose, artificial (saccharine, sorbitol, aspertame-NutraSweet).

REPLACEMENT: fruit, juice concentrate, apple butter, raisins, etc.

6. WHITE FLOUR

AVOID: White rice, pasta, sourdough, etc. Use only if whole grain is unavailable.

REPLACEMENT: Whole wheat flour products.

7. ALCOHOL

LIMIT: 4 oz (4 drinks) total per week.

8. CAFFEINE

REDUCE: Coffee, tea, soft drinks, decaffeinated drinks.

REPLACEMENT: Roasted grain drinks (Caro, Roastaroma, Pero, etc.).

9. TOBACCO

AVOID: SEE STOP-SMOKING SECTION

10. PROTEIN

AVOID: Excessive use of protein powder, liquid protein.

REPLACEMENT: Whole food!

11. SALT

AVOID: Salt added to food, soy sauce.

REPLACEMENT: Use other spices on food. Kikkoman salt-reduced soy sauce or one pickle. Use food where salt is listed near end of ingredients.

14

Composition Of Foods

There are many books written on how to control cholesterol and lose weight. However, many of these books fail when you get to the recipe section since they invariably contain foods that have cholesterol or fats in amounts that are undesirable. If you want to follow a program that can effectively lower your cholesterol and also can help you to control your weight, then this is the ideal program for you.

There is an easy way to remember whether a food contains cholesterol. Remember, if the food once had legs, wings, a tail, could wiggle or move, then it has cholesterol. Obviously chicken and turkey have wings and legs and fish have fins; therefore, they have cholesterol. If you ate a cockroach, it would have cholesterol in it. Don't laugh!! Some people eat fried grasshoppers and they have cholesterol, too!!

If you need to lose weight while you are trying to lower your cholesterol, then simply select the foods that emphasize the soups, a variety of vegetables and fruits, along with oat and corn bran, all of which will help you to lose weight while you lower your cholesterol. If you are trying to gain or maintain your weight, then be sure to select more of the whole grain dishes such as cereal, rice, beans and peas, while eating less of the soup, salad, and fruit dishes.

Select those foods that you enjoy most. Eat them on a frequent and regular basis. By doing so, you will automatically see improvements in your long-term efforts to control cholesterol. Your body will be getting rid of a minimum of 100 mg of cholesterol a day naturally. And, since you will be eating foods that have no cholesterol in them, you can count on that portion being excreted and not being replaced. Also, by selecting foods lowest in fat and calories, you can expect to reduce your body fat level and reshape your body.

By consuming foods that are high in soluble fiber (14 grams or more per day), you can excrete even more cholesterol than 100 mg per day. This will help you achieve more effective results than if you had resorted to medications for cholesterol control.

The old method of measuring crude fiber used in 1974 was an inaccurate laboratory estimate that has since been replaced by the term "plant fiber," also known as Dietary Fiber. Dietary Fiber is the cell wall components of plant foods not digested in the human small intestines, providing bulk to the stools and almost zero calories.

COMPOSITION OF FOODS

Soluble fiber (gums, pectin and mucilages) commonly found in oat bran, psyllium husk and black-eyed peas help to lower cholesterol and stabilize blood sugar levels when used in amounts equal to 14 grams or more per day.

Insoluble fiber (hemicelluloses or noncellulosic polysaccharides, cellulose and lignin) commonly found in wheat bran primarily helps to promote regularity and to accelerate weight loss.

The combination of soluble fiber and insoluble fiber equals total fiber. Your intake of "total fiber" should add up to at least 40 to 60 grams per day to promote regularity, proper bowel function and daily elimination.

Vegetables have a high water content and contain the least amount of fat, calories and sodium. This is why vegetables, including potatoes, should be eaten often if you're trying to lose weight. Vegetables also provide a small amount of complex carbohydrates for an efficient source of energy. Vegetables have zero cholesterol, making them safe to eat in unlimited amounts. Fiber is good for weight loss because it has almost no calories. Notice the good source of dietary fiber from onions, artichokes, brussel sprouts and yams. (Fiber remains intact and undigested, leaving valuable bulk to pass through the intestines). Vegetables provide some soluble fiber that helps to draw excess cholesterol out of our bodies.

Beans and peas are low in fat (except soybeans), low in sodium and have no cholesterol. For example, black-eyed peas are very high in total and soluble fiber. Beans, split peas, and black-eyed peas are high in concentrated food density, protein and calories. You should limit their use to smaller portions until you reach your ideal weight.

Fruits are the second lowest source of fat and calories. Fruit is the lowest source of sodium and they have no cholesterol. Certain fruits are high in fiber (berries, peaches, prunes). Fruit is good for weight loss and cholesterol and blood pressure reduction.

Cereal, bread and grains are usually low in fat (read labels to be sure there are no added oils or fat), have zero cholesterol and have moderate amounts of sodium and calories. Grains provide an ideal balance of protein for human needs, and they will become the center of your diet after you achieve your ideal weight. Grains are rich in fiber helping to prevent digestive disorders.

The highest source of fiber comes from bran. Turn to the section titled "Composition of Foods Chart." Notice that psyllium husk seed (Metamucil) has 8 times more soluble fiber than any other bran. If you add 3 to 6 Tbsp of psyllium a day to your cereal or drinks, you can significantly lower your blood cholesterol level. And if you use fiber in combination with a zero cholesterol diet, you'll get the most effective results. Limit the use of rice bran and wheat germ because they're higher in fat than other bran (3 - 5 grams of fat vs. 2 grams of fat).

Nuts and seeds should be limited to small handfuls a day, because they're very high in fat with 48 to 84 grams of fat per 4 ounces (cup serving). Nuts are the highest in calories of plant foods. Avocados and black olives are next highest in fat and calories.

Soups with 3 grams of fat or less per 10 oz can are great for weight loss because they're low in calories and the broth is filling. Some name brand soups are high in sodium (over 1000 mg per can serving), so make homemade soups whenever you can.

Sugar beverages tend to contribute excess calories and you should avoid them. Fruit juice diluted with mineral water or clean, filtered water are your best choices. Limit liquor to 4 oz a week or less.

You may be surprised to learn from the food composition list, that poultry and seafood have as much cholesterol as red meat. They are too high in protein (excess protein can cause osteoporosis, fatigue or kidney damage) and they have no fiber. Poultry and seafood are also concentrated in pesticides and toxic chemicals. Reduce or avoid chicken and fish whenever possible.

Salad dressings can be very high in fat, calories and sodium. Notice that some salad dressings are much better than others. Buy no-oil salad dressings.

Desserts are now available low in fat and with no dairy products added (sorbet, nonfat, dairy free Haagen Dazs and Tofutti Lite). Be careful to avoid high fat desserts (pound cake and cheese cake).

Red meat and organ meats contain a concentration of fat, calories and cholesterol. Be alerted that certain cuts of meat are even worse than others. A simple rule of thumb to follow would be to use meats only on limited occasions, and when they are used, only as flavoring and not as the main course. Beef producers are making available leaner cuts of meat. "Lean and Free" are cuts of steak from dairy bulls fed a high fiber, low fat ration (without growth hormones or antibiotics) and slaughtered before 11 months of age. However, this does not make lean cuts of meat an unlimited use item - because they still have from 35 to 50 mg of cholesterol per 3 1/2 ounces.

Dairy products, eggs and cheese are extremely high in cholesterol, fat, sodium and calories. They have no fiber and no complex carbohydrates. You need to become aware of the need to avoid these foods.

Fats, oils, margarine and butter are the highest hidden source of fat and calories. Don't be mislead by advertising that promotes "no cholesterol" and ignores the terrible concentration of fat.

Fast foods are high in fat, calories and sodium. Start ordering side dishes like bean burritos or potatoes without cheese. It will make a tremendous difference in the quality of your health.

The section titled "Composition of Foods Chart" needs to be studied carefully so you can make the best food choices while following **The Delgado Diet**.

15

Making the Delgado
Health Plan Your Way
of Life

All across America there is a new attitude about food. People care again about quality and freshness and are eagerly exploring new food tastes. They're preparing foods in a new way, using more fresh fruits, vegetables, herbs and spices to create a light, delicious fare. Scorned are the old culinary crutches of the unimaginative cook - greasy fats, salt and sugar.

This section will help you in learning to be a more informed and creative cook. Cooking without fat and salt will open a new world of foods, from old-fashioned regional American foods to international cuisine - plus we will show you how to invent your style of light and healthful cooking.

Begin with a positive attitude! Take pride in your efforts to learn a more healthful lifestyle. There is no need to feel deprived of your old-style foods. Once you begin to use our recipes, you'll know that this is a way of eating you can happily live with for a long and healthy life.

CLEAN OUT THE CUPBOARDS
This is it! Today is the day you're going to begin your new style of cooking. So grab an empty box and rid your cupboards, refrigerator and freezer of those health and vitality-robbing foods. Get rid of foods high in fat, sodium and sugar! Then stock up on the foods listed on our shopping guide!

BE A FOOD DETECTIVE
Government regulations require food manufacturers to list ingredients in order of descending predominance. It would seem to be a simple matter to determine if a food is high in fat, sodium or sugar. But, it is not that easy. Food manufacturers, increasingly aware of consumer concern, have responded not by cutting down unhealthful ingredients, but by making the public THINK that the product is healthier! Various marketing strategies are used to mask the actual levels of some ingredients, especially fat, salt and sugar. Buzz words such as "LITE" are tacked onto a product name, usually with little or no

reduction in the fat or caloric content. Sometimes an irrelevant statement is made, such as "NO CHOLESTEROL" boldly printed across a jar, as one nationally advertised peanut butter now proclaims. Of course there is no cholesterol in peanut butter. Cholesterol is only found in foods of animal origin. What they don't tell you is that peanut butter is about 80% pure fat. It's important to learn about label reading to choose foods wisely.

FATS

Studies show that lowering the amount of total fats in the diet has the beneficial effect of reducing the rate of heart disease, cancer, diabetes, stroke and hypertension. An obvious reason to cut down on fats is they are fattening! Fat has twice the amount of calories per gram compared with protein or carbohydrates. Animal foods, especially red meats and dairy foods, can increase the percent of fats in your diet. Up to 55% of your total daily calories come from fat - this is why the average American diet is so high in fat. Switching to smaller portions of lean animal proteins, such as skinless poultry, fish and nonfat dairy products, is one very effective way to cut down on fat. Another way to reduce fat would be to avoid all meats and dairy products completely. You can do this by focusing on the use of grains, vegetables, beans and fruits as the center of your meals.

Another source of excess fat in the average American diet is fried foods and snacks - potato chips, fried chicken and fish, and French fries. Salad dressings, cooking oils, mayonnaise and nut butters also contribute to a high fat intake. In processed foods, check and avoid foods containing anything but a minimum of these fats:

- Lard and shortening
- Beef fat
- Chicken fat, EPA fish liver oil
- Vegetable oils, coconut oil, cottonseed oil, olive oil, lecithin, safflower oil, sunflower oil, canola etc.

Review the fat content of the foods on your current shopping list. Do any of the foods need to be removed or limited? Next, go to your refrigerator and cupboards and note how many of the following fatty, greasy foods you are still eating. Note that any foods containing over 20% of their calories from fat and over four grams of fat per serving should be avoided or limited. You should always eat less than 22 grams and never more than 40 grams of fat per day.

FAT IN FOODS

Food	Percent Calories of Fat	Grams Fat in 1/2 Cup
Salad oil (corn, olive, etc.)	100	109
Butter	100	91
Margarine	100	90
Mayonnaise	100	87
Bacon	94	70
Cream cheese	91	43
Hamburger (ground beef)	89	16
Avocado	88	19
Peanut butter	85	65
Beef (T-bone steak)	82	20
Egg yolks	80	37
Lamb	76	13
Sunflower seeds	76	34
Cheddar cheese	73	25
Cashews	73	32
Whole eggs	65	14
Mackerel	50	10
Milk, whole	49	5
French fries	43	7
Grains, Beans, Fruits, and Vegetables	1-15	.1-3

HIDDEN SODIUM IN FOODS

Sodium is naturally found in whole foods such as grains, beans, fruits and vegetables. Unless your physician has advised you to eat a very low sodium diet, the sodium level of these foods need not concern you. A diet composed of these foods, eaten in their natural state, will supply you with just the right amount of sodium needed for body function. What we are investigating here is the sodium level of processed foods - those jars and bottles, boxes and bags in your cupboard and refrigerator!

You may consider yourself already educated about sodium. You've thrown away the salt shaker and you only buy foods that list salt as the last ingredient. You've made a good start! But it's just not possible to guess the sodium level in a package by reading a simple list of ingredients. The only way to be certain of the sodium content is if the manufacturer has included a nutritional disclosure statement. Guides, such as the Composition of Foods Section of our book, also can tell you the amount in many products. Don't assume that the sodium level is low just because it is listed last. Salt is concentrated, with 2,000 mg in one teaspoon. In proportion to other ingredients, it may be the smallest volume, yet still be much too high for your health. The United States government recently declared a standard for food manufacturers making nutritional claims. Foods advertised as "low sodium" may have no more than 135 mg sodium per serving. The manufacturer may claim "No Added Salt," but still use other compounds or ingredients already containing sodium.

OTHER SODIUM COMPOUNDS

Many other types of sodium compounds are used in food manufacturing. They can contribute significant amounts of unwanted sodium to your diet. They are often "hidden," because they don't necessarily taste salty. A prime example is monosodium glutamate (M.S.G.), commonly used in many processed foods. Some people even use it directly in food preparation. Oriental foods are notorious for its use. You may have used it under the trade name "ACCENT." But what are the other salty compounds?

SODIUM NITRATE - used in preserving and coloring processed meats such as ham, bacon and luncheon meats.

BAKING POWDER AND SODA - found in your pancake mix, biscuits, quick breads and cakes.

BRINE - used to preserve pickles, sauerkraut, corned beef and pastrami, also used in feta cheese.

DISODIUM PHOSPHATE - added to quick cooking cereals such as Instant Oatmeal packages; used as an emulsifier in cheeses, chocolates, beverages and sauces.

SODIUM ALGINATE - used in chocolate milk and ice creams to create smooth textures.

SODIUM BENZOATE - used as a preservative.

SODIUM HYDROXIDE - used to soften and loosen skins of olives, hominy and other fruits and vegetables.

SODIUM PROPIONATE - used to retard mold in bread and cheese foods.

SODIUM SULFITE - used to bleach maraschino cherries.

SODIUM SACCHARIDE - artificial sweetener.

In addition, the following ingredients found on labels are also high in sodium:

SOY SAUCE
TAMARI
AUTOLYZED YEAST
HYDROLYZED YEAST
MISO (different types can have varying amounts of sodium).

WHEN I SEA SALT, I SEE RED

Has anyone ever told you to use "sea salt" instead of regular salt!? This gimmick is misleading! Advertisements in some health food publications may have led you to believe that sea salt is somehow more healthful than ordinary table salt. While it's true that sea WATER is rich in magnesium, calcium and iodine, sea SALT is so refined that insignificant amounts of these nutrients are left. Sea salt is just as loaded with sodium as any other brand.

You just pay more to poison yourself!

WHAT ABOUT SALT SUBSTITUTES?

A look at the shelf on the "diet" or "health food" aisle of a supermarket will show you several types of salt substitutes on the market. The newest type, the ones we recommend, are creative blends of herbs and spices, with absolutely no salt or sodium chloride added.

Another type of salt substitute is potassium chloride (KCL). It is marketed under the trade names of K Salt Sub, No Salt, Lo Salt and Salt H. Because it is a crystal, like sodium chloride, it has the appearance of salt. Some people find its biting taste similar to salt's effect on the taste buds. Others find it bitter, or chemical, to the taste. We suggest you avoid this salt substitute based around potassium chloride. Also, potassium chloride should not be used by certain people. Although KCL is somewhat safe for people with healthy kidneys, it can cause a dangerous buildup of potassium in the bloodstream of people with impaired kidneys. It also must be avoided by individuals taking diuretics that cause the kidneys to retain potassium.

The third type of salt substitutes are somewhat new on the market. Morton's "Life" salt and others of its kind are 50/50 blends of potassium chloride and sodium chloride. While it is an improvement over regular table salt, this product still contains 1,000 mg of sodium in one teaspoon. These are not recommended if you want to control your high blood pressure without drugs.

PROTEIN

You need to limit the use of high protein animal foods if you want to avoid the following problems:

1. **OSTEOPOROSIS** - loss of bone: the greatest single cause of lost bone material in post-menopausal women is the overuse of protein in the diet, especially animal protein, which is more acidic and higher in sulfur than plant protein. Minerals including calcium are pulled out of your bones to neutralize the acid from animal proteins. If you want strong bones and teeth, cut down on the use of high animal protein foods like skim milk,

yogurt, cottage cheese, chicken and fish. You can gain bone density by maintaining your protein intake under 75 grams per day, especially if most of the protein comes from plant foods. By reducing the use of animal protein (meat, cheese, eggs) you can avoid:

2. **FATIGUE, DEHYDRATION, KIDNEY DAMAGE, GOUT & ARTHRITIS** - Foods high in protein leave waste products such as urea, uric acid and ammonia. This buildup of waste acts as a powerful diuretic, which leads to water dehydration of your body tissues and a loss of endurance. Tremendous stress is placed on your kidneys to remove waste, which could lead to failure of one or both kidneys, resulting in death. High uric acid is a well known cause of gout arthritis. To prevent this keep your total protein intake under 75 grams per day, with no more than 25 grams coming from animal sources. Limit animal proteins to less than one cup per day. For best results, don't use any animal protein (meat or dairy product).

ANIMAL PROTEIN: Limited Use Suggested

FOOD	GRAMS PROTEIN IN 1 CUP	CALORIES OF PROTEIN
Chicken	44	76
Pork	40	45
Beef	30	30
Cottage cheese	30	50
Cottage cheese, low fat	24	79
Cod fish	27	89
Egg whites	27	85
Skim milk	9	41
Whole milk	9	21

Remember that starch plant foods like grains, fruits and vegetables supply sufficient protein, as you can see from the following chart:

FOOD	PLANT PROTEIN: Ideal GRAMS PROTEIN IN 1 CUP	CALORIES OF PROTEIN
Pears	1	5
Mushrooms	2	38
Bananas	3	5
Orange	2	8
Sweet potatoes	4	6
Potatoes	3	11
Rice	5	8
Corn	5	12
Spaghetti	4	14
Kidney beans	14	26
Lentils	16	26
Split peas	16	26

SUGAR

Sugar is present naturally in many foods. There is sugar in fruit and milk, for instance. When sugar is refined from foods, however, it becomes an "empty calorie," with no other nutritional value other than calorie. To metabolize refined sugars, your body must actually draw vitamins and minerals from its storage sites.

Sugar is used as a flavoring and preserving agent in a host of processed foods, from breakfast cereals to ketchup and hot dogs. The highest percentage of sugar in the American diet comes from soft drinks (21), sweets (18), bakery goods (13) and milk products (10). A diet based on fast foods and convenience items is sure to be loaded with sugar, even if you avoid candy and other sweets. Consumers have been concerned about the sugar content of foods for a long time. Some companies in the food industry have responded by lowering the sugar content of their products, or offering non-sweetened versions. It is easy today to buy fruits canned in their juices, for example. Just as often, though, the sugar content of a product is simply disguised. A look at some "health foods" and some types of breakfast cereals will show you a few of the ways sugar is hidden. One way is to use another type of sugar, or to embellish the name, such as "clean raw sugar," or "turbanado" sugar. Some stores will promote products sweetened with honey instead of sugar. Honey is a highly refined sugar, processed courtesy of the bees. It has the same effect on the body as other sugars processed by man. A current marketing gimmick is to combine several types of sugars in one product. A label that might have read, "sugar, wheat, corn, salt, spices" can appear to be lower in sugar by using, "wheat, corn syrup, honey, corn, sugar, salt and spices. When reading an ingredient label, be aware of these other names for sugar:

- Raw sugar
- Brown sugar
- Turbanado sugar
- Molasses
- Honey
- Corn syrup, corn syrup solids
- Maple syrup, maple sugar
- Anything ending in -ose, such as fructose, mannose, etc.

Use any type of sugar as little as possible. The best way to sweeten your food is with fresh fruit, applesauce, unsweetened apple butter, small amounts of apple juice concentrate or rice milk. The recipe section of this book, *The Delgado Health Plan Recipes* will give you an abundance of additional ways to sweeten with a minimum of refined sugars.

FIBER IN THE DIET
WHAT IT IS AND WHY IT'S IMPORTANT

Fiber is the indigestible residue of certain foods, such as whole grains, fruits and vegetables. Meats and dairy foods contain almost no fiber. It is not a single substance, but is composed of cellulose, lignin, hemicellulose, pectin and gums. These five components of fiber all resist the digestive enzymes in your stomach.

WHAT WE KNOW ABOUT IT

Years ago, nutritionists believed that fiber lacked nutritional value. In recent years, however, our thinking has been revised about its benefits. We now know that dietary fiber has a positive effect on several health problems, and more health practitioners are suggesting that we increase our consumption of fiber-rich foods.

Dr. Denis Burkitt, the British physician, began the movement toward high fiber in the treatment of several diseases. He noticed that the Uganda natives he worked with seldom contracted heart disease, colon cancer or diverticular diseases of the bowel. Burkitt concluded their diet was responsible. It was high in vegetable fiber (primarily from whole grains) and low in animal protein, fats, refined grains and sugars. This is directly opposite of the typical English and American diet, with our heavy emphasis on meats, fats, white flour, and sugar foods and drinks. Other studies have shown that high fiber diets may:

- Lower blood cholesterol by reducing the amount of time food is in the digestive tract, thus limiting re-absorption of cholesterol in the bile salts during digestion.
- Improve blood sugar processing in the diabetic, through the gum and pectin components in fiber.
- Prevent constipation.
- Help weight control, by providing a full feeling, increasing chewing time and retarding the rate of ingestion.

CAN YOU GET TOO MUCH FIBER?

Yes, some people get too much fiber from added wheat or oat bran and can have some uncomfortable side effects. An excess can lead to painful intestinal gas, nausea and vomiting. You can prevent this if you maintain a sufficient fluid intake and experiment with the amount of fiber that suits your needs.

If you are eating whole grain breads, vegetables and fresh fruits, you are probably getting the right amount of fiber. You may not need to continue supplementing your diet with added bran after you've achieved your health goals of reduced cholesterol levels, weight loss and regularity.

GRAINS

Grains are high in complex carbohydrates, contain small amounts of fat and moderate amounts of protein and are cholesterol free.

Whole (i.e., unrefined) grains are high in B-vitamins, minerals, and fiber. A whole grain is composed of three parts:
- The germ, high in B-vitamins, vitamin E, minerals and essential fatty acids.
- The endosperm, primarily composed of starch, with trace amounts of vitamins and minerals.
- The bran, chiefly indigestible fiber, together with B-vitamins and minerals.

During the refining process, the germ and the bran are removed, and only four vitamins and one mineral are replaced. Therefore, whole grains are far more nutritious than their refined counterparts.

Grains are a good source of calories for those who wish to gain weight or maintain weight. If you've been trying to lose fat weight on our program, but your progress has been slower than you had hoped for (as measured by body composition testing), then you may need to reduce the amount of grain servings temporarily, while you increase the vegetables, soups, salads and fruit.

75 CALORIES PER SERVING

1/2 cup barley, cooked
1/3 cup brown rice, cooked
1 small dinner roll
3 Tbsp cornmeal
1 corn tortilla
1/2 cup cracked wheat
1/2 cup rye, cooked
1/2 cup triticale, cooked
1/3 cup Shredded Wheat
2 ounces pasta, cooked

3 Tbsp whole wheat flour
1/2 cup buckwheat, cooked
1 slice bread
1/2 whole wheat bagel
1/2 cup wheat, cooked
1/4 cup homemade granola, cooked
1/2 cup millet, cooked
1/2 cup oats, cooked
1/4 cup Grape-Nuts
1/2 large whole wheat pita bread

COOKING TIMES & PROPORTIONS
FOR DINNER GRAINS
GRAINS(1 cup dry measure)

Grains	Water	Time	Yield
Barley (whole)	3 cups	75 min.	3-1/2 cups
Brown rice	2 cups	1 hour	3 cups
Buckwheat (whole)	2 cups	15 min.	2-1/2 cups
Bulgur wheat	2 cups	15 min.	2-1/2 cups
Cracked wheat	2 cups	25 min.	2-1/3 cups
Millet	3 cups	45 min.	3-1/2 cups
Coarse cornmeal (polenta)	4 cups	25 min.	3 cups
Wild rice	3 cups	2 hours	4 cups
Whole wheat berries	3 cups	2 hours	2-2/3 cups

BEANS AND PEAS

Beans and peas are good sources of protein, carbohydrates, vitamins, minerals and fiber. They are low in fat and completely cholesterol free. High in calories, they are very helpful for those who are trying to gain weight, or having difficulty maintaining it. If you are trying to lose weight, then you may need to reduce your intake of beans, depending on your progress.

Serving sizes are measured after the beans have been cooked, rather than when dry.

125 CALORIES PER SERVING

1/2 cup azuki beans 1/2 cup black beans
1/2 cup black-eyed beans 1/2 cup garbanzo beans
1/2 cup kidney beans 1/2 cup lentils
1/2 cup lima beans 1/2 cup navy beans
1/2 cup peas, fresh or dried 1/2 cup pinto beans
1/2 cup white beans

COOKING TIMES & PROPORTIONS FOR BEANS
BEANS (1 cup dry measure)

Beans	Water	Time	Yield
Black Beans	4 cups	2-1/2 hrs.	2 cups
Black-eyed peas	3 cups	2 hours	2 cups
Garbanzos (chick peas)	4 cups	5 hours	2 cups
Kidney beans	3 cups	3 hours	2 cups
Great Northern beans	3-1/2 cups	4 hours	2 cups
Lentils/split peas	3 cups	1 hour	2-1/4 cups
Lima beans	2 cups	1-1/2 hours	1-1/4 cups
Baby lima beans	2 cups	1-1/2 hours	1-3/4 cups
Pinto beans	3 cups	4 hours	2 cups
Red beans	3 cups	5 hours	2 cups
Small white beans (navy, etc.)	3 cups	3 hours	2 cups
Soybeans	4 cups	4 hours	2 cups
Soy grits	2 cups	15 min.	2 cups

VEGETABLES

Vegetables are composed primarily of complex carbohydrates and water. They are high in vitamins, minerals and fiber. They contain small amounts of fat, moderate amounts of protein and are cholesterol free.

Most vegetables are low in calories and are an ideal food for those who are trying to lose weight.

Vegetables are best fresh or frozen, without added fats, oils, sauces or salt. Canned vegetables are high in salt and should be used only in moderation.

There is no upper limit to the number of servings you may have of the vegetables listed. However, if you want to gain weight, or have difficulty in maintaining it, then you should eat more vegetables from Category C and less from A and B. If you want to lose weight, then select the lower calorie veggies in Categories A and B while eating less from C.

CATEGORY A: 25 CALORIES PER SERVING

1 cup asparagus	1 cup cucumbers
1 cup bean sprouts	10 cherry tomatoes
1 cup bell pepper	1 cup leeks
1 cup green beans	1 cup cabbage
1 cup bok choy	1 cup zucchini
1 cup mushrooms	1 cup celery
1 cup snow peas	1 cup turnips
1 cup radishes	1 cup cauliflower
1 medium tomato	1 cup squash: summer, crookneck

CATEGORY B: 50 CALORIES PER SERVING

1 cup beets	1 cup carrots
1 cup onions	1 cup broccoli
1 cup eggplant	1 cup rutabagas
1 cup brussel sprouts	

CATEGORY C:
100 CALORIES PER SERVING

1 cup or cob corn	5 oz white potato
3 oz sweet potato or yam	1 cup parsnips
1 small white potato	1/2 medium yam
1/2 medium sweet potato	1 cup squash: acorn, butternut, hubbard

FRUIT

Fruits are a good source of vitamins A and C. Yellow fruits, such as apricots and cantaloupes, are high in vitamin A. Citrus fruits, cantaloupes and strawberries are high in vitamin C. Fruits are low in fat and cholesterol free. They are high in carbohydrates, including sugars and fiber.

Fruit juices and simple sugars are listed here as a sub-category. These are concentrated sources of sugar, with all the fiber removed. Sugars and fruit juices have an adverse effect on health when consumed in large quantities.

Choose several servings (three to eight) per day from the fruit group, with no more than two of them from the simple sugars and juices. Even two servings from simple sugars and juices may be too much for sensitive diabetics, and those with high serum triglyceride levels.

Servings: Three to eight per day, of which not more than two should be from the simple sugars and juices.

50 CALORIES PER SERVING

1 small apple
1/2 banana
3/4 cup papaya
10 large cherries
1 medium peach
1 small tangerine
1/2 cup pineapple
1 small fresh pear
2 dates
2 peach halves, dried
3 medium fresh apricots
1/2 cup berries: blackberries,
strawberries

1/4 cantaloupe
1/8 honeydew melon
1 cup watermelon
1 small nectarine
1 small orange
2 medium plums
1 pear half, dried
1 fig, fresh or dried
2 medium prunes
2 Tbsp raisins
6 med. apricot halves, dried
blueberries, raspberries,

SIMPLE SUGARS AND JUICES:
50 CALORIES PER SERVING

1/3 cup apple juice
1/2 cup apple sauce
1/3 cup grape juice
1 Tbsp molasses
1/2 cup grapefruit juice
1/3 cup peach or pear nectar
1 small glass of wine, 3 oz

1 oz juice concentrate
2 tsp honey
1 Tbsp sugar
1/2 cup orange juice
1 Tbsp jam or jelly
1/3 cup pineapple juice
6 oz beer, light preferred

DAIRY PRODUCTS

Dairy foods vary in their fat and cholesterol content. Nonfat dairy products are the lowest in fat and cholesterol. Low fat products are the next lowest, with whole fat products highest.

Whenever possible, nonfat products are your first choice, but because of the high protein content, do not exceed two servings per day. Keep in mind that if you are allergic to dairy products, as many people are, then you should avoid using them whenever possible. People who are allergic to dairy products usually find that they can still consume small amounts of yogurt, cottage cheese or Liteline cheese without a bad reaction. This is because yogurt and cheese are fermented, which compared to milk, are a little easier for your body to digest. However, since all the vitamins, minerals and protein your body needs are available in whole complex carbohydrate foods, there is no nutritional need to use dairy products. You should avoid all dairy products to be at the peak of health and feel your best.

Whole eggs and egg yolks are not listed, since they are extremely high in cholesterol. Egg whites are free of fat and cholesterol, and are included in this section.

Low fat, Rice Dream cheese, Lifetime cheese, or Liteline cheese can be used in place of high fat, hard, semi-soft, and soft regular cheeses. Low fat cheeses may be used as a substitute for a day's serving of meat, poultry or fish. The maximum serving of any cheese is one ounce per day.

Servings: Up to three times per week.

100 CALORIES PER SERVING

1 cup nonfat milk	1 cup buttermilk
1 cup nonfat yogurt	1 cup low fat yogurt
1/2 cup hoop cheese	6 egg whites
4 oz tofu, drained	5 tbsp nonfat powdered milk
1/2 cup evaporated skim milk	1/2 cup low fat cottage cheese

MEAT, POULTRY AND FISH

Meat, poultry and fish contain considerable amounts of cholesterol and fat.

Red meat is significantly higher in fat than are chicken and fish. The only red meat cut with a low fat content is flank steak, which is included here. Shrimp is the only shellfish with an exceptionally high cholesterol content, and has therefore been excluded.

All organ meats - liver, kidney, brain, etc. - are extremely high in cholesterol content, and have also been excluded.

Serving: No more than three times per week (three oz cooked)

100 CALORIES PER SERVING

albacore	abalone	clams	cod
cornish game hen	crab	flank steak	frog legs
haddock	halibut	lobster	oysters
perch	red snapper	rock fish	salmon
tuna in water	sea bass	swordfish	scallops
chicken, light meat no skin	turkey light meat no skin		

16

Food Selection
and Label Reading

Did you ever notice how easy it is to buy unplanned items at the supermarket? Snacks at the checkout counter, "specials" on the aisle-end gondolas and manager's super savers at the meat counters all seem to jump into your shopping cart. Supermarket marketing and merchandising is a very sophisticated, multibillion dollar industry. It's all too easy to be manipulated by packaging and advertising. Here are some pointers to make you supermarket smart:

- NEVER go shopping when you're hungry. People who shop on an empty stomach buy 10 to 20% more groceries than when they are full. This advice can save both your health and your bank balance!
- Think of the shopping cart as your stomach. What goes in the cart goes inside you. It's easier to resist temptation in the store than when the food is in your kitchen.
- Don't buy "bad" foods for the kids or guests. You know who will want just one bite! Make the treats you serve others real treats - wonderful fresh fruits or dishes you've made yourself.
- Generally, the foods on the perimeter of the store are the fresh foods - the produce fruits and vegetables. The less you wheel your cart down aisles of cans and boxes, the better.
- Plan your shopping after you've planned your menu. And plan your menus around complex carbohydrates - grains, beans, fruits and vegetables, not animal proteins.

SUBSTITUTION LIST

The following list will help you in preparing your shopping list to substitute for the items you discarded today.

GOODBYE TO:	BETTER BUY:
Table salt, Accent, Season Salt, M.S.G.	Lemon, Pepper, Spike, Mrs. Dash, Instead of Salt
Garlic salt	Garlic powder
Onion salt	Onion powder
Soy sauce, tamari	Low sodium soy sauce (use in very limited amounts), 500 mg in 1 Tbsp
Bouillon cubes	No salt added vegetable
Worcestershire sauce, A-1 steak sauce	Mrs. Dash, no salt added steak sauce
Canned soup	Low sodium, low fat, or homemade soups
Artichokes marinated in oil/salt	Artichokes canned in water low salt
Canned vegetables in salt	Fresh, frozen or canned, salt free
High oil/salt salad dressings	No oil/salt-free salad or homemade salad dressings
Non-dairy creamer	Lite soy milk, rice milk
Sugar	Fruit concentrates
Bacon, sausage, ham, luncheon meats	Wheat meat with spices
Pickles, relish	Salt-free pickles
Mustard, catsup	Salt-free mustard, catsup
Most cheeses	Non-fat cheeses
Whole milk, cream	Lite soy milk, rice milk
Cereals with salt or sugar added	Nutri-Grain, Shredded Wheat, Nutti Rice, etc.
Ice cream w/sugar	Nouvelle Sorbet, (at health food stores)
Jello, puddings	Add your own sweetener gelatin desserts
Jam, jelly, preserves, high in sugar	Low sugar or sugar-free fruit preserves
Soft drinks	Sparkling mineral water (except Vichy)

FOOD LABELS
HOW TO CALCULATE THE TOTAL
% OF FAT, PROTEIN AND CARBOHYDRATE

The calculations presented below can be used to determine what percent of a store-bought food product is fat, what percent is protein, and what percent is carbohydrate, so you can decide if the food is on **The Delgado Diet** or not. A general guideline is to limit anything greater than 18% protein and anything greater than 20% fat. Complex carbohydrates (but not sugars) are free!!

The data you need to memorize to do these calculations is:

- 1 gram of protein is approximately 4calories.
- 1 gram of carbohydrate is approximately 4calories.
- 1 gram of fat is approximately 9 calories.

Now you can tackle any label providing nutritional information. Here is how:

EXAMPLE 1.
NATURAL WHOLE GRAIN BREAD
Data given on the label:
140 calories per serving
6 grams protein per serving
25 grams carbohydrate per serving
2 grams fat per serving

A. PROTEIN:
   6 g. protein X 4 calories / g. protein = 24 calories divided by 140 calories X 100% = 17% protein
B. CARBOHYDRATE:
   25 g. carbohydrate X 4 calories / g. carbohydrate = 100 calories divided by 140 calories X 100% = 71 %
C. FAT:
   2 g. fat X 9 calories / g. fat = 18 calories divided by 140 calories X 100% = 13% fat
CONCLUSION: This whole grain bread would be okay to include in your diet because the total % of protein and fat are less than **The Delgado Diet** maximums listed.

EXAMPLE 2.
OATS, N' HONEY BREAD
Data given on the label:
150 calories per serving
6 grams protein per serving
23 grams carbohydrate per serving
4 grams fat per serving

A. PROTEIN:
6 g. protein X 4 calories / g. protein = 24 calories divided by 150 calories X 100% = 16% protein
B. CARBOHYDRATE:
23 g. carbohydrate X 4 calories / g. carbohydrate = 92 calories divided by 150 calories X 100% = 61 % carbohydrate
C. FAT:
4 g. fat X 9 calories / g. fat = 36 calories divided by 150 calories X 100% = 24% fat

CONCLUSION: This bread would be marginally   unacceptable because the % of fat is above the maximum.

EXAMPLE 3.
CHEDDAR CHEESE
Data from Nutrition Almanac or on some labels:
114 calories per serving
7 grams protein per serving.
.4 grams carbohydrate per serving
9.5 grams fat per serving

A. PROTEIN:
7 g. protein X 4 calories / g. protein = 28 calories divided by 114 calories X 100% = 26% protein
B. CARBOHYDRATE:
.4 gram carbohydrate X 4 calories / g. carbohydrate = 1.6 calories divided by 114 calories X 100% = 1.4% carbohydrate
C. FAT:
9.5 g. fat X 9 calories / g. fat = 86 calories divided by 114 calories X 100% = 75% fat

CONCLUSION: This cheddar cheese is 75% fat and only 1 oz.; has over 9.5 grams of fat. That means if you added this to a "20% calories from fat diet," you would push the total fat intake for the day to over 25% fat! Notice also this cheese has 26% protein, and that any food over 15% protein is excessive and can promote osteoporosis and fatigue. The

How to Look Great & Feel Sexy

carbohydrate content is only 1.4%, and this is far below the recommended 60% of calories from carbohydrate.

NOTE: Sugar should be considered a simple carbohydrate (not complex). The closer it is found to the beginning of the ingredient list the greater the % of sugar present. Though some labels are starting to list the amounts of simple vs. complex carbohydrates present, this is not always done and you will often have to make an educated guess about the total % of sugar present (more than 10% sugar is considered excessive).

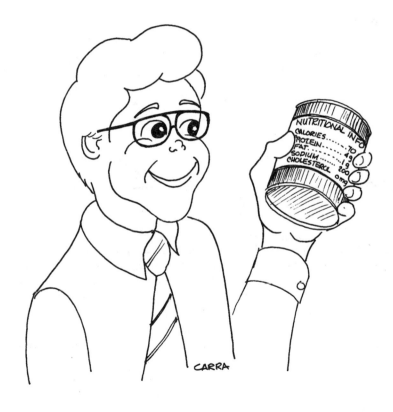

POINTS TO REMEMBER IN LABEL READING

This section will help a health conscious individual, such as yourself, to be informed about reading food labels at the supermarket. The intelligent food shopper can scrutinize labels and detect hidden fats, sugars, sodium and cholesterol.

- Ingredients are listed in order of descending predominance.
- If a product claims to be "low sodium," they must include the sodium content. Be sure to note the serving size.
- To determine the percent of fat in a product, multiply the grams of fat by 9, then divide by the total calories. *Look for items under 20% fat.
- Review the code names for fat, salt and sugar. Avoid foods with added sodium compounds, and high percentages of fat and sugar.

The food manufacturers decide the serving size for their product and give nutritional information on a "per serving" basis. Smaller serving sizes are sometimes used to try to make their foods appear to have less fat, sodium, etc.

Different sugars may be listed as different ingredients, very often making it difficult for most people to tell just how much sugar would be in that food. For example, in one food item, sugars could be listed as corn syrup, dextrose and brown sugar.

To make matters worse, a label is currently only required when a manufacturer makes a claim about the nutrient content of a food. This means about half of all foods have no nutrition labeling. For example, labeling is only required if the food has a written claim like "low calorie" or "low sodium," or when the food has been fortified with vitamins and minerals. When referring to sodium or calories, the FDA has only defined a few claims ("low" and "reduced"). If the claim is being made about fiber or fat, ambiguous terms generally are used such as "lite" or "natural." These terms allow the food manufacturers to say whatever they wish, without being forced to reveal an itemized label.

On your next trip to the market, you can make better decisions on which food products to purchase, because your decisions will be based on the quality of the food and not just on the taste. You also may have to cut back on, or avoid, many foods you have routinely bought in the past. Keep the following **Delgado guidelines** in mind in this order of importance:

1. "The first rule" would be to consume less than 100 mg of **CHOLESTEROL** in a day (zero cholesterol intake would be even better). High cholesterol accounts for more deaths in the U.S. than all other causes combined.

2. "The second rule" is to <u>keep your **FAT** intake between 10 and 20 grams per day</u> while you're trying to lose weight, and never more than 40 grams a day if you are at your ideal weight. It would be better to avoid any food with 4 or more grams of fat per serving.

3. "The third rule" is **PROTEIN** is the #3 enemy when used in excess. <u>Keep your protein intake between 40 and 80 grams a day.</u> If protein is the first ingredient of any food item, it is probably too concentrated for regular use. <u>Center your diet around complex carbohydrates (starches, fruits and vegetables) and not around protein from meat, chicken, fish, eggs, milk, cheese or nuts.</u>

4. "The fourth rule" is to cut back on excessive calories from **SUGAR**. If sugar is listed near the beginning of the ingredient list, or if sugar is listed under different names, then you should rarely use the product. <u>Simple carbohydrates (sugars) should be limited to less than 25 grams a day.</u>

5. "The fifth rule" is to <u>keep total **SODIUM** intake per day between 2000 to 4000 mg.</u> Use less than 200 mg of sodium per serving for *low sodium diets* and less than 600 mg for *moderate use.*

6. "The sixth rule" is to <u>reduce or avoid **CAFFEINE AND ARTIFICIAL ADDITIVES.**</u>

Not all additives are harmful, but many have not been thoroughly tested long enough on humans to assess their safety. Buy organic whenever possible, and if the label lists too many ingredients of which you are not sure, then it would be better to avoid that product.

The rules above are listed 1 through 6 in order of importance so that you realize it would be safer to cheat occasionally on a food with slightly more sugar or salt, than to cheat with foods higher in cholesterol and fat.

The final concept to follow when making food selections is to decide whether a food has redeeming value. Foods that are advertised as having "no cholesterol" or "low salt" may not have any positive value. You should ask the following questions to determine the food value: Does this food have fiber in it? (We need 40 to 60 grams of total fiber a day). Is the food unprocessed? Is the food high in complex carbohydrates? (Your body needs at least 200 grams or more of carbohydrates a day to operate efficiently).

How to Look Great & Feel Sexy

17

Save Your Life
Reduce Your
Cholesterol Level

Your cholesterol level will not affect your weight or your energy level; however, it is a problem that has been tragically overlooked for many years. Cholesterol and atherosclerosis are major problems in America and the overall degree of this problem is not fully understood by our society. We know the death rate from heart disease has decreased slightly; but, it still affects millions of Americans.

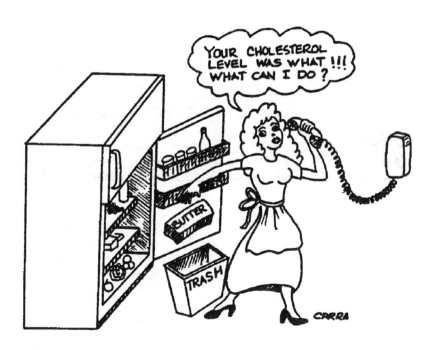

Consider the fact strokes are the second leading cause of death. Then combine heart attacks and the number of people who die of strokes and we have diseases that kill more than 50% of all Americans. The pain and the suffering these diseases cause our country is tragic and yet, we continue to ignore dietary treatment. As Americans, it is important that we have the information available to us about the low fat, zero cholesterol **Delgado Plan**.

Several years ago I worked with stroke victims in physical therapy in the critical care units. These people had lives just like you and I. They had families. They led happy and successful lives. Then, one unexpected day they had a stroke. Overnight their whole world crumbled and they became bedridden and in need of constant care.

Stroke rehabilitation is a laborious, slow process. It may take six months before a stroke victim can actually walk on their own, and even then many victims never regain full function. Half their body is paralyzed simply because arteries leading to the brain became severely clogged with cholesterol. Consequently, part of the brain dies due to lack of oxygen. Some stroke victims can no longer speak clearly, if that part of the brain was affected. Think about it - the brain never stops working. When you go to sleep, your brain is still functioning and coordinating your whole body.

These are very serious problems: cholesterol, heart disease and strokes. There is a tendency for Americans to ignore something they cannot see. I have conducted over 3,000 seminars in the last 20 years and I spent most of the seminar time educating people about the importance of cholesterol control. When a patient comes to the seminar overweight, fatigued and lacking energy, they immediately know what they want. They want to lose weight and increase their energy. Since we have a solution for them, these people are easy to work with because they will follow the guidelines for losing weight and increasing energy. However, the people with high cholesterol levels don't believe it's a problem.

Cholesterol is the silent killer. Since there are no nerve endings in the arteries, you don't know cholesterol is building up. Unfortunately a massive heart attack or stroke is the first symptom some people will experience. Then you'll seek treatment, but at that point, there is already irreversible damage.

Special interest groups such as the meat, egg and dairy industries are trying to divert attention from their high cholesterol foods by placing the blame on saturated fats. These groups claim palm oil and coconut oil, which are high in saturated fat, are the cause of elevated cholesterol levels. People are now buying vegetable oils high in monounsaturated and polyunsaturated fats mistakenly believing these are better for them.

In the Journal of American Medical Association, March 23, 1990, Vol. 263, Dr. David Blankenhorn of U.S.C. reported his studies on the effects of fats and the development of atherosclerotic lesions in human coronary arteries. The results shocked the margarine and oil industry since it was proven all fats including polyunsaturated, monounsaturated, saturated and fatty acids (lauric, oleic and linoleic acids) more than 26% of calories from fat caused cholesterol lesions in the heart arteries in less than two years. Those people who were protected from cholesterol lesions ate the least amount of all types of fats.

The public is also misled by believing if they avoid saturated fats they can continue to eat their high cholesterol foods. I can't tell you how many people who come to the clinic still eat at least one or two eggs a week, and think it's safe for them. Of course, we know eggs are one of the most potent sources of cholesterol. You should never eat more than one or two eggs per year. That would be only if you were unaware they were in a recipe, such as a bakery item.

I believe part of the reason people continue to eat high cholesterol foods comes from watching television and the brain-washing that conditions them.

A study showed that the average person during their lifetime spends:

2 weeks	Speaking with their child (30 sec per day)
3 weeks	Brushing their teeth
1/3 year	Conversing with spouse (4 min per day)
1/2 year	Sitting at red lights
3/4 year	Opening junk mail
1 year	Searching for things they lost
2 years	Exercising (if they exercise one-half hour a day)
3 years	Attending meetings
4 years	Cleaning their house
5 years	Waiting in lines
6 years	Eating
7 years	In the bathroom
23 years	Watching television (ASTONISHING!)

The dairy and meat industries promote their products and bombard us with advertising. The average child will watch over 100,000 commercials by the time they're a teenager. These commercials claim eggs, meat and cheese build strong bodies and "milk has something for every body." Commercials about beer, Pepsi, Coke and candy will complete the child's' nutritional education. Spokespersons paid by these special interest groups mislead the public into believing they can eat as much meat, eggs, and cheese as they wish. Deliberately eating these products ignores the fact cholesterol kills more people in America than any other cause of death.

Dr. Wong and Dr. Gold reported the results of their study on over 1,000 youngsters age 2 to 20 (November 1990 American Heart Association Meeting). They found over 53 % of children with a dangerously high cholesterol level (200 mg or higher) watch television two or more hours per day. Those who watched four or more hours per day were four times as likely to have high cholesterol levels.

Cholesterol building up in the arteries is a leading cause of senility. By the age of 60, many senior citizens in our country are completely senile and end up in nursing homes needing constant care. If we look at the issues, we know that cholesterol is the culprit. Even a two-year-old who is fed high cholesterol foods can develop a build-up. By the time he is three, he'll already have fatty streaks in his arteries. That is how early it starts.

In Finland they have the highest cholesterol level in the world and the highest death rate from heart attack and stroke. Their infants are born with a higher cholesterol level than the worldwide averages because the mothers are eating a very high cholesterol diet. In this country our teenagers eat a high cholesterol diet of cheeseburgers, fried foods, beef burritos with added cheese. With all this cholesterol, it's inevitable that a teenager will develop clogged arteries. When they reach 30 or 40 years old, the first heart attacks appear. Every day 3,425 people across the country have a heart attack (1,250,000 per year), and over half these people will die immediately. Heart attacks occur in teenagers, but we don't hear much about them because they're not as frequent as in a 40-year-old. So, we have to start this nutritional plan of zero cholesterol and low fat intake.

In the last ten years there has been a significant decrease in the number of deaths from atherosclerosis (cholesterol plaques in the arteries). One study estimated that over 180,000 people are alive today in the U.S. because they learned how to lower their cholesterol level, and keep it down. Stop Smoking campaigns have also helped to decrease the death rate. However, the number one causes of death in the U.S. are still heart disease, stroke and cancer.

DEATHS IN 1987
(Most recent year for complete statistics)

Heart Disease, Stroke	908,000
Cancer	476,700
Accidents	92,500
Obstructing lung disease	78,000
Pneumonia & Flu	68,600
Diabetes	37,800
Suicide	29,600
Cirrhosis of Liver	26,000
Atherosclerosis	23,100
AIDS - drug related abuse	4,400

At Healthy Studios, we are often asked "What is the difference between fat and cholesterol? Fat provides calories; yet, in excess it is the major contributor to obesity and to many diseases that affects our culture. A high fat diet of oils, margarine, whole milk, cheese, meat, etc. can increase the levels of fat in your blood (triglycerides) which leads to the risk of:

1. **HIGH BLOOD PRESSURE** (blood thickened by fat)

2. **ARTHRITIS** (low oxygen from fat causing destruction of joints)

3. **DIABETES** (fat desensitizing insulin causing poor glucose control)

4. **BREAST AND COLON CANCER** (fat causing excessive production of cancer causing hormones and chemicals)

5. **CHRONIC FATIGUE** (high fat levels in the blood that reduces the oxygen carrying capacity of red blood cells to the brain)

6. **GLAUCOMA** (fat increases cortisone levels in the eyes causing swelling, restriction of fluid flow that can result in damage to the retinal nerves of the eye and blindness)

7. **MULTIPLE SCLEROSIS** (fat damages the nerves of the body from reduced oxygen carrying capacity of the blood)

8. **ATHEROSCLEROSIS** (low oxygen levels caused by fat forces more cholesterol deposits into the arteries)

In comparison, cholesterol is much different from fat. First because cholesterol cannot cause you to gain weight since it lacks calories. Unlike fat, you can't see cholesterol in food, since it's permeated equally throughout all animal tissue. This is why there is just as much cholesterol in the white part of chicken or fish as there is in the skin or fat portions. High cholesterol levels can lead to:

1.   **ATHEROSCLEROSIS** or narrowing of arteries and capillaries.
2.   **HEART ATTACK** from cholesterol blocked arteries to the heart.
3.   **STROKE** (clogged and weakened arteries to the brain)
4.   **SENILITY** (loss of brain function due to clogged arteries).
5.   **IMPOTENCY** (loss of male sexual function due to cholesterol clogging arteries to the penis).
6.   **PROSTATE CANCER** (cholesterol build up in the prostate gland restricts oxygen to the gland inducing mutated cancerous cells).
7.   **CATARACTS** (lens of the eye fills with cholesterol causing blindness).
8.   **GANGRENE** (restricted blood flow to the extremities: fingers, toes, hands and feet, leading to numbness, tissue death and amputation caused by cholesterol build up).
9.   **KIDNEY FAILURE** (clogged arteries to the kidneys).

In my book, _Fatigue to Vitality,_ and in my CD-ROM, audio cassette and video tape series, you can learn more about how to prevent and even reverse diseases such as diabetes, cancer, arthritis, kidney and heart disease. Please see the end of the book for further details, and ordering information. Please contact me in care of Healthy Studios for inquiries and orders.

If you are a user of electronic mail and have access to the Internet you may prefer to send inquiries; orders through the Internet. Please address requests to Healthy Studios in care of Nick Delgado Ms., Ph.D. to NickDelgado@msn.com (E-Mail).

MAILING ADDRESS:

HEALTHY STUDIOS
25422 Trabuco Road, #105-141
Lake Forest,, CA 92630
Or call: 800-631-0232

18

Composition of Foods Chart

NOTE: Foods with less than .1 mg or .1 gm in any category (fat, protein, etc.) are listed as 0. If the information is not available, the notation will be "-". Additional information on vitamins and minerals is available through the U.S. Government Composition of Foods; however, we have provided the information that is most pertinent to your goals of weight loss and cholesterol reduction.

We have listed the foods in order of lowest fat, calories, and cholesterol in the beginning on up to the highest, most harmful foods at the end. Abbreviations for food categories are CAL (calories), CHO (carbohydrates), PRO (protein), NA (sodium), TF (total fiber), SF (soluble fiber), CHOL (cholesterol). All measurements are in grams, except cholesterol and sodium which are measured in milligrams.

VEGETABLES
1 cup serving, raw
(unless otherwise noted)

	FAT	CAL	CHO	PRO	NA	TF	SF	CHOL
Watercress, 1 sprig	0	0	0	.1	1	1	.4	0
Parsley, 10 sprigs	0	3	.7	.2	4	2	.7	0
Romaine lettuce, 4 lvs	0	8	.8	.8	4	.6	.2	0
Iceberg lettuce, 4 lvs	0	12	2	.8	8	.6	.2	0
Onions	0	48	11	2	0	5	3	0
Beets, cooked	0	52	12	2	84	4	1	0
Water Chestnuts, 8	.1	38	9	.5	10	.4	-	0
Radish,10	.2	7	2	.3	11	1	.2	0
Endive	.2	8	2	.6	12	1	.5	0

VEGETABLES Con't.	F A T	C A L	C H O O	P R O O	N A	T F	S F	C H O L
Alfalfa Sprouts	.2	10	1	1	2	4	-	0
Cucumber	.2	14	3	.6	2	1	.4	0
Cabbage	.2	16	4	.8	12	1	.8	0
Celery	.2	16	2	.6	70	3	.8	0
Green Peppers	.2	18	4	.6	4	2	.5	0
Cauliflower	.2	24	5	2	14	3	2	0
Eggplant, cooked	.2	26	6	.8	12	4	2	0
Zucchini,	.2	28	7	1	4	4	2	0
Pumpkin, cooked	.2	48	12	2	4	4	1	0
Okra, cooked	.2	50	12	3	8	5	2	0
Carrots	.2	50	11	2	50	5	2	0
Artichoke 1	.2	53	12	3	79	15	2	0
Swiss chard	.3	26	2	3	125	1	-	0
Red peppers	.3	31	7	1	4	2	.8	0
Tomato	.3	33	7	2	4	.8	.2	0
Dill Pickle, 1	.4	11	2	.7	1428	.7	.3	0
Turnips, cooked	.4	28	8	1	88	3	2	0
Turnip greens	.4	30	6	2	42	2	.7	0
Leeks, cooked	.4	32	8	.4	5	3	1	0
Kale	.4	34	6	2	30	4	2	0
Collards	.4	36	7	3	2	2	1	0
Bamboo shoots	.4	36	7	4	6	1	-	0
Spinach, cooked	.4	42	6	6	126	4	.9	0
Green snap beans	..4	44	10	2	4	3	.8	0
Sauerkraut	.4	44	10	2	1560	5	2	0
Rutabaga, cooked	.4	58	13	2	30	3	2	0
Summer squash	.6	36	8	2	2	1	.5	0
Asparagus	.6	44	8	5	8	5	1	0
Brussel sprouts	.6	66	12	7	36	8	3	0
Winter squash	.8	78	18	2	2	7	.7	0

VEGETABLES Con't.	F A T	C A L	C H O	P R O	N A	T F	S F	C H O L
Mushrooms, 10	.1	50	8	4	10	4	.5	0
Broccoli	.2	24	4	2	24	5	2	0
Potato, cooked	.2	134	31	2	8	3	2	0
Yams	.2	158	36	2	12	8	4	0
Green peas	.6	122	21	9	3	3	-	0
Parsnips, cooked	.8	126	30	2	16	6	.8	0
Corn cooked	2	180	42	6	28	8	3	0

BEANS/PEAS
1 cup serving, cooked

	F A T	C A L	C H O	P R O	N A	T F	S F	C H O L
Lentils	0	212	39	16	26	4	2	0
Split peas	.3	230	42	16	26	10	3	0
Pinto beans	.6	204	37	13	13	11	4	0
Lima beans	.6	208	40	12	28	9	2	0
Kidney beans	.8	206	36	14	6	12	5	0
Navy beans	1	224	40	15	13	3	-	0
Black-eyed peas	1	198	30	14	8	25	11	0
Garbanzo beans	4	396	49	16	35	3	-	0
Soy beans	12	254	20	22	26	3	-	0

FRUITS
1 cup serving
(unless otherwise noted)

	F A T	C A L	C H O O	P R O	N A	T F	S F	C H O L
Loquat, 1	.1	5	1	.1	.1	1	-	0
Kumquat, 1	.1	12	3	.2	1	1	-	0
Grapes, 10	.1	15	4	.2	.1	.4	.1	0
Peach, 1	.1	37	10	.7	.1	5	1	0
Passion fruit, 1	.2	18	4	.4	5	2	-	0
Lime, 1	.2	20	7	.5	1	.3	-	0
Fig, 1	.2	37	10	.4	1	.6	-	0
Tangerine, 1	.2	37	9	.6	1	2	.5	0
Grapefruit, 1/2	.2	38	10	.8	.1	2	.6	0
Casaba melon, 1/10	.2	43	10	2	20	1	-	0
Honeydew melon, 1/10	.2	46	12	.6	13	1	-	0
Cranberries	.2	46	12	.4	1	4	1	0
Orange, 1	.2	62	15	1	.1	1	.3	0
Crabapple, 1	.3	83	22	.4	1	.7	-	0
Lemon, 1	.4	22	11	1	3	6	1	0
Rhubarb	.4	26	6	1	4	4	1	0
Kiwi fruit, 1	.4	46	11	.8	4	1	-	0
Boysenberries, frozen	.4	66	16	1	2	5	-	0
Plum, 1	.5	36	9	.6	.1	.6	.2	0
Guava, 1	.5	45	11	.8	2	5	-	0
Apricot, 3	.5	51	12	1	1	2	1	0
Apple, 1	.5	81	21	.3	1	3	1	0
Strawberries	.6	45	10	1	2	1	-	0
Blackberries	.6	74	18	1	.2	9	1	0
Blueberries	.6	82	20	1	9	5	.6	0
Cherries, 10	.7	49	11	.9	.1	1	.3	0
Watermelon	.7	50	12	1	3	-	-	0

FRUITS Con't.	F A T	C A L	C H O	P R O	N A	T F	S F	C H O L
Pear, 1	.7	98	25	.7	1	5	1	0
Cantaloupe, 1/2	.8	94	22	2	23	1	-	0
Gooseberries	.9	67	15	1	1	7	1	0
Applesauce, unsweetened	.2	106	28	.4	5	4	1	0
Dates, 10	.2	228	61	2	2	2	-	0
Persimmon, Japanese	.4	118	31	1	3	3	-	0
Plantain, cooked	.4	178	48	1	8	-	-	0
Pomegranate, 1	.5	104	27	2	5	.3	-	0
Papaya, 1	.5	117	30	2	8	4	1	0
Prunes, 10	.5	201	53	2	3	12	4	0
Banana, 1	.6	105	27	1	1	2	.6	0
Mango, 1	.6	135	35	1	4	2	.5	0
Elderberries	.8	105	27	1	.2	10	-	0
Raisins	.7	434	115	5	17	16	4	0
Olives, green - 6	5	45	1	.6	936	1	-	0
Olives, black - 6	12	121	2	1	550	1	-	0
Avocado	30	306	12	4	21	-	-	0

CEREALS
1 ounce serving, cold

	F A T	C A L	C H O	P R O	N A	T F	S F	C H O L
Puffed Rice, 1 C.	.1	57	13	.9	0	.2	.1	0
Grape Nuts, 1/4 C.	.1	101	23	3	197	2	.5	0
Kellogg's Corn Flakes, 1 C.	.1	110	24	2	351	.4	.1	0
Corn Chex, 1 C.	.1	111	25	2	271	.4	.2	0
Special K, 1/2 C.	.1	111	21	6	265	.8	.2	0
Rice Chex, 1 1/8 C.	.1	112	25	2	237	.1	-	0

CEREALS Con't.	F A T	C A L	C H O	P R O	N A	T F	S F	C H O L
Product 19, 3/4 C.	.2	108	24	3	325	1	.3	0
Golden Grahams, 3/4 C.	.2	109	24	2	364	.2	-	0
Rice Crispies, 1 C.	.2	112	25	2	340	.1	-	0
Shredded Wheat, 1 lg. biscuit	.3	83	19	3	0	3	.4	0
Grape Nuts Flakes, 7/8 C.	.3	102	23	3	218	2	.5	0
Nutri-Grain, wheat	.3	102	24	3	193	2	.3	0
Trix, 1 C.	.4	109	25	2	27	.1	-	0
All Bran, 1/3 C.	.5	71	21	4	320	9	2	0
Wheaties, 1 C.	.5	99	23	3	354	3	.5	0
Life, 2/3 C.	.5	104	20	5	148	1	.3	0
Total, 1 C.	.6	100	22	3	352	3	.5	0
Wheat Chex, 2/3 C.	.7	104	23	3	190	3	.5	0
Honey Nut Cheerios, 3/4 C.	.7	107	23	3	257	-	-	0
Kix, 1 1/2 C.	.7	110	23	3	339	.2	-	0
Kellogg's Raisin Bran, 3/4 C.	.7	115	28	4	269	1	-	0
Bran Chex, 2/3 C.	.8	91	23	3	263	6	1	0
Corn Bran, 2/3 C.	1	98	24	2	244	6	2	0
Cheerios, 1 1/4 C.	2	111	20	4	307	2	.7	0
C.W. Post, 1/4 C.	4	126	20	3	49	-	-	0
Nature Valley Granola, 1/3 C.	5	126	19	3	58	-	-	0
Quaker 100% Natural, 1/4 C.	6	133	18	3	12	-	-	0

HOT CEREAL 1 cup serving, w/o salt								
	F A T	**C A L**	**C H O**	**P R O**	**N A**	**T F**	**S F**	**C H O L**
Cream of Rice	.1	126	28	2	2	-	-	0
Farina	.2	116	25	3	1	-	-	0
Malt-o-Meal, plain or chocolate	.3	122	26	4	2	-	-	0
Cream of Wheat, reg.	.5	134	28	4	2	-	-	0
Cream of Wheat instant	.6	153	32	4	6	-	-	0
Wheatena	1	135	29	5	5	-	-	0
Oats, reg., quick or instant	2	145	25	6	1	4	2	0
Maypo	2	170	32	6	9	-	-	0

BREADS without eggs or dairy products 1 serving								
	F A T	**C A L**	**C H O**	**P R O**	**N A**	**T F**	**S F**	**C H O L**
Rye bread, 1 slice	.3	63	13	2	144	.9	.3	0
Pumpernickel, 1 slice	.3	64	14	2	148	4	.6	0
Corn tortilla, 1	.5	32	6	.8	3	-	-	-
Whole Wheat bagel	.6	152	32	5	360	-	-	0
Whole Wheat bread, 1 slice	.8	63	12	3	137	1	3	0
White bread, 1 slice	.8	70	70	2	132	.5	.2	0
Soda cracker, 4	1	35	6	.7	88	-	-	-
Saltine cracker	1	52	9	1	132	-	-	0
Whole Wheat English muffin, 1	2	130	26	5	171	-	-	0
Whole wheat pancake	3	74	9	3	0	-	-	0
Graham cracker, 2	3	107	20	2	188	3	.5	0
Bran muffin, 1	5	126	20	5	178	-	-	0
Buckwheat pancake, 1	5	135	18	5	338	-	-	0
Waffles, 2	5	204	32	6	599	-	-	0
Plain pancake, 1	6	62	22	5	417	-	-	0

GRAINS
1 cup serving, no salt added
(unless otherwise noted)

	F A T	C A L	C H O	P R O	N A	T F	S F	C H O L
White rice, 2/3 C, cooked	.1	149	33	3	10	.2	.2	0
Wild rice, 2/3 C. cooked	.2	78	17	3	11	-	-	0
Popcorn	.4	31	6	2	.2	-	-	0
Macaroni, cooked	.6	154	32	5	1	1	.3	0
Spaghetti, cooked	.6	155	32	5	1	2	.5	0
Brown rice, 2/3 C. cooked	.8	156	33	33	16	3	.3	0
Whole wheat pasta, cooked	1	174	37	7	2	-	-	0
Egg noodles, cooked	2	200	37	7	1	-	-	50
Bulgur, dry	2	628	139	15	7	-	-	0
Pot/Scotch barley, dry	2	696	154	19	8	-	-	0

BRAN
1 ounce, (6 tbsp.)

	F A T	C A L	C H O	P R O	N A	T F	S F	C H O L
Psyllium (Metamucil)	-	180	-	-	1	20	16	0
Corn Bran	-	-	-	-	-	6	2	0
Wheat bran	2	40	16	4	0	14	2	0
Oat bran	2	110	16	6	0	4	2	0
Wheat germ	3	108	14	8	1	-	-	0
Rice bran	5	100	9	4	tr	10	3	0

NUTS/SEEDS
4 oz serving

	F A T	C A L	C H O	P R O	N A	T F	S F	C H O L
Chestnuts, roasted	2	280	60	4	4	-	-	0
Pumpkin seeds	48	592	15	38	652	-	-	0
Sunflower seeds	56	648	21	26	4	-	-	0
Peanuts, roasted, salted	56	660	21	30	492	9	.1	0
Almonds, roasted, salted	58	888	28	9	668	14	2	0
Pistachios, roasted, salted	60	688	31	17	888	-	-	0
Cashews, roasted, salted	64	652	37	18	728	-	-	0
Walnuts	64	688	14	28	0	5	1	0
Pecans, roasted, salted	74	748	25	9	888	7	1	0
Brazil nuts	75	744	14	16	0	9	1	0
Filberts, roasted, salted	75	752	20	11	888	8	1	0
Macadamias	84	796	16	10	4	-	-	0

SOUPS
10 ounces, canned

	F A T	C A L	C H O	P R O	N A	T F	S F	C H O L
Beef broth, bouillon	.5	16	.1	3	782	-	-	0
Chicken broth	1	39	.9	5	776	-	-	0
French Onion, Knorr	1	56	-	-	1156	-	-	0
Minestrone, Maneschewitz	1	83	-	-	108	-	-	0
Pritikin soups	1	130	-	-	200	-	-	0
Vegetable, Health Valley	1	133	-	-	613	-	-	0
Campbell's Home Cookin'	1	150	-	-	1050	-	-	0
Gazpacho	2	57	.8	8	1183	-	-	0
Chicken w/ rice, Campbell's	3	80	8	5	1030	.1	.1	9

SOUPS Con't.	F A T	C A L	C H O	P R O	N A	T F	S F	C H O L
Vegetarian vegetable, Campbell's	3	100	15	4	975	.1	.1	0
Tomato, Campbell's	3	113	20	4	838	-	-	0
Minestrone Progresso	3	168	28	7	767	.3	.2	0
Clam Chowder, Snow's	4	160	22	11	875	0	0	8
Lentil, Progresso	4	179	24	11	819	4	2	4
Cream of Mushroom, Lipton	5	118	14	4	1263	0	0	2
Black Bean, Health Valley	5	213	33	9	573	4	1	0
Split Pea w/ham Campbell's	5	222	32	12	997	5	2	4
Ham w/bean, Campbell's	9	260	-	-	1097	-	-	-

BEVERAGES
1 cup serving
(unless otherwise noted)

	F A T	C A L	C H O	P R O	N A	T F	S F	C H O L
Club soda	0	0	0	0	75	0	0	0
Diet soda	0	0	.4	0	76	0	0	0
Ginger ale	0	113	29	0	25	0	0	0
Seven-up	0	144	36	0	4	0	0	0
Cranberry juice	0	147	37	0	5	0	0	0
Cola drink	0	151	38	0	15	0	0	0
Tea	0	0	0	0	29	0	0	0
Coffee, 6 ounces	0	3	.5	0	2	0	0	0
Grape juice	0	89	22	.1	0	0	0	0
Apple juice	0	92	23	.7	12	0	0	0
Orange juice	0	92	23	.8	58	0	0	0

LIQUOR

	F A T	C A L	C H O	P R O	N A	T F	S F	C H O L
Red/white wine, 3 1/2 ounces	0	70	1	0	7	0	0	0
Gin, whiskey, rum, vodka, 1 ounce	0	97	0	0	.4	0	0	0
Beer, 12 ounces	0	151	13	1	25	0	0	0
Cordials, liquors, 1 ounce	.1	74	8	0	1	0	0	0

POULTRY
3 1/2 ounces serving, roasted
(organ meats are stewed)
(unless otherwise noted)

	F A T	C A L	C H O	P R O	N A	T F	S F	C H O L
Goose liver, 1	4	125	6	15	132	0	0	-
Pheasant	4	133	0	24	37	0	0	-
Chicken gizzard, 1	4	153	1	27	67	0	0	194
Quail	5	134	0	22	51	0	0	-
Duck liver, 1	5	136	4	19	-	0	0	-
Chicken, white meat w/o skin	5	173	0	31	77	0	0	85
Chicken drumstick, 1	6	112	0	14	47	0	0	48
Chicken liver, 1	6	157	1	24	51	0	0	631
Turkey liver, 1	6	169	3	24	64	0	0	626
Chicken wing, 1	7	99	0	9	28	0	0	29
Chicken heart, 1	8	185	.1	27	48	0	0	242
Turkey white meat	8	197	0	29	63	0	0	76

POULTRY Con't.	F A T	C A L	C H O	P R O	N A	T F	S F	C H O L
Chicken, dark meat w/o skin	10	205	0	27	93	0	0	93
Chicken, white meat	11	222	0	29	75	0	0	84
Turkey, dark meat	12	221	0	28	76	0	0	89
Chicken, dark meat	16	253	0	26	87	0	0	91
Goose	22	305	0	25	70	0	0	91

SEAFOOD
3 ounce serving; baked,
broiled or steamed
(unless otherwise noted)

	F A T	C A L	C H O	P R O	N A	T F	S F	C H O L
Shrimp	.9	102	2	20	133	0	0	167
Sturgeon, caviar, teaspoon	2	26	.7	5	352	0	0	55
Crab, hard shell	2	89	.5	16	422	0	0	95
Scallops	3	85	3	13	425	0	0	29
Cod	3	100	.3	17	331	0	0	50
Flounder	3	101	.3	17	340	0	0	50
Haddock	3	102	.4	18	322	0	0	59
Snails	3	111	2	18	31	0	0	57
Abalone	3	120	4	19	15	0	0	55
Perch	4	110	.3	18	341	0	0	55
Pike	4	110	.3	18	313	0	0	55
Bass	4	117	.4	20	376	0	0	56
Clams	5	93	2	10	326	0	0	40
Lobster	5	111	.2	15	398	0	0	78
Frog legs, 2	6	121	9	8	239	0	0	78

SEAFOOD Con't.	F A T	C A L	C H O	P R O	N A	T F	S F	C H O L
Oysters	6	134	10	9	372	0	0	46
Tuna	6	155	.3	25	299	0	0	56
Swordfish	7	148	.4	20	369	0	0	56
Catfish	7	149	.5	19	491	0	0	59
Salmon	7	149	.4	21	380	0	0	36
Carp	9	161	.5	19	472	0	0	59
Sardines, canned in oil	9	172	0	20	700	0	0	102
Halibut	9	214	0	31	168	0	0	75
Trout	14	217	.3	21	342	0	0	55
Mackerel	15	213	.3	19	336	0	0	94
Herring	15	222	.4	19	377	0	0	95
Eel	22	286	5	15	88	0	0	51

SALAD DRESSINGS/SAUCES
2 ounce serving

	F A T	C A L	C H O	P R O	N A	T F	S F	C H O L
Vinegar	0	8	4	0	0	0	0	0
Good Seasons No Oil Italian Mix	0	12	-	-	60	0	0	0
Weight Watcher's French	0	15	-	-	345	0	0	36
Pritikin No Oil	0	24	-	-	20	0	0	0
Soy sauce	0	44	6	6	4416	0	0	0
Horseradish	0	24	6	.8	56	0	0	-
Catsup	.4	64	15	1	624	0	0	0
Kraft Catalina Reduced Calorie	1	32	-	-	240	0	0	0
Barbecue sauce	1	47	8	1	5	0	0	0
Wish Bone Lite Russian	1	50	-	-	280	0	0	0
Wish Bone Lite French	4	60	-	-	140	0	0	36
Mustard	4	60	4	4	780	0	0	0

DRESSINGS/SAUCES Con't.	F A T	C A L	C H O O	P R O O	N A	T F	S F	C H O L
Oriental Chef Tangy Soy	8	70	-	-	480	0	0	0
Wish Bone Lite Ranch	8	90	-	-	300	0	0	16
Kraft 1000 Island	10	110	-	-	305	0	0	16
Kraft Catalina French	12	140	-	-	360	0	0	36
Seven Seas Viva Italian	14	140	-	-	640	0	0	0
Hidden Valley Ranch	16	160	-	-	280	0	0	16
Newman's Own	18	160	-	-	160	0	0	0
Homemade Vinegar/Oil 2 parts oil, 1 part vinegar	19	166	-	-	0	0	0	0
Mayonnaise	44	396	2	.8	314	0	0	32

DESSERTS

	F A T	C A L	C H O O	P R O O	N A	T F	S F	C H O L
Honey Hill Nonfat Frozen yogurt, 3/4 C.	0	120	-	-	0	0	0	6
Angel food cake, 1 piece (1 12)	.1	146	33	3	73	2	1	0
Fig bars, 1	.9	57	12	.6	40	4	1	8
Dole fruit sorbet, peach, 4 ounces	1	110	27	1	10	2	1	0
Tofutti Lite, 3/4 C.	1	135	-	-	-	-	-	0
Chocolate chip cookie	2	47	7	.5	40	-	-	1
Sugar cookie, 1	2	71	12	.8	41	-	-	4
Oatmeal cookie, 1	3	54	6	.8	30	-	-	5
Shortbread cookie, 1	3	75	10	1	9	-	-	12
Chocolate cake, 1 piece	4	131	23	2	146	-	-	29
Sponge cake, 1 piece	4	193	36	5	113	-	-	172

DESSERTS Con't.	F A T	C A L	C H O	P R O	N A	T F	S F	C H O L
Brownie, 1	5	50	21	2	50	-	-	13
Boston cream pie, 1 piece	6	207	34	4	175	-	-	64
Banana cake, 1 piece	7	247	43	3	180	-	-	38
Rice Dream, 3/4 C.	8	205	-	-	-	-	-	-
Ice Bean, 3/4 C.	14	235	-	-	-	-	-	-
Pound cake, 1 piece	14	351	49	6	271	-	-	149
Fruitcake, 1 piece	15	433	71	6	170	-	-	37
Apple pie, 1 piece	22	457	67	4	355	-	-	0
Haagen Dazs., 3/4 C.	24	395	-	-	-	0	0	-
Cheesecake, 1 piece	25	406	37	5	531	-	-	92
Carrot cake, 1 piece	28	478	53	5	170	-	-	92

MEATS
3 ounce serving; broiled, lean cuts
(unless otherwise noted)

	F A T	C A L	C H O	P R O	N A	T F	S F	C H O L
Sweetbreads	3	143	0	28	99	0	0	396
Vienna sausage, 1	4	45	.4	2	152	0	0	8
Pork sausage, 1 link	4	48	.1	3	168	0	0	11
Canadian bacon, 2 slices	4	86	2	11	719	0	0	27
Leg of lamb	4	117	0	18	44	0	0	56
Beef liver, braised	4	137	3	21	60	0	0	331
Veal cutlet	4	140	.7	26	247	0	0	106
Lamb chop, loin	5	116	0	17	186	0	0	58
Ham, lean	5	133	.1	21	1128	0	0	47
Venison	5	153	0	25	338	0	0	70
Veal liver	5	158	5	22	83	0	0	340

MEATS Con't.	FAT	CAL	CHO	PRO	NA	TF	SF	CHOL
Round steak	7	165	0	24	54	0	0	70
Beef bologna, 1 slice	8	89	.6	3	284	0	0	16
Pork loin chop	8	166	0	23	56	0	0	71
Tenderloin steak	8	176	0	24	54	0	0	72
Rabbit	8	182	0	25	231	0	0	90
Bacon, 3 slices	9	109	.2	6	303	0	0	16
T-bone steak	9	182	0	15	56	0	0	68
Porterhouse steak	9	185	0	24	56	0	0	68
Beef frankfurter, 1	13	145	1	5	76	0	0	22
Flank steak	13	207	0	22	70	0	0	60
Lean ground beef	15	238	0	24	76	0	0	68
Short ribs	15	251	0	26	50	0	0	79
Ground beef	17	248	0	23	79	0	0	86
Knockwurst 1 link	19	209	1	8	687	0	0	39
Liverwurst	24	279	2	12	732	0	0	135
Chuck roast	24	301	0	23	50	0	0	84
Kielbasa	31	264	2	12	915	0	0	57

DAIRY AND EGGS
4 ounce serving
(1/2 cup)

	FAT	CAL	CHO	PRO	NA	TF	SF	CHOL
Egg white, 1 large	0	16	.4	3	50	0	0	0
Skim milk	.6	90	12	8	126	0	0	6
Buttermilk	2	100	12	8	258	0	0	8
Low fat fruit yogurt	2	226	42	10	122	0	0	10
Plain low fat yogurt	2	144	16	4	160	0	0	20
Sherbet	4	270	58	2	88	0	0	14

DAIRY AND EGGS Con't.	F A T	C A L	C H O	P R O	N A	T F	S F	C H O L
Egg yolk, 1 large	6	63	.04	3	8	0	0	213
Whole egg, 1 large	6	79	.6	6	69	0	0	213
2 % low fat milk	6	120	12	8	122	0	0	36
Ice milk	6	184	30	6	106	0	0	18
Plain yogurt	8	140	10	8	104	0	0	28
Whole milk	8	156	10	8	120	0	0	36
Chocolate milk	8	208	26	8	150	0	0	30
Goat milk	10	168	10	8	122	0	0	28
Human milk	10	172	10	8	122	0	0	28
Ice cream	14	268	32	4	116	0	0	58
Evaporated milk	20	338	24	18	266	0	0	74
Eggnog	20	342	38	10	138	0	0	150
Sweetened, condensed milk	26	982	166	24	390	0	0	104
Half and half	28	316	10	8	98	0	0	90
Sour cream	28	492	10	8	124	0	0	102

CHEESES
4 ounce serving

	F A T	C A L	C H O	P R O	N A	T F	S F	C H O L
Low fat creamed cottage cheese	2	102	4	15	459	0	0	9
Part-skim ricotta	10	170	6	14	154	0	0	38
Mozzarella, part skim	18	328	3	28	528	0	0	64
Feta cheese	24	300	5	16	1264	0	0	100
American cheese spread	24	328	9	16	1524	9	9	60
Swiss cheese	24	332	2	24	852	0	0	80

CHEESES Con't.	F A T	C A L	C H O O	P R O	N A	T F	S F	C H O L
Edam	24	404	3	28	1092	0	0	100
Camembert	28	340	.4	22	954	0	0	81
Processed Swiss	28	380	2	28	1552	0	0	96
Gouda	28	404	2	28	928	0	0	128
Parmesan	28	444	4	40	1816	0	0	76
Provolone	30	400	2	28	992	0	0	80
Brie	31	380	.4	24	713	0	0	112
Romano	31	440	4	36	1360	0	0	116
Colby	32	380	2	24	684	0	0	92
Bleu cheese	32	400	3	24	1583	0	0	84
Muenster	32	416	1	28	712	0	0	108
Monterey jack	34	424	.8	28	608	0	0	101
Roquefort	36	420	2	24	2054	0	0	104
American cheese processed	36	420	1	24	1624	0	0	108
Cheddar	38	456	2	28	704	0	0	119
Cream cheese	4	396	2	8	332	0	0	124

FATS AND OILS
1/2 cup

	F A T	C A L	C H O O	P R O	N A	T F	S F	C H O L
Margarine	91	813	..6	1	1224	0	0	.1
Butter	92	810	0	1	993	0	0	247
Chicken fat	102	920	0	0	0	0	0	88
Vegetable shortening	102	920	0	0	0	0	0	0
Olive oil	109	952	0	0	0	0	0	0
Peanut oil	109	952	0	.1	0	0	-	-
Corn oil	109	960	0	0	.1	0	0	0
Safflower oil	109	960	0	0	.1	0	0	0
Soybean oil	109	960	0	0	0	0	0	0
Sunflower oil	109	960	0	0	.1	0	0	0
Wheat germ oil	109	960	0	0	0	0	0	0

FAST FOODS 1 serving	F A T	C A L	C H O O	P R O O	N A	T F F	S F F	C H O L
McDonald's vanilla shake	8	352	60	9	201	0	0	-
chocolate shake	9	383	66	10	300	0	0	9
hot cakes with butter and syrup	10	500	94	8	1070	-	-	59
French fries	11	220	26	3	109	-	-	9
Filet-of-Fish	26	435	36	15	799	-	-	45
Big Mac	35	570	39	25	979	-	-	83
Wendy's chicken sandwich	10	320	31	25	500	-	-	59
breakfast sandwich	19	370	33	117	770	-	-	200
baked potato w/broccoli/cheese	25	500	54	13	430	5	2	22
Taco Bell taco	9	162	9	12	-	-	-	-
bean cheese burrito	11	350	48	15	-	-	-	-
Cheese pizza, 1/2 of 12" pie	12	653	96	39	1347	-	-	-
Arby's roast beef sandwich	15	350	32	22	880	-	-	45
Jack in the Box								
Fajita Pita	8	292	29	24	703	1	3	34
Super Taco	17	288	21	12	765	-	-	37
Egg Rolls (5)	32	675	70	26	1505	-	-	50
Jumbo Jack with cheese	40	677	46	32	1665	-	-	110
Ultimate Cheeseburger	69	942	33	47	1176	-	-	127
Kentucky Fried Chicken, 2 piece combo	35	643	46	35	1441	-	-	180
Burger King onion rings	16	270	29	3	450	-	-	-
Whopper with cheese	45	740	52	32	1435	-	-	-

How to Look Great & Feel Sexy

Summary of Research

How to Look Great & Feel Sexy

Summary of Research:

DHEA-Dehydroepiandrosterone benefits:
- Decrease body fat, appetite & increases lean muscle mass
- Increases metabolism, stabilizes blood sugar & diabetes
- Prolong life expectancy, male & female sex hormones
- Menopause, depression, memory & learning problems
- Immune system, less infection, Epstein-Barr, Lupus, herpes
- Chronic Fatigue Syndrome, Alzheimer's, osteoporosis
- Lower cholesterol, atherosclerosis, cancer

Estrogen & Progesterone benefits:
- Menopausal symptoms: hot flashes, night sweats
- Prevent vaginal dryness, aging skin
- Reduced Alzheimer's, more alert, better memory
- Increased bone density, prevent osteoporosis
- Less heart disease, less colon cancer

Human Growth Hormone-benefits
- Enhanced sexual performance, firmer, larger penis
- Increase energy, better exercise performance (in some studies)
- Better cardiac output, stronger bones, heals wounds
- Muscle mass gain 8.8%, body fat reduction 14.4%
- Less cellulite and wrinkles, thicker skin-collagen
- Sharper vision, better memory, improved mood
- Organ regrowth: liver, spleen, kidneys, heart
- Lower cholesterol-LDL, lower blood pressure

Note-You must be under a doctors care and have a prescription to take Human Growth Hormone. Take small dosages of 3 IU in the day and 2 IU at night to avoid side effects; carpal tunnel syndrome, fluid retention, headaches, joint swelling. A safer alternative is to use the homeopathic IGF-1, DHEA and Avena Sativa to increase your body's natural production of Human Growth Hormone and IGF-1.

Melatonin benefits:
- Free radical scavenger antioxidant in cells
- Younger, vigorous and sexually rejuvenated
- Natural sleeping pill, REM dream sleep
- Reduces jet lag resets biological clock
- Retards tumors, prevents Parkinson's disease
- Reduces incidence of Alzheimer's, Down's syndrome, asthma
- Lowers cholesterol, prevents heart disease, cataracts

Testosterone & Free Testosterone
- Promotes libido (sexual desire)
- Improves and maintains erection
- Promotes muscle growth, slows protein catabolism
- Enhances immune system
- Sperm production, nourishes male urinary

Testing/Diagnostic Procedures:

Wellness Lab screen
- Lipid (HDL, LDL, VLDL, Cardiac risk), glucose
- Blood morphology, Blood clumping, CBC
- Free Radical damage -- ROTS in dry blood cells
- Carotid artery ultrasound
- Chemistry panel, liver enzymes, kidney BUN
- PSA (Prostatic Acid Phosphate)

Saliva tests for hormones:
1. DHEA
2. Free Testosterone
3. Progesterone
4. Estradiol
5. Melatonin

Blood tests for Hormones:
1. IGF-1 (Insulin Like Growth Factor) Somatomedin
2. Human Growth Hormone
3. Thyroid Panel T3, T4, TSH
4. Total testosterone

Nutritional and Lifestyle Suggestions:

Nick Delgado anti-aging Supplements
- DHEA
- Melatonin
- Avena Sativa -- Green Oats, Nettle, Saw Palmetto increase total testosterone, unbind Free Testosterone
- Pro-gest cream Wild Yam (women: PMS, bone density)
- Es-Gen cream (women: hot flashes, mood swings)
- Kelp, sea veggies, iodine for Thyroid/avoid Dairy
- Human Growth Hormone-Saizen 4 IU Somatropin
- Homeopathic IGF-1

Nick Delgado Supplements, Diet, Exercise
- Antioxidants A, E, C, B complex
- Colloidal minerals filter free of "heavymetals"
- Soluble fiber, psyllum or metamucil
- Filtered water, veggie juice
- Vegan low fat, dairy free, meat free diet
- Workouts-high intensity, 3 sets per exercise to failure
- Aerobics-dancing, treadmill, stair stepper
- Sex, cuddling, holding, kissing 1-2 x day

How to Look Great & Feel Sexy

How to Look Great, Feel Younger, Stronger and Sexier in 90 days*

"How to Look Great & Feel Sexy!" Only $31.95
Did you know that there are eight natural hormones in our bodies that control everything from our energy levels and libido to how fast we age? In fact, many of the complaints associated with aging such as decreased vitality and sex drive, increased body fat, and slower mental processing can be alleviated just by restoring these hormones to youthful levels!

Read this book by Dr. Nick Delgado, sought after speaker, talk show host, presenter of over 3,500 seminars, and an expert on aging and nutrition. He'll reveal how these hormones are helping thousands discover the secret of "The Fountain of Youth" - often within 90 days! And his simple techniques guarantee even the busiest people can get immediate results.
The book "How to Look Great & Feel Sexy!" explains:

- Amazing facts about diet programs to avoid like the Zone, Slim Fast, Weight Watchers, and Phen Fen.
- Ways to reduce the risk of heart attacks and strokes and improve the immune system in only 9 days.
- How testosterone and DHEA renew strength, reduce body fat, and improve sexual potency past age 40.
- How to determine the levels of each of these hormones in your own body.
- Where to find the best natural hormones rather than prescribed synthetics.
- How to improve mental acuity in 30 days with a combination of hormones, diet, and exercise.

Dr. Delgado, former director of the Nathan Pritikin program, conducts programs for Tony Robbins at Mastery University. This book, "How to Look Great & Feel Sexy!" discusses the latest on nutrition, exercise, vitamins, minerals, and hormones. You will learn techniques for achieving optimal mental attitude to achieve maximum health! Enjoy 600 tasty recipes, including Italian, Chinese, Mexican, Thai, and American cuisine's. 400 pages.

"Mastering the Powers of Your Inner Health" Only $19.95
This book gives you the secrets of how to live life to the fullest, beginning with practical information on nutrition for infants and the nursing or pregnant mother. You will find out the best drug free ways to build up muscle and reduce body fat. "Mastering the Powers of Your Inner Health" shows you how to enhance the immune system and overcome allergy symptoms. Discover how to establish health as a priority within your values and goals.

"Reverse Aging" Series 12 Cassette Tapes. Only $129
You will hear the essence of the best interviews conducted by Dr. Nick Delgado on his television program. Discussions cover slowing the aging process with nutrition, natural hormones, herb's, exercise, stress reduction and smoking cessation. Tapes on humor, happiness, fitness and discipline for busy people, how to preserve the earth's resources, senile brain damage from meat, male sexual impotency, and the reversal of atherosclerosis. Also learn relief for neck and back pain, improving circulation, skin rejuvenation, oxygen therapy, cosmetic procedures, supplements, homeopathy and allergies.

"Look and Feel Great" 8 audio tapes. Only $89.95
These tapes explain how to establish new winning habits, helping you to lose unwanted body fat and gain lean muscle tissue. This program will bring you high-energy living. Discover how to reduce cholesterol, triglycerides and achieve ideal body weight. Shop at the supermarket and order healthfully dinning out at almost any restaurant. Learn the cause and prevention of heart disease, diabetes, arthritis, cancer, osteoporosis, hypertension, hearing loss, digestive problems, ulcers, hernia, gallstones and varicose veins.

CD-ROM "Live Long & Love It!" $29.95
Dr. Delgado's plan provides an entertaining and informative multi-media experience. A dynamite addition toward personalizing your health & fitness plan. PC Minimum Requirements: 486/25Mhz w/10MB available on hard drive, 4MB RAM, SVGA, CD-ROM, Sound Card, Mouse, Windows™ 3.1, DOS 5.0 or higher and MPC Level 1 complaint.

"Wellness" video $23.95
Nick's dynamic video tape of his most popular nutrition presentation will stimulate and motivate you to stay on the health track. Filled with information that you can see and use now.

"Good Safe Sex" video and audio. Only $69
You'll appreciate the candor of this helpful discussion on sex. The audio: Sex is the Sizzle in Relationships. The video: Tasteful discussion of love-making techniques that will improve your sexual intimacy and transcend your relationship.

Special $229: "Reverse Aging" 12 audio tapes + "Look & Feel Great" 8 audio tapes and "Wellness" video.

* Money Back Guarantee - Study this program for 90 days, keep a wellness record of your body fat, cholesterol lipid level, exercise, supplements and 24 hour food recall once a week. If this program helps you to improve your health beyond your present level you will have met the Delgado challenge. If not satisfied, just send in a record of your tests and wellness diary and a refund minus shipping and handling costs will be returned without question.

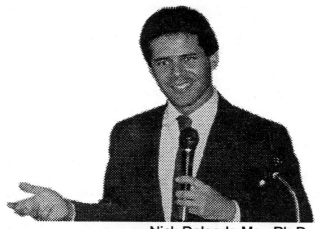

Nick Delgado Ms., Ph.D.

 **HEALTHY STUDIOS ®**
25422 Trabuco Road, #105-141
Lake Forest, California 92630

Inquiries; Orders **800-631-0232**

Change the Course of Your Life Experience with the Best Health that
You Can Attain.

USE THIS HANDY ORDER FORM

Qty	Description	Unit Price	Total
	Special 20 Audio Tapes, 1 Wellness Video	$229.00	
	Reverse Aging Series - 12 Audio Tapes	$129.00	
	Delgado Diet and Exercise Plan - 8 audios	$89.95	
	Sex Series - 1 video, 1 audio tape	$69.00	
	"How to Look Great; & Feel Sexy"	$31.95	
	Nick's book titled "Fatigue to Vitality"	$22.95	
	"Mastering the Powers of Your Inner Health" Book	$19.95	
	Wellness - video	$23.95	
	Diet and Exercise Plan - CD ROM	$29.95	

Postage & Handling		
Order Total Postage	SubTotal	
Up to $35.............................$5	Postage and Handling	
Over $35.............................$9	Add 8% State Tax	
	TOTAL ENCLOSED	
Canada and Europe........Add $18		
Australia and Asia.........Add $35		

Allow 4 weeks for delivery.
_____*PAL video tapes add $10 per video*

Mail To: Nick Delgado, Ms. Ph.D.
Healthy Studios
25422 Trabuco Rd., #105-141
Lake Forest, CA 92630

FAX Orders **714-951-7013**
For Credit Card Orders Call
800-631-0232
(Leave detailed message of order, credit card #& expiration date.)

Today's Date:_____

Send to:

Name _____

Address _____

City/St/Zip _____

Daytime Phone_____

MasterCard _____ Visa _____ AmEx_____

CC# _____ Exp. Date_____

Signature _____

THE DELGADO HEALTH PLAN RECIPES

Appetizers
&
Beverages

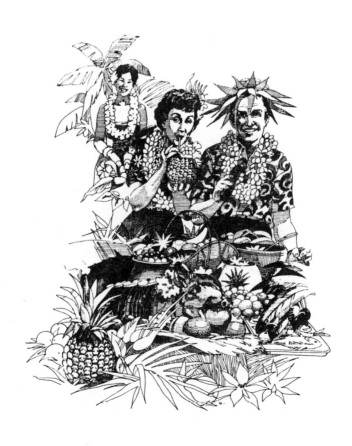

How to Look Great & Feel Sexy

BEAN SALSA DIP

1(30 oz.) can Rosarita   (8oz.) jar Pace Picante sauce
Vegetarian Refried Beans

Blend together and serve with homemade tortilla chips.

BLACK BEAN DIP

8 oz. dried black beans, cooked and   1 clove garlic, minced
    drained   1 tsp paprika
1 lg. onion, chopped   1 tsp dried mustard
1 jalapeno pepper, seeded and sliced   3 parsley sprigs, chopped
1 sm. green pepper, chopped   chili powder to taste
1 shallot bulb, chopped   2 lg. scallions, chopped

Combine all ingredients in blender, making certain that they are evenly distributed. If mixture becomes too thick while blending, add water. Refrigerate in glass or plastic containers until ready to serve.

CHILI SAUCE DIP - Fast Weight Loss

1(12 oz.) bottle chili sauce   2 Tbsp horseradish
3 Tbsp lemon juice   1/4 c. finely chopped celery
3 drops Tabasco sauce   1 Tbsp minced parsley

Combine all ingredients and chill. Serve with tortilla chips or fresh raw veggies. Yield: About 1 ½ cups.

BARBECUE SAUCE

1 c. tomato paste (low-salt)   1 tsp garlic powder
3 Tbsp honey or other sweetener   Dash of red cayenne pepper or
1 tsp horseradish   Tabasco sauce
1 Tbsp onion powder   1/4 tsp ground cloves
1 Tbsp low-sodium Dijon mustard   1/2 tsp liquid smoke

Combine all ingredients in jar and mix well. Store in refrigerator.

CRANBERRY SAUCE

1 c. grape juice concentrate   2/3 c. dates
1/2 c. orange juice   1 (12 oz.) pkg cranberries
1/2 c. apple juice concentrate   (fresh or frozen)

Combine all ingredients in blender and blend for 2 minutes at high speed. Chill and serve. Yield: About 3 cups.

CUCUMBER ONION DIP

1 sm. avocado
1 can split pea soup
2 c. cucumber: peeled & chopped fine
1/4 tsp pepper
1/2 tsp onion powder

4 Tbsp dried onion
1/2 tsp paprika
1 tsp Worcestershire sauce
2 tsp lemon juice
Dash of Tabasco sauce

Place avocado, split pea soup, 1/2 cup cucumber, pepper onion powder, 2 tablespoons dried onion, and remaining ingredients in blender and mix until smooth. Stir in remaining cucumber and onion; chill for several hours. Serve as topping for baked potatoes or serve with whole wheat crackers or fresh vegetables. Yield: 3 cups.

FRIED ZUCCHINI - Fast Weight Loss - Microwave

1/3 c. Butter Buds
1/3 c. Italian style seasoned
   bread crumbs

1 tsp paprika
3 zucchini, sliced
1 tsp basil

Prepare Butter Buds. In a plastic bag, combine bread crumbs, basil, and paprika. Dip zucchini in Butter Buds. Shake in crumb mixture to coat evenly. Arrange vegetables on a dish; cover with a paper towel. Microwave on full power 2 minutes. Rearrange, moving outside pieces to center of dish. Cook on full power 1 more minute. 16 servings.

GARBONZO SPREAD

1/2 c. red onion, chopped
1/2 bunch parsley, chopped finely
1 tsp basil
2/3 c. toasted sesame seeds (optional)
Salt to taste (optional)

1/2 tsp cumin
1/4 tsp garlic powder or 2
   cloves garlic, fresh
3 c. cooked, mashed garbanzo
   beans

Blend all ingredients together. Makes about 3 cups. Use as vegetable or cracker dip, sandwich spread, or with falafels. Cook 1 cup dry garbanzo beans with 4 cups water for 3 to 4 hours. Yield: 2 cups.

GARBONZO "NUTS"

Soak dried garbanzo beans in water overnight. Drain well, then place on non-stick baking sheet in a single layer. Sprinkle on onion and garlic powder to taste. Bake in 350 degree oven for 1 1/2 hours until beans are brown and crisp. Great for snacking. Unique nutty flavor.

GARBONZO BEAN SPREAD - HUMMUS

1/2 onion, chopped
1/4 c. parsley, finely chopped
1 Tbsp basil
1 Tbsp oregano
2 Tbsp curry powder or to taste

2 Tbsp toasted sesame seeds
1 sm. clove garlic, minced
Juice of 1 lemon
3 c. well-cooked garbanzo
   beans, mashed

Sauté onions in a non-stick pan until transparent. Add a small amount of stock or water if needed to keep the onions from sticking. Add all of the other ingredients except garbanzos and sauté until parsley is soft. Add mixture to garbanzos and mix well. Serve cold as a sandwich spread or dip.

HUMMUS BEAN DIP-QUICK

1 (6 oz). box Hummus dip mix   (any brand)

Mix in a bowl with 1 full cup of water. If too thick, add a little more water until you get desired smoothness. Dip fresh raw vegetables, like carrots, celery, broccoli, etc.

MOCK CAVIAR - Fast Weight Loss

1 lg. eggplant
1 onion, chopped fine
1 clove garlic, minced
1/2 c. bell pepper, finely chopped

1 1/2 Tbsp lemon juice
Ground pepper
Pam non-stick spray

Slice eggplant in half and spray each half with Pam non-stick spray. Place halves, cut side down on baking pan. Broil on middle rack of oven for 20 to 25 minutes. Cool slightly, then scoop out pulp and mash with fork. Sauté onion and garlic in non-stick pan (use non-stick spray). Stir onion and garlic into eggplant pulp with remaining ingredients. Chill for 2 to 3 hours. Sprinkle with chopped parsley and serve with bread rounds or toast. Yield: About 2 1/2 cups.

LENTIL DIP

1/2 c. dry lentils
1/4 c. minced onions
1 clove garlic, minced
3 c. water

1 tsp ground cumin
4 tsp green taco sauce
1/4 c. tomato sauce

Place lentils, onion, and garlic in water. Bring to a boil, then reduce heat to low. Cook until lentils are soft, about 30 minuses. Drain and save liquid for stock. Put mixture into blender or food processor. Add cumin, lemon juice, chili powder, taco, and tomato sauces. Puree until smooth. Chill. Yield: 1 1/2 cups.

MARINATED MUSHROOMS I - Fast Weight Loss

1 lb. bite sized mushrooms
2 green peppers, cut into
3/4 inch pieces
1 sm. onion, cut into wedges and
   then separated

1 c. water
1 Tbsp honey
2 tsp dry mustard
2 tsp low-sodium soy sauce
1 c. red wine vinegar

Preparation time: 15 minutes. Chilling time: 2 to 3 hours.

Prepare mushrooms by cleaning and trimming stems. Set aside with green pepper and onions in a bowl. Combine water, vinegar, honey, mustard, and soy sauce in a pan. Bring to a boil. Pour over mushrooms, green peppers, and onions. Cover. Marinate in refrigerator for several hours.

Before serving, thread on small bamboo skewers. Serve as appetizer.

MARINATED MUSHROOMS II - Fast Weight Loss

20 lg. mushrooms
2 Tbsp fresh chopped parsley
2 Tbsp sherry
1/2 c. defatted chicken broth

1/2 c. no oil Italian dressing
1/4 tsp tamari
Garlic powder to taste

1. Sauté mushrooms and parsley in sherry in a sauté pan for a few minutes.
2. Remove from heat, transfer to a bowl, add the rest of the ingredients, and marinate for 1 hour. Makes 4 servings. Each serving contains 40 calories. 7% fat, 121 mg sodium, and 0 mg cholesterol.

MUSHROOM ANTIPASTO

1 1/4 c. tomato puree
1/2 c. water
2 Tbsp red wine vinegar
1 tsp toasted dehydrated onion flakes
2 cloves garlic, minced
1/2 green pepper, seeded and diced
1/2 red pepper, seeded and diced

1/4 c. chopped fresh parsley
1 tsp salad herbs or Italian
   herb blend
2 Tbsp apple juice concentrate
1/4 tsp freshly ground nutmeg
1 lb. sm. fresh mushrooms
   quartered

1. Combine tomato puree and water.
2. Then combine with all other ingredients, except mushrooms, and mix thoroughly. Pour over mushrooms and marinate overnight. Serve as hors d'ocuvres or antipasto.
   Makes 4 servings. Each 1 cup serving contains 75 calories. 6% fat, 26 mg sodium, 0 mg cholesterol.

MUSHROOMS & SPICY CHILI - Fast Weight Loss

1/2 c. vinegar
1 c. water
1 Tbsp bell pepper, diced
2 Tbsp peppercorns or cracked black
   pepper

1 Tbsp garlic, minced
2 sm. whole hot dried red chili
   peppers
1 lb. sm. whole mushrooms
   (fresh or canned)

Mix vinegar bell pepper, peppercorns, garlic, and chilies together in a quart jar or small saucepan.

Add mushrooms to mix and microwave for 4 minutes at 70% power or heat in small saucepan over medium heat until just below boiling.

Strain into a quart jar. Add mushrooms back to strained marinade and cool to room temperature, then refrigerate.

Marinate at least 4 to 6 hours before serving. Mushrooms are best the next day, but will keep refrigerated for up to 2 weeks. Serving size: 8 servings, 4 to 5 mushrooms each. Per serving: 25 calories. 25 mg sodium.

POTATO BALLS

2 c. leftover mashed potatoes or use
   Potato Buds

1/2 c. bread crumbs

Preparation time: 10 minutes. Cooking time: 20 minutes

Form potatoes into balls about 1 1/2 inch in diameter. Roll in bread crumbs. Place on a non-stick baking sheet and bake at 350 degrees about 20 minutes until browned. Turn once or twice for even browning.

POTATO POPPERS

1/4 onion chopped
1 c. cooked brown rice
1 c. whole grain bread crumbs

1 c. mashed potatoes
2 Tbsp tomato sauce

Preheat oven to 350 degrees. Simmer onion in a small amount of water.
Combine all ingredients and form into 1 1/2 inch balls. Place on a non-stick
baking sheet and bake until slightly browned, about 15 minutes.

LOW - SODIUM CATSUP

1 c. tomato paste (low-salt)
3 Tbsp lemon juice
2 Tbsp honey or other sweetener
1 tsp horseradish
1 Tbsp low-sodium Dijon mustard

1 Tbsp onion powder
1 tsp garlic powder
Dash red cayenne pepper or
    Tabasco sauce
1/4 tsp ground cloves

Combine all ingredients; store in refrigerator.

POTATO CHIPS(FAT FREE) - Fast Weight Loss

3 med. baking potatoes or sweet
    potatoes
Salt-free vegetable or Italian seasoning

ground pepper, or dried
    herbs(optional)

1. Preheat oven to 375 degrees. Line a baking sheet with cooking parchment
   or one side of a brown paper bag. Scrub or peel potatoes.
2. In a food processor, using the fine slicing blade (1 mm), slice potatoes. Or,
   slice potatoes paper thin by hand.
3. Place potato slices in a single layer on the paper and sprinkle with
   seasonings, if using. Bake for 7 minutes, then turn the chips and bake for
   another 7 to 10 minutes, or until golden brown and crisp. Check often and
   remove any chips that brown too quickly.
4. Let chips cool on the baking sheet, then store in a paper bag. Makes 2
   servings, approximately 100 chips.

How to Look Great & Feel Sexy

FRIES, CAJUN STYLE - Fast Weight Loss

No stick cooking spray | 1 lemon
4 baking potatoes | 2 tsp Cajun seasoning

Serves 4. Preheat the oven to 425 degrees. Spray a cookie sheet with no stick cooking spray. Cut the unpeeled potatoes into thin, long strips. Place in a bowl of ice water with the juice of 1 lemon to prevent potatoes from browning. Drain the potatoes. Distribute evenly over the cookie sheet and sprinkle with Cajun seasoning. Bake for 20-25 minutes turning potatoes several times. Potatoes will be cooked and lightly browned. Serve immediately. Each serving: 0 mg cholesterol, 125 cal..

HOME FRIES - Fast Weight Loss - Microwave

3 potatoes, peeled, cut in cubes or slices | 1/2 tsp garlic powder
1 pkg. Butter Buds, prepared | 1/4 tsp dill weed
1/4 c. chopped onion | 1/4 tsp thyme
1/2 tsp browning sauce | 1/2 tsp paprika

In a 1 1/2 quart casserole dish, combine all ingredients. Make sure potatoes are evenly coated. Microwave on full power 9 minutes or until potatoes are fork tender. 4 servings.

ZUCCHINI PIZZA HORS D'OEUVRES

4 zucchini, cut into 1/4 inch thick slices | 1/3 c. green onions, sliced
1 1/2 c. mushrooms | 1 c. pizza sauce
1/2 c. olives, chopped

Arrange sliced zucchini on baking sheets. Top with 1 to 2 teaspoons pizza sauce, a few olive pieces, and green onions and a sprinkling of mushrooms. Broil about 6 inches from heat until lightly browned (4 to 6 minutes). Serve hot. 5 dozen hors d'oeuvres.

SEASON "SALT"

2 tsp sesame seeds | 1 1/4 tsp corn starch
1/2 tsp paprika | 1/2 tsp celery powder
3/4 tsp red dried bell peppers | 1 tsp onion powder
1/4 tsp thyme | 1 tsp garlic powder
1 can Schilling vegetable flakes

Grind all ingredients that are not fine in food processor and blend with remaining ingredients. Vary ingredients according to taste.

SESAME KOMBU

Soak in water to cover for 15 minutes 20 inch piece of kombu or wakame. Wipe kombu off with paper towel and cut in small squares.

Bring 1/2 cup water to a boil. Drop in 6 to 8 scallions, sliced in 1/4 inch rounds and cook for 1 minute. Drain, rinse with cold water, and squeeze out excess liquid. Mix together in a bowl:

2 Tbsp light miso   **1/3 c. water**
2 Tbsp tahini

Add scallions and kombu to miso mixture. Serve as a side dish at room temperature or chilled. Yield: About 1 cup. Per 2 tablespoon serving: 40 calories, 1 gm protein, 3 gm carbohydrates, 5 gm fat.

VEGETABLE HUMMUS POCKET SANDWICHES

1/2 c. finely chopped green onions   **1/8 tsp red pepper**
1/2 c. finely chopped green bell pepper   **1 (15 oz.) can garbanzo beans,**
3 Tbsp fresh parsley   **rinsed drained**
1 Tbsp sesame seeds   **4 (6 inch) whole wheat pita**
1/2 tsp whole oregano   **bread rounds, cut in**
1/2 tsp mint flakes   **half crosswise**
1/2 tsp garlic powder   **1 med. tomato, cut into 8 (1/4**
2 c. alfalfa sprouts   **inch)slices**

Combine first 8 ingredients in a 1 quart casserole. Cover with a heavy duty plastic wrap and turn back one corner to vent. Microwave on high for 3 minutes. Place bell pepper mixture and garbanzo beans in blender or food processor for 1 minute or until smooth. Spoon about 1/4 cup bean mixture (hummus) into each pita bread half. Cut tomato slices in half, open sandwiches and place 2 tomato slices and 1/4 cup alfalfa sprouts into sandwich half. Serve immediately. Serves 8.

BANANAS IN COCONUT MILK...Kluay Buat Chee

5 ripe bananas, peeled and quartered   **2 Tbsp apple juice concentrate**
1 1/2 tsp perfumed thick coconut milk*   **2 Tbsp roasted mung beans,**
1/2 tsp salt   **crushed**

This dish is not widely known to foreigners, even those in Thailand. Among the Thai it is seldom served to guests. Siamese Buddhist nuns dress in white, from whence comes the Thai name for the dish, Kluay Buat Chee; exactly translated: Nun Bananas.

In a 2 quart coated saucepan, place all the ingredients, except the mung beans. Bring to a boil, then simmer for 2 minutes. Pour into a serving dish and sprinkle with mung beans. Serve warm or chilled. 4 to 5 servings.
*Add 2 to 3 drops jasmine essence (Yod Nam Malee).

SMOOTHIES

2 bananas
1/2 c. apple juice

1/2 c. frozen fruit (raspberries, strawberries, blueberries, etc.)

OR

2 frozen bananas
1/2 c. frozen and crushed pineapple

1/2 c. apple juice

Blend using a Vita Mix which retains the whole food and fiber until smooth. To freeze bananas, peel, wrap in plastic wrap, and place in freezer for 6 hours.

TROPICAL SMOOTHIE

2 c. unsweetened pineapple juice
2 bananas

1/2 c. oat bran
8 ice cubes

Place all ingredients in blender and blend for about 1 minute at high speed. Serves 4.

FRUIT SHAKE

2 peeled oranges
2 peeled bananas
2 c. crushed ice

1 1/2 c. apple juice
Dash of cinnamon

Blend in blender (add ice gradually). Sprinkle cinnamon on top.

STRAWBERRY SHAKE

4 c. orange juice
2 c. frozen strawberries

1/2 tsp almond extract

Place all ingredients in blender and serve cold. Serves 4.

CRANBERRY DELIGHT

1 c. cranberry juice, chilled
1 Tbsp lemon juice

1 egg white
1/2 c. crushed ice

Blend all ingredients until foamy. Serve immediately. Serves 2.

CRANBERRY TEA PUNCH - Fast Weight Loss

5 herbal tea bags or 5 tsp loose tea
1/4 tsp ground cinnamon
1/4 tsp ground nutmeg
2 1/2 c. boiling water

2 c. cranberry juice
1 1/2 c. water
1/2 c. orange juice
1/3 c. lemon juice

Steep tea and spices in hot water in covered teapot for 5 minutes. Remove tea bags and strain. Cool mixture; when cooled, add remaining ingredients. Chill and pour over ice cubes. Serves 6 to 8.

CRANBERRY SPRITZER - Fast Weight Loss

3 c. cranberry juice, chilled
1 c. unsweetened pineapple juice, chilled
Lime slices (optional)

1 (33 oz.) bottle club soda, chilled
1/2 c. lemon juice chilled or orange juice, chilled

Combine juices in pitcher as above. Repeat process as above for each serving. Garnish with lime slices, if desired. Serves 6 to 8

CRANBERRY GLOG

1 (40 oz.) bottle cranberry-apple juice
1/2 c. raisins
1/4 c. cranberries
1/2 tsp cardamom (optional)

4 orange slices, each studded with 2 whole cloves
1/2 tsp or 1 stick cinnamon

Combine all ingredients in a medium saucepan. Bring to a boil, then simmer for 30 minutes. Let stand 1 hour. Serve hot in mugs. Serves 6.

PEACHY SPRITZER

2 (21 oz.) cans peach nectar, chilled
1 c. unsweetened orange juice, chilled
1/2 c. lemon juice, chilled
Crushed ice

1 (33 oz.) bottle club soda, chilled
Orange slices (optional)

Combine juices together in a large pitcher, stirring well. Pour 1/2 cup mixture over crushed ice in a tall glass; add 1/2 cup club soda. Repeat for each serving; garnish with orange slices, if desired. Serves 6 to 8.

How to Look Great & Feel Sexy

LEMON COOLER

4 c. apple juice
1/2 c. lemon juice
Lemon wedges for garnish

2 Tbsp frozen pineapple juice
concentrate, thawed

Place all ingredients in blender and process for 2 minutes. Serve ice cold and garnish with lemon wedges. Serves 4.

ORANGE DELIGHT

1 c. orange juice
1 banana
1 tsp honey (optional)

1 c. apple juice
1 c. crushed ice
Shake of cinnamon

Blend at high speed until frothy. Serves 2 to 3.

CARROT - APPLE JUICE

2 oz. fresh apple juice
2 oz. fresh carrot juice

1 sm. apples, coarsely
chopped
3 ice cubes

Combine in blender and liquify. Serves one.

PINEAPPLE - CUCUMBER JUICE - Fast Weight Loss

3 oz. cucumber, peeled
1 oz. fresh pineapple
3 ice cubes

1/2 fresh apple, coarsely
chopped
2 parsley sprigs

Combine in blender and liquify. Serves one.

SPIKED TOMATO JUICE - Fast Weight Loss

4 c. tomato juice
4 long stems or green onions

Trim and wash stems. Sip juice through stem.

STRAWBERRY JUICE

1 c. apple juice
1 c. frozen apple juice concentrate
2 Tbsp arrowroot
2 Tbsp tahini

2 Tbsp honey
2 c. fresh strawberries
2 tsp vanilla

Combine juice and juice concentrate in a saucepan. Blend in arrowroot. Cook until thickened, stirring constantly. Place in blender or food processor and blend with remaining ingredients. Pour mixture into a shallow metal tray and freeze for 1 to 2 hours until edges are firm but center is still slushy. Stir well and return to freezer until firm. Process in food processor or beat with an electric mixer until smooth. Serves 8.

HARVEST PUNCH

1 gal. apple cider
4 to 8 whole cloves
4 tsp allspice
6 cinnamon sticks

1 c. orange juice
Dash of honey (optional)
Juice of 1 lemon

Bring all ingredients to a slow boil and simmer about 10 minutes. Strain and serve hot. Serves 20.

HOT CAROB THIRST QUENCHER

1/2 c. cold water
1/2 c. rice milk
1/3 c. carob powder

2 tsp dry Postum
2 c. boiling water

Place the cold water, rice milk, carob powder, and Postum in a blender. Blend until the dry ingredients look wet. Add the boiling water and blend at high speed for about 30 seconds or until mixture becomes frothy and all the ingredients are well blended. Serve immediately. Makes 2 servings.

HOT FRUIT TEA PUNCH

8 c. boiling water
4 cinnamon sticks, broken
1 Tbsp whole cloves
Few dashes nutmeg
4 herbal tea bags

Juice of 2 lemons
1 lg. can unsweetened pineapple juice
1 (6'1/4 oz.) can frozen grapefruit juice
or orange juice or 1 (48 oz.) can
apple juice

Bring water to a boil in a large stainless steel or enamel saucepan. Add spices and tea bags. Remove tea bags after 3 minutes of steeping; let remainder of spices simmer about 20 minutes. Add lemon juice, pineapple juice, and one other juice. (If frozen juice is used, prepare according to directions.) Bring to a boil; leave on lowest heat to keep warm. For a larger crowd, add another can of pineapple juice. Serves 30.

HOT SPICED CIDER

1 (32 oz.) bottle apple cider
4 sticks cinnamon

1 strip lemon peel
4 whole cloves

With sharp knife, peel a strip of lemon peeling from ripe lemon. In saucepan, slowly heat all ingredients. Simmer at least 10 minutes. Serve with stick of cinnamon in each mug. Serves 4 (8 ounces).

HOT SPICED CIDER II

1 qt. apple cider
1/2 tsp whole cloves

1/2 tsp allspice
2 sticks cinnamon

Combine all ingredients in 2 quart casserole. Heat in microwave oven on full power for 9 minutes. Then simmer on low for 4 minutes. Remove spices and serve.

SNAPPLE

4 c. fresh apple cider or juice
1/4 c. cinnamon sticks
1 Tbsp whole cloves
1/8 tsp ginger

1/8 tsp allspice
1 whole vanilla bean or dash
of vanilla extract

Place all but 1/4 cup of cider in a saucepan. Wrap cinnamon sticks in a clean piece of cheesecloth and place in saucepan. Mix powdered spices in blender with remaining 1/4 cup of cider and add to pan. Finally, add whole vanilla bean or dash of vanilla to mixture. Heat over low flame until warm. Remove cheesecloth mixture and vanilla bean and serve warm.

Variation: Add dash of orange or lemon extract in place of or in addition to vanilla. Serves 4.

WHITE LIGHTNING

3 c. white grape juice
1 c. grapefruit juice

1 (40 oz.) bottle cranberry
juice
1 lemon, sliced

Combine juices and lemon in a large saucepan. Bring to a boil. Cover and simmer for 10 minutes. Remove slices and serve hot in mugs. Serves 16.

SUPER NACHOS

1 onion, chopped
2 cans vegetarian refried beans
1 (4 oz.) can diced California
green chilies
3/4 c green taco sauce

8 c. tortilla pieces
1/4 c. chopped green onion
1 c. olives, sliced
1 c. Seitan wheat meat,
shredded

Spread beans in a shallow 10 x 15 inch oven-proof dish. Sprinkle chilies over beans, then cheese, then taco sauce. Bake, uncovered, at 400 degrees for 20 minutes. Remove from oven and add 1/4 cup chopped green onion and 1 cup pitted sliced olives. Arrange tortilla pieces around edges of bean mixture and serve at once. Serves 10.

ANGELED EGGS

6 hard boiled eggs, peeled
1 baked or boiled potato, cooled
(1/2 c. at least)
1 stalk celery, minced
1/4 c. minced onion

1Tbsp chutncy (salt free)
1 tsp curry powder
1 to 2 Tbsp Mayonnaise (no
cholesterol, less fat imitation
found in Health Food Stores)

Cool and peel hard boiled eggs. Cut in half lengthwise. Remove and discard egg yolks (high cholesterol). In small bowl mash potatoes, celery, onions curry powder, chutney, and mayonnaise. Add a little more mayonnaise if too dry. With teaspoon, stuff mixture into the center of egg halves. Sprinkle with paprika and chill 1 hour before serving. Yield: 12 egg halves.

How to Look Great & Feel Sexy

Breakfast

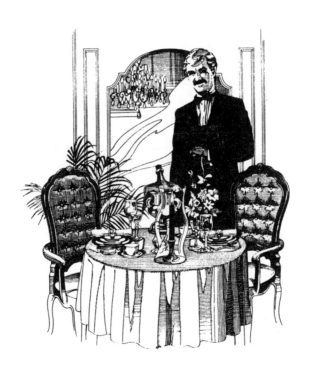

How to Look Great & Feel Sexy

BREAKFAST POTATOES

15 sm. red potatoes, cubed	1 tsp onion powder
1 med. onion, chopped	1/4 tsp black pepper
1 red bell pepper, chopped	1/2 tsp oregano
1/2 green bell pepper, chopped	1/2 to 1 c. water
1 tsp garlic powder	1 packet Butter Buds mixed
	with water

Place 1/2 cup water and Butter Buds in non-stick skillet and heat. Add potatoes and cook for about 5 minutes. Add remaining ingredients and simmer until tender.

BREAKFAST SAUSAGE

1 lg. jar Seitan's wheat meat	1/2 tsp basil
1 packet Butter Buds	1/2 tsp thyme
1/4 tsp cumin	1/2 tsp sage
1/4 tsp marjoram	1/2 tsp garlic powder
1/4 tsp oregano	1 Tbsp oat bran
1/4 tsp cayenne pepper	

Sprinkle wheat meat with spices and oat bran and refrigerate for several hours. Bake in 400 degree oven until done or cook in non-stick pan. Serves 8.

OMELETTE

1 sm. tomato, diced	2 Tbsp chili salsa
1/2 yellow onion, chopped	6 egg whites, beaten
1 zucchini, sliced and quartered	4 pieces whole wheat toast
3 oz. fresh mushrooms, sliced	Dash of pepper to taste
1/4 c. green bell pepper, chopped	

In a non-stick skillet, sauté first 5 ingredients (use non-stick spray). Add salsa and pepper. While mixture simmers, pour egg whites into pan, stirring while it cooks to keep from sticking. Cook until egg whites are set. Spoon over toast. Serves 2 to 3.

OMELET WITH STRAWBERRIES

4 egg whites
3 Tbsp water
1/2 c. strawberries

1/4 tsp cream of tartar
Pam spray

Beat egg whites, water, and cream of tartar until egg whites are stiff. Spray browning skillet with Pam spray. Pour omelet mixture into skillet. Cook on medium high for 3 1/2 minutes or until knife inserted in center comes out clean. Spread half of the strawberries on omelet. Fold omelet over and spread remaining strawberries over top before serving.

VEGETARIAN OMELET

12 egg whites
1/2 c. salsa
1 c. cauliflower, sliced
1/2 lb. Italian green beans
1 pkg. frozen, chopped spinach, thawed
8 oz. tofu
1 Tbsp Butter Buds

1/2 tsp basil
1/2 tsp oregano
1/2 tsp Veg-It seasoning
1 onion, chopped
2 cloves garlic, minced
1/4 lb. mushrooms

Steam fresh beans and cauliflower over boiling water until crisp tender (4 to 5 minutes). Drain tofu and cut into 3/4 inch cubes. Heat Butter Buds in a frying pan over medium heat. Add onion, garlic, and mushrooms; cook until onion is soft. Add beans, cauliflower, spinach: basil, oregano and Veg-It seasoning. Cook until heated through. Add egg whites. Add tofu. Cook until eggs are set. Pour salsa on top.

CREPES

1 c. whole wheat flour
1 1/2 c. apple juice

4 egg whites, stiffly beaten
1 Tbsp apple juice
    concentrate

Blend egg whites with apple juice. Then add apple juice concentrate and blend in the flour. Pour 1/3 cup batter into heated Silverstone (nonstick pan). (Be sure to spray pan with Pam and wipe with damp paper to remove excess.) Brown crepe on both sides to golden. Note: Crepes may be served as breakfast pancakes alone or with fruit or other toppings.

HUEVOS RANCHEROS I

1 steamed corn tortilla	1/4 c. green chilies
1 egg white, poached	1/4 c. salsa

Top steamed corn tortilla with poached egg white, chilies, and salsa. Makes 1 serving. Each serving contains 93 calories.

Variation: You may also add ½ cup cooked beans (vegetarian refried) or no oil.

6% fat, 156 mg sodium, 0 mg cholesterol.

YEAST CREPES

2 c. whole wheat pastry flour	1 tsp salt
1/3 c. nutritional yeast flakes	3 c. soy milk or water
(saccharomyces cerevisiae)	1/2 tsp baking powder

Served plain, these are little eggless omelets. Try rolled around ratatouille or filled with mushrooms.

Combine all ingredients in blender or beat well by hand. Batter can rest for 30 minutes in the refrigerator. Heat a 9 inch skillet and put a few drops of oil on the bottom. Rotate pan to coat bottom. Pour 1/4 cup of batter into pan and immediately tilt and rotate pan so batter forms an even layer over the whole bottom. Cook over medium high heat until the top starts to dry up and edges loosen. Slide pancake turner under the crepe, flip over and cook the other side.

Nutritional yeast tastes cheesy in spreads, sauces, salad dressings, crackers, breading meal, and on vegetables and popcorn. Added to soups, gravies, and glutton, it has a good nutty flavor. You can add it to your baby's food, too. Store in a cool, dark place.

Do not use brewer's yeast or torula yeast in this recipe. Use only Saccharomyces cerevisiae (a rich source of Vitamin B12 and B-complex). It comes in golden or bright yellow flakes or powder. If you use any other kind, this recipe will not taste the same.

HUEVOS RANCHEROS II

2 corn tortillas   3 egg whites

SAUCE
2 lg. onions   1 (14oz.) can tomatoes
1 green bell pepper   1 (14oz.) can chicken broth

GARNISH
Fresh cilantro   2 thin slices of avocado
Chopped green onion   2 slices low-fat, low-
                                                       cholesterol cheese

Place 1 to 2 cooked tortillas on a plate. Scramble egg whites and place on top of tortillas. Add ½ cup of sauce and garnish with fresh cilantro, chopped green onions, avocado, and low fat cheese.

To prepare sauce: In a frying pan, sauté onions and green pepper in a little water until soft. Add tomatoes and broth. Boil, uncovered, stirring to prevent sticking, until sauce is reduced to about 2 ½ cups.

FRENCH TOAST

4 slices whole grain bread   1/2 tsp vanilla
1 c. apple juice   1 Tbsp date pieces
1 Tbsp tapioca granules   1 ripe banana
1/2 tsp cinnamon

Put all ingredients except bread, into blender in order given. Process 3 minutes. In a bowl dip bread into mixture and bake on a non-stick riddle (use a non-stick spray). Cook until browned. Serve with homemade fruit spread. Serves 4.

FRENCH RAISIN TOAST

2 slices whole wheat raisin bread   1/2 tsp cinnamon
2 egg whites   1/2 c. apple juice or rice milk
1 tsp vanilla extract   2 Tbsp apple juice concentrate

In a shallow bowl. Beat egg whites together with other ingredients. Dip both sides of bread in batter until soaked with mixture. Spray griddle with non-stick spray; brown on both sides. Serve with fruit topping or apple butter.

APPLE - SPICED OATMEAL

1 /2 c. old fashion rolled oats   2 Tbsp raisins
1 1/2 c. water   1/2 tsp cinnamon
2 Tbsp apple juice concentrate

Bring water to a boil. Stir in oats and other ingredients. Simmer stirring occasionally, for 15 to 20 minutes or until oats are cooked and mixture has thickened. Serves 1.

CORNMEAL HOT CEREAL

1 c. whole grain cornmeal   1/2 tsp cinnamon
1 1/2 c. water   1/4 c. raisins or currants
1 c. unfiltered apple juice

In a saucepan, add all ingredients and stir constantly over medium heat until it thickens. Remove from heat and serve. Serves 2 to 4.

OAT BRAN CEREAL - Weight Loss

2/3 c. oat bran   1/2. tsp cinnamon
1 c. water   1/4 c. raisins or currants
1 c. unfiltered apple juice   (optional)

In a saucepan, add all ingredients, stirring constantly to blend. Cook 2 minutes approximately over medium heat until desired thickness. Serves 2.

GRANOLA I

5 c. uncooked rolled oats   7 Tbsp frozen concentrated
4 c. Grape Nuts cereal (not the flakes   apple juice
   or Nutty Rice)   1/2 tsp coconut extract
1 c. brown rice flour   2 1/2 tsp vanilla extract
6 lg. apples, peeled and grated   1/2 tsp almond extract
     3 tsp cinnamon

Combine all ingredients in a large bowl. Spread mixture on a flat non-stick pan or cookie sheet. Bake at 275 degrees for about 45 minutes (until mixture is dry and rather crumbly).

Microwave: Combine all ingredients in a bowl as above. Place bowl in microwave and cook on high for 10 minutes. Makes 20 servings.

GRANOLA II

3 1/2 c. old fashioned rolled oats
1 c. chopped walnuts
1 c. shredded coconut
1 c. chopped almonds
1/2 c. sesame seeds
1 tsp cinnamon

1/2 tsp ground cloves
1/4 c. honey
2 Tbsp grated orange peel
1/2 c. dried apricots
1/2 c. raisins

Combine all ingredients. Spread mixture in 2 large baking pans. Bake, uncovered, at 200 degrees for 55 minutes. Cool completely, then stir in 1/2 cup raisins and 1/2 cup chopped dried apricots. Cover and store at room temperature. (For Quick Granola try Muesli.) Makes 8 cups.

TROPICAL MUESLI

4 c. rolled oats
1 1/3 c. flaked coconut
4 oz. banana chips

3/4 c. Brazil nut pieces
4 oz. candied pineapple
1 c. bran

Mix all ingredients together making sure they are evenly distributed. Store in a large screw-top jar. Yield: About 6 cups.

BANANA PANCAKES

1 c. whole wheat pastry flour

2 tsp baking powder
1 1/2 c. nut milk, rice milk, or
fruit juice

2 Tbsp unsweetened
applesauce
1 med. banana (firm but
ripe), finely chopped

Mix flour and baking powder together. Mix liquid with applesauce. Add to dry ingredients and stir until just moistened. Fold in banana. Spoon batter onto a non-stick griddle. Turn when bubbles appear.

BANANA BUCKWHEAT PANCAKES

1/2 c. Fearn buckwheat pancake mix
1/2 c. wheat and soya pancake mix
1/2 c. oat bran
1 Tbsp cinnamon

1 egg white
1 1/4 to 1 1/2 c. water
1 banana, mashed
1/4 c. raisins

Mix dry ingredients together. Add egg white and mix. Add water, a little at a time, until there is a thick creamy texture. Stir in banana and add raisins. Cook on non-stick pan. Flip pancakes when bubbles begin to pop. Makes about 9 medium sized pancakes.

BUCKWHEAT PANCAKES

1 c. Aunt Jemima buckwheat
pancake mix
4 egg whites

1 c. rice milk or
soy milk

Spray a non-stick skillet with non-stick coating. Place on a medium heat to warm pan. Mix all ingredients. Pour batter onto hot pan. Turn when tops are covered with bubbles. Turn only once. Serve with fresh fruit spreads, apple butter, or fresh fruit slices.

OATMEAL PANCAKES

2 c. old fashioned rolled oats
2 c. water
1/2 c. whole wheat pastry flour

2 stiffly beaten egg whites
1 tsp vanilla
8 Tbsp apple juice concentrate

Chop rolled oats coarsely, using low speed on blender. A food processor is even better if you have one. Mix rolled oats and water; let stand for 5 minutes. Stir in flour; add remaining ingredients. Fold in stiffly beaten egg whites. Bake on a non-stick skillet, using high heat at first and turning down heat as bubbles appear. Makes 15 (4 inch) pancakes.

WHOLE WHEAT PANCAKES

3/4 c. whole wheat flour
1 tsp baking powder
1/3 c. ground toasted almonds
2 Tbsp coarsely chopped toasted
almonds
2 Tbsp Butter Buds

2 Tbsp honey
2 egg. whites
Pinch of cream of tartar
1/2 c. rice milk, soy milk,
or nut milk

Sift flour and baking powder into medium bowl. Add ground and chopped almonds. Lightly whisk rice milk, Butter Buds, and honey in another bowl. Add to dry ingredients and mix just until moistened. Beat whites with cream of tartar in large bowl until stiff but not dry. Gently fold whites into batter. Let stand 10 minutes. Heat non-stick griddle or skillet over medium heat. Ladle batter onto griddle. Cook until bubbles begin to appear. Turn and cook other side. 12 pancakes.

ZUCCHINI PANCAKES

3 c. shredded zucchini
1/3 c. minced onion
6 egg whites
3/4 c. whole wheat flour
3/4 tsp baking powder

1/4 tsp pepper
1/2 tsp oregano leaves
Grated Parmesan cheese
  (optional)

Blend all ingredients, except Parmesan cheese. In a non-stick skillet, spoon about 3 tablespoons of the zucchini mixture for each pancake Cook 4 pancakes at a time, turning once, until golden brown on each side Sprinkle the Parmesan cheese. 4 servings.

HERB PANCAKES

3/4 c. whole wheat flour
1 4 tsp baking powder
1/2 c. water
3 Tbsp Butter Buds
2 egg whites

1 Tbsp minced fresh basil
1 1/2 tsp minced fresh thyme
1 1/2 tsp minced fresh
  rosemary
1 1/2 tsp minced fresh sage

Mix all ingredients together. Heat non-stick griddle or skillet. Ladle batter onto griddle. Cook until bottom side is brown, about 2 minutes. Flip over. Makes 1 dozen pancakes.

WAFFLES

3 c. water
2 c. rolled oats
1 c. barley flour

1/2 c. whole wheat pastry
  flour
1 Tbsp unsulphured molasses
  or malt syrup

Combine all ingredients in blender and blend until smooth. Let batter "rest" for 15 minutes. Ladle onto preheated waffle iron. Use about 1 cup of batter for a 4 section waffle. Lightly spray with a non-stick spray to prevent sticking. Makes about 4 large waffles.

APPLESAUCE

1 c. water	1 Delicious apple
1 lemon, juiced	1/2 tsp cinnamon
2 Pippin apples	2 tsp cornstarch

Put 3/4 cup water into a heavy saucepan. Add lemon juice. Heat water to gently simmer. Wash and slice applies. Place in hot water. Add cinnamon. Cook for 8 to 10 minutes until apples are barely soft. Turn off heat. Mix cornstarch with 1/4 cup water. Add to apple mixture, stirring constantly. Remove from heat when apple mixture thickens. May be used to spoon over pancakes.

EASY BLUEBERRY SAUCE

2 c. apple or mixed berry juice	Pinch cinnamon or nutmeg
1 (10 oz.) jar blueberry preserves	1 tsp vanilla
2 to 3 tsp kudzu or arrowroot	1 pt. blueberries (fresh or
1/2 c. cold water	frozen)
Pinch of sea salt	1 to 2 tsp lemon juice (optional)

This sauce is a perfect replacement for the butter and maple syrup that usually top pancakes. It is also delicious on cake (instead of fat dense frosting) or with muffins or cornbread.

Pour juice into a saucepan and slowly bring to a boil. Add blueberry preserves and continue to simmer. Dissolve kudzu or arrowroot in cold water and add to simmering sauce. Stir until the sauce thickens and becomes clear and shiny . Stir in salt, cinnamon or nutmeg and vanilla. Add blueberries and lemon juice, if desired. Stir. Lower flame and keep warm until ready to serve. Serves 8. Helpful Hint: Extra sauce can be stored in the refrigerator for several days. Per serving: 57 calories, 0.3 g protein, 0.3 g fat, 14 g carbohydrates, 9 mg cholesterol, 0 mg sodium.

FRUIT SYRUPS

2 pkgs. frozen fruit	1 c. apple juice
1/2 c. apple juice concentrate	2 Tbsp cornstarch

Mix frozen fruit with unsweetened apple juice and apple juice concentrate. Add cornstarch; mix until blended and heat to thicken. Especially delicious with strawberries or blueberries. Other variations include peaches apples, cherries, apricots, strawberry-banana, grape, and pineapple. Delicious over pancakes or as a spread on toast.

ORANGE APPLE MARMALADE

2 c. very thinly sliced oranges
  w/peelings
3 c. dried Golden Delicious apples
  ground

2 1/2 c. apple juice
  concentrate
3 c. water
1 c. orange juice concentrate

Put all ingredients in large pot. Cook slowly about 1 hour or until oranges are tender. Vary orange and apple juice to taste.

BLUEBERRY JAM

2 c. blueberries

24 pitted dates (1/3 lb.)

Blend blueberries. Add dates, a few at a time. Blend until smooth. Put in jars. May be kept up to 3 days if refrigerated. Other jams can be made, substituting other fruit for the blueberries: Strawberries, peaches, apples, etc. Makes 1 pound or 1 1/2 cups.

PEACH JAM

2 Tbsp frozen orange juice
  concentrate

2 1/2 c. mashed sweet peaches
3 tsp pectin

Mix juice concentrate with peaches; stir in pectin and let stand 30 minutes. Stir 3 times vigorously. Serve fresh or may be frozen to retain fresh taste.

PEACH OR APRICOT JAM

3 c. diced fresh peaches or apricots
1 1/2 tsp fresh lemon juice

1 1/2 tsp unflavored gelatin
2 Tbsp apple juice
  concentrate

Place peaches or apricots in saucepan. Cover and cook over very low heat without water for about 10 minutes. Remove lid and bring the juice to the boiling point. Boil for 1 minute and remove from heat. Soften gelatin in lemon juice for 5 minutes. Pour some of the hot juice from the fruit into the gelatin mixture and stir until the gelatin is completely dissolved. Stir the dissolved gelatin into the fruit. Add 2 tablespoons apple juice concentrate. Allow to cool to room temperature and store in the refrigerator. 35 calories in 1 level tablespoon.

APRICOT BREAKFAST BARS

1/2 c. apple juice
1 banana
1 egg white
1/2 tsp lemon extract
1/2 tsp cinnamon

1/2 c. oat bran
1/2 c pitted dates
4 fresh apricots, pitted
1 tsp vanilla extract

Combine first 6 ingredients in blender. Pour into a non-stick 10 x 1 1/2 inch baking dish (use non-stick spray). Bake at 350 degrees for 30 minutes. While mixture is baking, blend dates, apricots, and vanilla in blender. You may have to stop blender and press mix away from blades as mixture is sticky. Top bars with this apricot mixture after 30 minutes and bake 10 minutes more at 400 degrees. Serves 4.

BARLEY BREAKFAST PUDDING

1 c. cooked barley
1/4 c. unfiltered apple juice
1/2 c. diced apples
1/8 tsp nutmeg

1/4 tsp cinnamon
1/2 tsp vanilla
3 Tbsp raisins
1 Tbsp chopped walnuts

Mix all ingredients together and bake in a non-stick pan (use Pam) for 30 minutes at 350 degrees. Serves 2.

BREAKFAST CHERRY COBBLER

3 c. frozen cherries (unsweetened)
3/4 c. Old Fashioned oats
1/2 c. Grape Nuts, Nutty Rice, or
  Nuggets

1/2 c. chopped walnuts or, pecans
6 oz. cherry cider or apple cider
1/2 tsp pure vanilla extract
1/2 tsp cinnamon

In an 8 x 10 inch glass baking dish, sprayed with non-stick spray, spread cherries on bottom (evenly). Sprinkle each dry ingredient evenly over cherries to form a topping. Combine cherry cider and vanilla together and pour evenly over top. Bake at 350 degrees for 20 to 30 minutes. Delicious.

CINNAMON PRUNE STICKS

1 box Sunsweet pitted prunes
1 c. spicy apple cider

2 cinnamon sticks

In a medium saucepan, empty the box of prunes, add cider and cinnamon sticks. Simmer on low for 30 minutes. Enjoy these spiced prunes hot or cold; 3 or 4 daily is recommended. Makes 8 to 10 servings.

How to Look Great & Feel Sexy

Breads, Muffins & Desserts

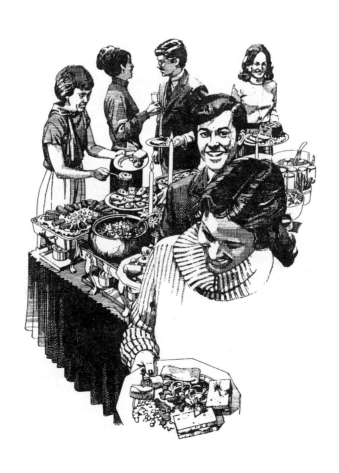

How to Look Great & Feel Sexy

BANANA BREAD I

1 1/2 c. whole wheat flour
1/4 c. wheat germ or oat bran
1 tsp cinnamon
2 tsp baking powder
1/2 tsp baking soda
1/2 c. chopped nuts

1/4 c. Butter Buds
1/2 c. honey
3/4 tsp vanilla
1 c. mashed banana
2 egg whites

Preheat oven to 350 degrees. Combine dry ingredients, including nuts. Combine wet ingredients and stir into dry mixture until thoroughly blended. This will make a thick batter. Spread in a floured 8 1/2 x 4 inch loaf pan. Bake for 45 to 50 minutes or until a toothpick inserted comes out clean. After cooling for 10 minutes in the pan, transfer to a cooling rack. Allow banana bread to cool completely before cutting. Note 1: To save time, obtain a bread maker by Dax or Panasonic or similar unit that mixes dough and cooks bread to completion. Note 2: For any bread recipe that calls for oil, just replace oil with the equivalent volume of applesauce, water, or rice milk (amazake).

BANANA BREAD II

1 pkg. Fearn banana cake mix
   (available in health food stores)
1 Pkg. Butter Buds
1/2 c. honey

2 mashed bananas
2 egg whites
1/3 c. rice milk
1 c. walnuts, chopped

Preheat oven to 350 degrees. Mix Butter Buds and honey. Add bananas and egg whites; mix again. Add contents of cake mix and rice milk alternately, ending with mix. Add nuts and stir until uniform. Turn into a 1 pound loaf pan. Bake for 60 minutes. (After 30 minutes, loosely place a sheet of foil over top of bread to prevent crust from browning excessively.)

CARROT BREAD

1 c. whole wheat pastry flour
1 c. oat bran
1 tsp baking soda
2 tsp baking powder
1 tsp Cinnamon
1/4 tsp nutmeg
4 egg whites

2 c. grated carrots
1 pkg. Butter Buds, made
   into liquid
1/3 to 1/2 c. pineapple
   concentrate
1/2 to 1 c. raisins

Combine all ingredients and mix well. Bake in non-stick loaf pan at 325 degrees for 45 minutes.

GARLIC BREAD

Whole wheat bread without
sugar or milk

Fresh or powdered garlic
Butter Buds

Mix 1 packet of Butter Buds in 1/2 cup hot cup of water sit in refrigerator for 5 to 10 minutes. Brush on bread and sprinkle with garlic. Broil in oven.

PUMPKIN BREAD

1/3 c. prepared Butter Buds
1/2 c. orange juice concentrate
4 egg whites
1 c. mashed pumpkin (canned)
1 tsp baking soda

1 tsp cinnamon
1/2 tsp nutmeg
1/8 tsp ginger
1 3/4 c. whole wheat flour

In a blender, process Butter Buds, juice concentrate, and egg whites. While blending, add pumpkin, soda, cinnamon, nutmeg, and ginger. Gradually add flour until you get a doughy consistency. Bake in a non-stick loaf pan (use non-stick spray) in a preheated 350 degree oven for 45 to 60 minutes. Toothpick should come out clean when done. Makes 1 loaf.

SOUR DOUGH BREAD

STEP A:
1 c. Sour Dough Starter
1 c. warm water

1 1/2 c. whole wheat flour, spooned
into cup and mixed with 3 tsp
. baking powder

STEP B:
1 c. whole wheat flour

In a large bowl, mix ingredients for Step A.

Blend 1/2 minute on low speed, then 3 minutes at medium speed, scraping the bowl all the time. Gradually stir in ingredients for Step B. Dough should remain soft and slightly sticky. Turn dough onto well floured board and sprinkle with flour so it doesn't stick to hands. Knead about 250 turns, adding flour as required. Shape for placing in loaf pan. Place in 9 x 5 x 3 inch loaf pan that has had cornmeal sprinkled on the bottom. Let rise in a warm place until doubled in size, about 1 hour. Gently slash top of dough with razor blade or sharp knife.

Bake in preheated oven on lowest rack position. See instructions below for oven temperature and baking time. Cool about 5 minutes on cake rack until bread shrinks from sides of pan. Remove from pan and cool on rack. Bake at 400 decrees for approximately 35 minutes.

Extra Quick Version: After placing dough in baking pan, bake immediately at 400 degrees approximately 45 minutes.

SPROUTED WHEAT BREAD

2 c. wheat or rye berries   1 1/2 c. water

Soak the berries in the water for 12 hours in a 2 quart jar. Pour off the excess water after soaking. Drink the water or feed it to your plants. This sprouting wheat does not need to be rinsed in the winter, but rinse it once or twice a day in the summer to keep it moist. However, do not rinse it on the day of use. This will prevent the wheat from becoming too moist.

After wheat has sprouted to the length of the wheat berry itself (about 2 days) grind in meat grinder*. Form into a 2 1/2 inch high by 8 inch long loaf by patting with Pam sprayed hands in a 9 inch Pam sprayed pie pan. Bake at 250 degrees for 2 hours.

*If dough seems too moist, add freshly ground whole wheat flour to desired texture. For a fruit bread, stir in the following after the wheat sprouts are ground: 1/2 cup chopped almonds, dates, raisins, currants, dried apricots, figs, prunes, etc.

DELICIOUS CORNBREAD

1 1/2 c. whole grain cornmeal   1 egg white
1/2 c. Millet   1/2 c. unsweetened
1 tsp baking soda   applesauce or creamed corn
1 c. "lite" soy milk or rice milk   3 Tbsp honey or apple juice

In a large bowl, combine all ingredients and mix well. Pour into muffin tins sprayed with non-stick spray. Bake at 425 degrees for 15-20 minutes. Very good and healthy.

SWEET CORNBREAD

1 1/2 c. yellow whole grain cornmeal   3/4 c. unsweetened applesauce
1 tsp baking soda   3 Tbsp unfiltered apple juice
1 egg white   1 c. rice milk
1/2 c. millet (optional)

In a large bowl, combine all ingredients and mix well. Pour into glass baking dish sprayed with non-stick spray. Bake at 400 degrees for 20 to 25 minutes. Serves 6.

TEXAS CORNBREAD

1 pkg. Old Mill cornbread mix	1 tsp cumin
(or other whole grain mix)	1 tsp chili powder
1/4 c. diced green chilies	1/4 c. corn kernels

Follow directions for cornbread, omitting egg yolk (add 2 tablespoons water if dry). Mix in remaining ingredients. Bake in non-stick, sprayed bakeware. Serves 6.

SWEET POTATO BREAD

1 c. mashed sweet potato or	1/4 tsp Nutmeg
yam, cooled	1 env. active dry yeast,
3/4 c. water	dissolved in 1/2 c.
1/2 c. frozen apple juice concentrate	lukewarm water
1 tsp soy sauce	4 c. whole wheat pastry flour
1 Tbsp cinnamon	1 Tbsp rice milk

Here's another use for leftover baked or boiled sweet potatoes or yams, when you get tired of putting them in your lunch.

Blend potato, rice milk, apple juice, soy sauce, and spices in food processor or blender. Transfer the mixture to a large bowl and stir in dissolved yeast. Slowly add 3 1/4 cups of flour, stirring to combine well. Knead for 3 to 5 minutes, gradually adding rest of the flour. Shape into a non-stick loaf pan (dough will be sticky) and set the pan in a warm oven. (Preheat the oven to 150 degrees, then turn off heat just before setting pan in it.) Let dough rise for 1 hour. Bake at 425 degrees for 10 minutes, then prick the surface with a fork in several places and brush with the tablespoon of rice milk. Lower heat to 375 degrees and continue baking for 35 to 40 minutes. Cool before slicing. Cover with foil or plastic wrap to keep moist. Makes 1 loaf, about 16 slices.

ZUCCHINI BREAD

3 c. whole wheat flour	2 tsp cinnamon
3 c. grated zucchini	1 c. chopped nuts
1 1/4 c. oat bran	4 egg whites
4 1/2 tsp baking powder	1 3/4 c. applesauce
1 tsp nutmeg	2 tsp vanilla extract

Preheat oven to 350 degrees. Mix together the flour, oat bran, baking powder, nutmeg, cinnamon, and nuts. In another bowl, mix the egg whites, applesauce, and vanilla extract. Stir in the grated zucchini. Add the flour mixture to the zucchini mixture; gradually stirring until blended. Turn the batter into 2 (8 1/2 x 4 1/2 inch) loaf pans and bake.

BISCUITS

1 c. whole wheat pastry flour   1/2 c. water
1 pkg. Butter Buds

Mix thoroughly. With wet hands, form into small biscuits. Bake on non-stick cookie sheet at 400 degrees for 6 minutes.

BURGER BUNS

1/4 c. warm water   1 tsp barley malt syrup or
1 Tbsp yeast   honey

In a large bowl, combine the above list of ingredients and let foam. Stir in, using your hands as dough gets stiff:

3 to 3 1/2 c. whole wheat flour   2 to 2 1/2 Tbsp toasted
1 c. water   sesame seeds
                                       1/2 tsp sea salt

Knead for about 10 minutes on lightly floured surface. Spray a clean bowl with Pam; turn dough around to coat. Cover bowl with a warm, damp towel and let rise until double in a warm draft-free place. Toast in a 350 degree oven in a flat pan for 10 minutes:

2 Tbsp toasted sesame seeds

Press dough down; divide into 8 balls. Flatten into 1/2 inch thick rounds, pressing top of dough into the seeds. Place, seed side up on a lightly oiled sheet. Lay a piece of waxed paper loosely over the top of the rolls; let them rise double. Heat oven to 376 degrees and bake buns 16 to 18 minutes. Remove to rack to cool. Per bun: Calories 175, protein 6 gm, carbohydrates 33 gm, fat 3 gm.

APPLE CORN MUFFINS

3/4 c. whole grain flour   2 stiffly beaten egg whites
2/3 c. whole grain cornmeal   1/2 c. unfiltered apple juice
1 tsp Rumford baking powder   1/4 c. pureed dates or date
1 apple, finely grated   powder

Blend all ingredients together; mix well. Pour into non-stick muffin pan 2/3 full and bake in preheated oven for 15 to 20 minutes or until done. Makes 8 muffins.

BRAN MUFFINS

2 egg whites, beaten
1 c. apple juice concentrate
1/2 c. unbleached flour
1/2 c. whole wheat flour
1 c. oat bran
3 tsp cinnamon
1 1/2 tsp baking powder

1 tsp ground cloves
Grated orange rind
1/2 c. unsweetened pineapple
1/4 c. chopped pecans or
   walnuts
1/4 c. raisins

Mix all dry ingredients. Add raisins, nuts, and spices; mix well. Add orange rind, apple juice, and egg whites. Bake at 400 degrees for about 25 minutes. Makes 12 muffins.

FRUIT AND NUT BRAN MUFFINS

2 Tbsp Butter Buds
3 Tbsp apple juice concentrate
2 egg whites
3/4 c. rice milk
1 c. bran

1 c. whole wheat flour
2 tsp baking powder
1 c. chopped cashews
3/4 c. raisins

Preheat oven to 425 degrees. In a large bowl, mix Butter Buds, apple juice concentrate, and egg whites. Add rice milk and bran. Stir. Add flour and baking powder; stir. Quickly fold in nuts and raisins. Fill muffin pans sprayed with Pam 2/3 full. Bake 20 minutes. 12 muffins.

OAT BRAN MUFFINS

2 egg whites
1 c. apple juice concentrate
1 c. whole grain pancake mix
1 c. Mother's Oat Bran by Quaker

2 tsp cinnamon
1/2 c. unsweetened crushed
   pineapple
1/4 c. chopped pecans or
   almonds

Beat the egg whites in a bowl with a mixer. Mix in the apple juice concentrate. In a separate bowl, mix the pancake mix, oat bran, and cinnamon. Mix dry and liquid ingredients together until well blended. Do not beat. Add the crushed pineapple and pecans. Divide into 12 equal sized muffins. Bake in a non-stick muffin pan at 400 degrees for 15 minutes. Note: Paper muffin cups do not work well with this recipe. Teflon muffin tins improve the texture greatly.

OAT BRAN PINEAPPLE MUFFINS

2 1/2 c. oat bran
2 to 3 Tbsp honey
1 Tbsp baking powder
1/2 c. rice milk

2 egg whites, beaten
1 lg. can crushed pineapple
  (with juice)
1/4 c. raisins (optional)

Mix dry ingredients. Add liquid and mix well. Bake at 425 degrees for 17 to 20 minutes. Makes 16 muffins.

PRUNE MUFFINS

1 c. concentrated apple juice
1 egg white
1 tsp cinnamon
1 c. pitted prunes

1 c. grated zucchini
1 c. oatmeal
3/4 c. oat bran
1/4 c. whole wheat flour

In blender, combine first 4 ingredients. In a bowl, combine rest of ingredients with blender mixture. Pour into non-stick muffin pans (use non-stick spray) and bake at 350 degrees for 30 minutes. Makes 12 muffins.

WHOLE WHEAT PUMPKIN MUFFINS (Microwave or Oven Method)

3/4 c. canned pumpkin
4 egg whites
1/2 c. honey
1/2 c. apple juice concentrate
1 1/2 c. whole wheat flour

1 tsp pumpkin pie spice
3/4 tsp baking powder
1/2 tsp baking soda
1/2 c. walnuts, chopped
1/2 c. raisins

Combine pumpkin, egg whites, honey, and apple juice concentrate. Add to combined dry ingredients in large mixing bowl. Mix until just blended. Stir in nuts and raisins. Spoon 2 tablespoons of batter into plastic muffin tray lined with paper liners. Bake on full power for 1 minute.

Oven Method: In a large bowl, combine all ingredients and mix well. Pour into muffin tins sprayed with non-stick cooking spray. Bake at 425 degrees for 15 to 20 minutes. Very good.

APPLESAUCE OATMEAL COOKIES

1/2 c. unsweetened applesauce
1 c. unfiltered apple juice
1 egg white
1 tsp vanilla extract
3 c. old fashioned oats

1/2 c. whole wheat flour
1/2 c. oat bran
1/2 tsp baking soda
1/3 c. chopped nuts and/or
  raisins

Combine all ingredients in a mixing bowl and blend well. Drop by rounded teaspoons onto cookie sheets sprayed with non-stick cooking spray. Bake at 350 degrees for 12 to 15 minutes. Serves 24.

APPLE SPICE COOKIES

3 egg whites
2 c. unsweetened applesauce
1 c. frozen apple juice concentrate
1 c. frozen orange juice concentrate
4 c. whole wheat flour

1 tsp nutmeg
1 1/2 tsp cinnamon
1/2 c. Grape Nuts cereal
1 c. raisins

Beat egg whites until foamy. Add applesauce and juices to egg whites. Combine dry ingredients. Drop onto non-stick baking sheet by teaspoon. Bake at 400 degrees for 8 to 10 minutes. Makes 4 to 5 dozen.

BANANA COOKIES

1 c. banana puree (2 med. bananas)
1/2 c. date pieces
1/4 c. chopped almonds

1 tsp vanilla
1 1/2c. uncooked oatmeal

Pour banana puree into a bowl and add remaining ingredients. Mix well; drop by tablespoons onto a non-stick cookie sheet (use non-stick spray). Bake at 375 degrees for 20 minutes. Makes 2 dozen.

BANANA RAISIN COOKIES

1 1/4 c. rolled oats
1 c. whole wheat flour
1 tsp cinnamon
l/2 c. apple juice

2 ripe bananas, mashed
3/4 c. raisins
1 tsp vanilla

Preheat oven to 350 degrees. Combine all dry ingredients in a large bowl. Add remaining ingredients; mix well. Batter should be a little stiff. Drop by teaspoon onto non-stick cookie sheet and flatten slightly. Bake for 15 minutes. Makes 15 to 18 cookies.

SOFT PUMPKIN COOKIES

1 3/4 c. whole wheat flour
1/4 c. oat bran
1 Tbsp non-aluminum baking powder
1 tsp cinnamon
1/2 tsp nutmeg
2/3 c. chopped nuts (optional)
2/3 c. sunflower seeds (raw) (optional)

1/2 c. raisins
1/2 c. unfiltered apple juice
1/2 c. unsweetened
   applesauce
1 1/2 c. mashed pumpkin

Preheat oven to 350 degrees. Combine ingredients in order given, mixing wet ingredients well. Stir batter until well blended. Drop by tablespoon onto non-stick cookie sheets sprayed with Pam. Bake 10 to 12 minutes until firm and lightly browned. Makes 2 dozen.

HARVEST APPLE COOKIES

1 1/4 c. whole wheat flour
1/ tsp non-aluminum baking powder
1/2 tsp cinnamon
1/2 c. prepared Butter Buds
1/4 c. unsweetened applesauce
1/2 c. unfiltered apple juice

1/2 c. chopped dates or date
   nuggets
1 c. apple, chopped and
   peeled
1/2 c. old fashioned rolled oats
1/4 c. oat bran

Preheat oven to 350 degrees. Combine dry ingredients; mix wet ingredients into dry. Mix batter until smooth. Drop by teaspoons onto non-stick cookie sheet sprayed with Pam. Bake 15 to 20 minutes until lightly browned. Makes 24.

OATMEAL COOKIES

1 env. (1/2 c.) prepared Butter Buds
1 c. unfiltered apple juice
1 egg white
1 tsp pure vanilla extract
1/2 tsp soda

3 c. old fashion oats
1 c. whole grain flour (whole
   wheat or any whole grain)
1/3 c. chopped nuts and/or
   raisins (optional)

Combine all ingredients in a mixing bowl and mix well. Drop rounded teaspoons onto sprayed (non-stick spray) cookie sheets. Bake at 350 degrees for 12 to 15 minutes. Voila, a natural delicious cookie with no cholesterol and no sugar.

WHOLE WHEAT COOKIES

1 1/2 c. whole wheat flour
1/2 c. apple juice concentrate
1 pkg. Butter Buds
2 Tbsp orange juice
1/2 tsp vanilla extract

1/2 tsp baking soda
1/2 tsp cinnamon
2 egg whites, lightly beaten
1 c. walnut pieces
1 c. golden raisins

Preheat oven to 375 degrees. Mix Butter Buds and apple juice concentrate until smooth. Beat in orange juice and vanilla. Combine flour, baking soda, and cinnamon; add to the creamed mixture alternately with the beaten egg whites. Stir in nuts and raisins. Drop by rounded teaspoonfuls onto an ungreased baking sheet. Bake for 10 to 12 minutes until golden. Transfer to a rack and cool. Makes 2 dozen 2 inch cookies.

CAROB BROWNIES

2 egg whites
1 Tbsp honey
1 1/2 tsp vanilla extract
1 c. grated zucchini

3 Tbsp carob powder
1/2 c. oat bran
1/2 c. apple juice
1/2 c. chopped dates

Beat egg whites, honey, and vanilla for 1 minute. Slowly while beating, add remaining ingredients. Bake in a non-stick 9 inch square pan (use non-stick spray) for 30 minutes at 350 degrees. Serves 8 to 10.

RAISIN CHEWS

3 egg whites, beaten slightly
12 oz. frozen apple juice concentrate
1/4 tsp cloves
3 tsp ground coriander
1 c. Nutty Rice cereal or equivalent
2 c. raisins

1 tsp allspice
3 tsp anise
1/2 tsp vanilla
2 c. whole wheat flour
1/2 c. oat bran

Preheat oven to 350 degrees. Combine the above list of ingredients in a mixing bowl:

If mixture is too wet to form, drop cookies. Add 1 to 2 cups oatmeal as needed. Drop by spoonfuls onto ungreased cookie sheet. Bake at 350 degrees for 5 to 10 minutes or until cookies start to spring back when you touch them. Makes about 50 cookies, 61 calories each.

APPLE SPICE CAKE

4 c. finely diced apples (5 to 6 apples)	2 1/2 tsp cinnamon
1/2 c. frozen apple juice concentrate	1/4 tsp nutmeg
1/2 c. water	1/4 tsp allspice
1/2 c. raisins	4 egg whites
1 1/4 c. rice flour	1 tsp vanilla extract
1 1/4 c. whole wheat pastry flour	2 tsp baking powder
1 c. Grape Nuts cereal	2 tsp baking soda

Combine the diced apples, apple juice, water, and raisins in a bowl. Cover with plastic wrap and store in refrigerator for 4 to 6 hours. Sift both flours, baking powder, baking soda, cinnamon, nutmeg, and allspice into a large bowl. Beat the egg whites until soft peaks form and then fold into the flour mixture. Add the apple raisin mixture (including the juice). Add vanilla extract and the Grape Nuts; stir well. Pour into a non-stick bundt pan. Bake at 325 degrees for 1 1/2 hours. Turn the cake out of the pan onto a large sheet of aluminum foil. Wrap the cake completely in foil and let sit for several hours. Makes 12 servings.

BLUEBERRY CAKE

6 c. apple juice	2 c. couscous (precooked
1 tsp lemon rind	semolina wheat product)
1 tsp vanilla	1 pt. blueberries

Bring first 3 ingredients to a boil in a medium pan. Add couscous; reduce heat and stir until almost thick, about 5 minutes. Add the blueberries to the hot mixture (berries will burst, leaving streaks and cake will be very colorful). Remove from heat.

Rinse a 9 x 9 inch square glass baking dish with cold water. Pour mixture into pan and chill in refrigerator until set, about 45 to 60 minutes. Remove from refrigerator; place a serving platter over baking dish and turn upside down. Cut into squares. Can be garnished with chopped nuts or Whipped Tofu Cream. Serves 10 to 15.

CRUNCHY CARROT CAKE

3 egg whites, whipped
1 c. grated carrots
1 (20 oz.) can crushed pineapple, in
   its own juice
1 tsp baking soda
1 tsp cinnamon

1 c. unfiltered apple juice
1 c. oat bran
1 c. whole grain pastry flour
1/2 c. raisins
1/2 c. chopped walnuts

Combine dry ingredients together. Combine liquid ingredients together. Blend together; mix well. Pour into non-stick baking dish. Bake at 350 degrees for 45 minutes. Serves 15.

CARROT CAKE

2 c. shredded raw carrots
1 c. raisins
1 1/2 c. apple juice concentrate
1/3 c. Butter Buds
2 c. whole wheat flour
1 1/2 tsp baking soda

1/2 tsp ground cloves
1/2 tsp ground allspice
1 tsp nutmeg
1 tsp cinnamon
1 c. chopped walnuts

Place carrots, raisins, apple juice concentrate, and Butter Buds in a 3 quart pan and bring to a simmer over medium heat. Simmer 5 minutes; remove from heat and let cool.

In a bowl, sift together flour, baking soda, cloves, allspice, nutmeg, and cinnamon. Stir into carrot mixture until flour is moist. Add vanilla and walnuts. Spoon into a 9 inch square baking pan, sprayed with Pam. Bake in a 350 degree oven for 35 minutes. 12 servings. **Carrot Cake Frosting:** In a saucepan, cook and stir 1 cup apple juice with 3 tablespoons tapioca until thickened. When cooked, add 1 teaspoon vanilla. Spread frosting on cake and serve.

COFFEE CAKE

1 c. raisins
4 1/2 c. whole wheat pastry flour
2 Tbsp baking powder
1 1/2 Tbsp carob powder
2 tsp cinnamon
1/2 tsp cardamom
1/2 tsp nutmeg
4 egg whites

2 lg. bananas, mashed
10 oz. frozen apple juice
  concentrate
1 Tbsp vanilla
3 Tbsp mineral water
3/4 c. water
3 Tbsp dry sherry (optional)

Cover raisins with hot water to soak. In a large bowl, sift together the flour, baking powder, carob powder, and spices. Mix together the remaining ingredients, except the egg whites. Stir this mixture into the dry ingredients. Beat the egg whites until stiff peaks form and fold them into the batter. Add the drained raisins and stir well. Pour the batter into a large non-stick baking pan. Sprinkle streusel topping evenly over the cake. Bake in a preheated 350 degree oven for 50 to 60 minutes. Cool cake completely. Store covered.

COFFEE CAKE TOPPING:

1 c. Grape Nuts cereal
2 Tbsp frozen apple juice concentrate
1 tsp vanilla extract

1/2 tsp cinnamon
1/4 tsp nutmeg
1/2 tsp cardamom

Process Grape Nuts in the blender just long enough to reduce the coarseness of the cereal. Add the other topping ingredients and sprinkle on the cake.

LEMON APPLESAUCE CAKE

1 c. Stone Buhr 7 Grain cereal,
  uncooked
1 c. unsweetened applesauce
1 c. whole wheat flour
1/2 c. oat bran
1 Tbsp baking powder
1 tsp cinnamon

1 tsp lemon rind, grated
1/2 c. unfiltered apple juice
1 env. prepared Butter Buds
2 egg whites
1/2 c. raisins
1/2 c. chopped nuts

One hour before starting, combine cereal and applesauce. Mix, cover, and set aside at least 1 hour or overnight. Preheat oven to 350 degrees.

In medium bowl, combine apple juice, Butter Buds, egg whites, raisins, and nuts; mix well. Add in dry ingredients and applesauce mixture, mixing well. Pour into 8 or 9 inch cake pan sprayed with non-stick cooking spray. Bake at 350 degrees for 30 minutes. Cool before slicing. Serves 14.

PINEAPPLE UPSIDE - DOWN CAKE

TOPPING:

6 slices canned unsweetened
pineapple rings
Pecan or walnut halves

2 Tbsp Butter Buds
1/4 c. honey

CAKE:

4 egg whites

2 Tbsp pineapple juice

1/2 c. whole wheat flour

1/2 tsp baking powder

1/2 c. honey

Preheat oven to 350 degrees. Line a 9 inch layer cake or square pan with wax paper.

For Topping: Melt Butter Buds, combine with honey, and spread over the paper. Arrange pieces of pineapple artistically in the pan. Place nuts in the open spaces.

To make the Cake: Mix honey and juice. Sift flour and baking powder over the juice mixture and fold to completely blend. Beat egg whites stiff and fold into flour batter. Spread batter over pineapple in baking pan. Bake for 30 minutes until golden. Cool for 10 to 15 minutes in the pan; invert and peel off paper. Cool completely. Don't worry if the cake sinks a little.

PUMPKIN SPICE CAKE

3 c. pumpkin
1 c. unfiltered apple juice
1/2 c. raisins
2 c. whole grain pastry flour
1 tsp baking soda
1 tsp baking powder
2 tsp cinnamon

1/4 tsp nutmeg
1/4 tsp allspice
4 egg whites, whipped
1 tsp pure vanilla extract
1 c. Grape Nuts
1/4 c. honey or applesauce

Combine dry ingredients together. Combine wet ingredients together, then blend both (mixing well). Pour into non-stick baking dish. Bake at 350 degrees for about 45 minutes. Serves 15.

WHOLE WHEAT FRUITCAKE

2 c. coarsely chopped dried figs

2 c. chopped dried apricots

1/2 c. chopped candied lemon peel

1 1/2 c. golden raisins

1 1/2 c. chopped dates

2 c. chopped pecans

2/3 c. green candied cherries, halved

2/3 c. red candied cherries, halved

1/2 tsp baking soda

1 1/2 c. whole wheat flour

1 1/2 c. brown rice flour

3/4 tsp nutmeg

1/2 tsp cinnamon

1/2 tsp ground cloves

1/2 tsp ground cardamom

2 pkgs. Butter Buds

12 egg whites

1 1/2 c. apple juice
concentrate

2 Tbsp water

1 tsp baking powder

1 c. red wine

Brandy

In a large bowl, combine the figs, apricots, lemon peel, raisins, dates, pecans, and cherries. In another bowl, sift together the flours, baking powder, spices, and Butter Buds. Add the flour mixture to the fruit and toss them together until all the bits of fruit are separated and coated. Beat the egg whites with the apple juice concentrate. Stir in the wine. Dissolve the baking soda in the water and stir it in too. Combine the egg mixture with the flour and fruit mixture and thoroughly stir them together.

Pour into 6 medium-small (7 1/2 x 3 1/2 inch) loaf pans. Bake the cakes in a preheated oven at 275 degrees for 2 hours. Allow the cakes to cool and remove them from the pans. Wrap each cake in several layers of cheesecloth and soak the cloth with as much brandy as it will absorb. Wrap the cake again, in foil or plastic wrap, to retain the moisture. To allow the fruit cakes to develop their full flavor, store them in a cool place for 4 weeks. Makes 6 medium sized fruitcakes.

DATE CAKE

3 egg whites

1/3 c. honey or apple juice

1 tsp baking soda

1/2 c. grated carrots (2 sm. carrots)

1 c. grated zucchini (1 sm.)

1 tsp cinnamon

1 c. water

1 c. oat bran

1 c. whole grain pastry flour

1 c. date pieces

Combine together in order given; blend with hand mixer. Pour into cake pan sprayed with non-stick cooking spray. Bake in preheated 350 degree oven for 30 minutes. When the cake reaches warm or room temperature, frost with "Date Frosting". *Please see next recipe.* This outstandingly delicious cake can be served at warm or at room temperature. Serves 15.

DATE FROSTING

1 c. apple juice
1/2 c. date pieces

1 tsp vanilla
3 Tbsp tapioca granules

Place all ingredients in blender and process for 2 minutes. Cook in saucepan 5 minutes over low heat, stirring constantly. Cool down to a warm temperature and frost cake. This delicious frosting can be served at room temperature not only on the date cake but also on the cake of your choice.

CHOCOLATE BANANA BROWNIES

No stick cooking spray
4 Tbsp cocoa powder
3/4 c. water
1 very ripe banana
1 c. white sugar or pitted dates or
   apple juice concentrate
2 lg. egg whites
1 tsp vanilla extract

1 tsp baking powder
1/4 tsp salt
1 c. all-purpose flour or
   whole wheat flour
1/2 c. oat bran (for best
   results, use an oat bran
   that is coarsely milled)

Preheat the oven to 350 degrees. Spray an 8 inch round or square cake pan with no stick cooking spray.

Place the cocoa, 1/4 cup water, and the banana, into a large blender cup or into the bowl of a food processor that has been fitted with a steel blade. Blend until it is smooth. Add sugar, egg whites, vanilla extract, baking powder, and salt; blend until the mixture is smooth. Add the flour, oat bran, and 1/2 cup water (a little at a time) and blend again until smooth.

Pour the chocolate mixture into the prepared pan. Bake at 350 degrees for 20 to 25 minutes. Wait until the brownies have cooled to cut into servings. Store brownies in the refrigerator. Each brownie: 0 mg cholesterol, 123 calories.

APRICOT PIE

For oat nut crust, whiz in blender until a coarse meal:
1 1/2 c. rolled oats

Mix in a bowl with:
1/2 c. walnuts: chopped fine   **1/4 c. water**
1/4 c. apple juice

Let stand 30 minutes. Oil a 9 inch pie pan and press mixture firmly into bottom and sides, using the back of a large spoon. Bake at 350 degrees for 30 minutes until edges begin to brown.

For filling, snip into small pieces with scissors dipped in cold water:
1 c. dried apricots

Place apricots in saucepan; add:
1 1/2 c. apple juice

Bring to a boil, reduce heat, and simmer 15 minutes until fruit is soft. Sprinkle on top to dissolve.
2 Tbsp kanten flakes

Stir in and cook over medium heat, stirring 3 minutes. Set off heat to cool. When it begins to set, pour into baked pie shell. Chill. This dessert can be made the day before. Yield: 8 servings. Per serving: 227 calories, 6 gm protein, 38 gm carbohydrates, 6 gm fat.

BANANA PECAN PIE

CRUST:
1 1/2 c. Grape Nuts   **1 tsp cinnamon**
1 1/3 c. apple juice concentrate

Mix above ingredients into 9 inch pie pan. Press to form shell. Bake at 350 degrees for 10 minutes.

FILLING:
1 pkg. Hain Natural banana pudding   **2 ripe bananas, sliced**
mix or banana tapioca mix   **1/2 c. apple juice concentrate**
Pecans   **1/2 c. water**

Empty contents of package into 1 quart saucepan and add liquids. Slowly bring to boil, stirring frequently. (Filling will not thicken until cooled.) Add bananas. Pour into pie shell. Top with a few pecans and chill.

BANANA CREAM PIE

In blender, add:

1/2 c. tightly packed cooked
brown rice

1/3 c. apple juice concentrate

Blend until thick and smooth. Add:

2 1/4 c. water
1 tsp Butter Buds
1 Tbsp cornstarch

4 Tbsp flour
1/4 c. sugar or honey
(occasional use)

Continue to blend until thoroughly mixed. Pour contents of blender into saucepan. Bring to a boil, stirring constantly. Remove from heat and allow to cool 15 minutes. Slice 2 large ripe bananas and stir into mixture. Pour into a prebaked crust. (Use one of our crust recipes.) Refrigerate for at least 2 hours. When ready to serve, top with a few banana slices and pecan halves. Makes 1 large 11 inch pie.

CRUMB TOPPED FRUIT PIE

CRUST:

1 1/3 c. fine whole wheat bread
crumbs, mixed with 1/3 c. bran
1 Tbsp each pectin and arrowroot

1 tsp coriander
1/2 tsp lemon extract
1 Tbsp vanilla extract

FILLING:

3 c. sliced fruit or berries of choice

1/3 c. frozen apple juice
concentrate

TOPPING:

1 c. fine whole wheat bread crumbs
1 Tbsp cinnamon

1 tsp vanilla extract

To Make Crust: Place ingredients in a bowl, mixing well. Using a rubber spatula, press the mixture into the non-stick pie pan firmly (bottom and sides) to form an even crust. Bake the crust at 350 degrees for 15 minutes until lightly browned. Remove from oven and allow to cool.

To make Filling: Place filling ingredients in a saucepan. Bring to a boil, then lower the heat and simmer for a few minutes, stirring frequently until the mixture is thickened. Pour the fruit filling into the prepared crust. Combine the topping ingredients, mixing well. Sprinkle the topping over the filling, lightly pressing it in the fruit with a spatula. Bake at 375 degrees for 15 minutes. Let pie cool, then slice to serve. Serves 6 to 8.

FRUIT PIE

1 1/2 c. Grape Nuts or Nuggets	1 env. unflavored gelatin
1/3 c. apple juice concentrate	2 sm. bananas
1 tsp cinnamon	2 c. strawberries, sliced
1 (8 oz.) can pineapple chunks	2 kiwi fruit, peeled and sliced
(juice pack)	1 3/4 c. unsweetened
	pineapple juice

Mix Grape Nuts, apple juice concentrate, and cinnamon together. Press into 9 inch pie pan. Bake at 350 degrees for 10 minutes.

In a small saucepan, stir together pineapple liquid and gelatin. Let stand 5 minutes. Cook and stir over low heat until gelatin dissolves. Cover and chill to the consistency of unbeaten egg whites.

Slice bananas. Arrange over cooled crust, then top with 2/3 cup of glaze. Arrange strawberry slices over glaze. Stir together pineapple pieces and remaining glaze, then spoon over strawberries. Chill for 2 to 4 hours. Just before serving, then spoon over strawberries.

The kiwi fruit contains enzymes that breaks down the gelatin, so be sure to put it on at the last minute.

FRENCH APPLE PIE

CRUST:

2 c. Grape Nuts or Nutty Rice	1/3 c. apple juice concentrate
Cinnamon	Additional water

Mix ingredients into a large pie pan and press to form shell. Sprinkle with cinnamon.

FILLING:

4 med. Granny Smith apples	2 tsp lemon juice
Cinnamon	

Arrange sliced apples in shell. Sprinkle with lemon juice and cinnamon. Cover with foil and bake for 45 minutes at 350 degrees.

GLAZE:

1/2 c. apple juice concentrate	1/2 c. water
1 Tbsp cornstarch	

Combine cornstarch and liquids in saucepan. Cook and stir until mixture thickens and becomes clear. Pour or spoon over pie. Chill.

MOCK CHOCOLATE PUDDING PIE

14 Medjool dates, remove pits
1 very ripe sm. banana
3/4 c. apple juice concentrate
3 c. water
4 Tbsp carob powder
1 tsp Postum
1 tsp cinnamon

1 tsp vanilla extract
1/2 tsp almond extract
  (optional)
1 1/2 tsp arrowroot or
  cornstarch
1 1/2 env. unflavored gelatin
1 c. water

In blender and in stages for easier liquefying, add dates, banana, apple juice, and water; blend well. Add the next 6 ingredients and continue to blend thoroughly.

In large saucepan, dissolve gelatin in water following directions. Add contents of blender to pan and cook 15 minutes, mixing periodically . Let cool 15 minutes. Pour over baked crust. Refrigerate until firm, approximately 8 hours. Top with sliced bananas and chopped walnuts, if desired. Makes 1 large pie and 1 small pie.

Pour into a glass a small amount of mixture from blender, tastes like a malt!

PEARADISE PIE

3 1/2 c. flaked whole grain cereal
1/4 c. toasted wheat bran
1/4 c. Butter Buds
1 (12 oz.) can pear nectar
1 Tbsp cornstarch
1 tsp vanilla
Whole strawberries (optional)

2 Tbsp lemon juice
1 Tbsp water
2 sm. bananas
2 c. fresh strawberries, sliced
1/2 of a sm. cantaloupe,
  seeded, sliced, and peeled

For Crust: Crush cereal into fine crumbs. Measure 1 1/4 cups crumbs; combine with wheat bran and Butter Buds. Press onto bottom and up sides of a 9 inch Pie plate to form a firm, even crust. Bake in a 375 degree oven for 4 to 6 minutes. Cool on a wire rack.

Meanwhile, for Glaze: Combine nectar and cornstarch. Cook and stir over medium heat until thickened and bubbly. Cook and stir 2 minutes longer . Stir in vanilla; set aside.

To assemble pie: In small bowl, combine lemon juice and water. Dip in banana and pear slices, being careful not to mash the bananas. In crust, layer 1/4 cup of the glaze, the banana slices, another 1/4 cup of the glaze, the sliced strawberries, and another 1/4 cup of the glaze. Arrange pear and cantaloupe slices atop. Top with remaining glaze. Chill 2 to 4 hours. Makes 8 servings.

How to Look Great & Feel Sexy

PINEAPPLE - LEMON MERINGUE PIE

CRUST:

1 1/4 c. whole wheat bread crumbs	1 tsp vanilla extract
3 Tbsp frozen apple juice concentrate	1/8 tsp lemon extract

Place ingredients in a bowl, mixing well. Using a rubber spatula, press the mixture firmly into the non-stick pie pan (bottom and sides) to form an even crust. Bake the crust in a 350 degree oven for 15 minutes until lightly browned. Remove from oven and allow to cool. Fill as directed below.

FILLING:

1 (20 oz.) can unsweetened (juice packed)	1 env. plus 2 tsp unflavored gelatin
1 1/3 c. rice milk	2 tsp arrow root
1/2 c. frozen apple juice concentrate	Dash of turmeric (for color)
3 Tbsp lemon juice	1 1/2 tsp lemon extract
2 Tbsp frozen orange juice concentrate	1 1/2 tsp vanilla extract
	3 egg whites

Place the filling ingredients, except for the flavor extracts and egg whites, into a blender and blend at high speed for 5 minutes. Set a large strainer over mixing bowl and pour mixture through strainer; discard residue in strainer (this insures a smooth pie filling). Transfer the filling mixture to a double boiler; cook for about 5 minutes, stirring with a wire whisk until mixture is very hot. Stir in lemon, and vanilla extracts. Let filling cool slightly, then pour into prepared crust. Beat egg whites until stiff peaks form. Swirl the beaten egg whites gently over the filling. Place the pie in the oven on a middle rack under a hot broiler. Watch meringue carefully, brown just lightly, then remove from oven. Chill pie for several hours or overnight until firm. Serves 6 to 8.

SWEET POTATO PIE

3 to 4 sweet potatoes, baked
1 (16 oz.) can crushed pineapple in
  own juice
1/4 c. chopped nuts (pecans, walnuts,
  or almonds)

1/3 c. Nutty Rice or Nuggets
  cereal
1 tsp pure vanilla extract
1/2 tsp pumpkin pie spice
1/3 c. unsweetened coconut,
  shredded

Spray a glass pie pan with non-stick spray. Peel sweet potatoes; dice and mash in a large mixing bowl. Add can of pineapple with juice, vanilla extract, and pumpkin pie spice. Beat thoroughly with mixer whipping until smooth. Pour into the pie pan or any glass baking dish and top with coconut, chopped nuts and Nutty Rice cereal. Bake at 350 degrees for 25 minutes.
A natural delicious dessert with fiber and no sugar. Enjoy.

PUMPKIN PIE I

CRUST:

1 1/2 c. Nuggets or Grape Nuts
  cereal
1 tsp cinnamon

1/3 c. apple juice concentrate

Mix above ingredients in a 9 inch pie pan. Press to form shell.

FILLING:

3/4 c. apple juice concentrate
1/4 c. honey
1/2 tsp cinnamon
3/4 tsp ginger
1/4 tsp nutmeg
3 Tbsp sweet dark rum

1/4 tsp ground cloves
2 c. pureed cooked pumpkin
6 egg whites
3 Tbsp crystallized ginger,
  chopped
1 Tbsp molasses

In a bowl, combine the apple juice concentrate, honey, molasses, spices, and pureed pumpkin. In another bowl beat the eggs with the rum. Combine the 2 mixtures and blend thoroughly. Sprinkle the crystallized ginger over the bottom of the pie crust. Carefully ladle the filling over the ginger. Bake the pies in the preheated 400 degree oven for 35 to 40 minutes or until a knife inserted comes out clean.

How to Look Great & Feel Sexy

PUMPKIN PIE II

CRUST:

1 1/2 c. Grape Nuts cereal
1 tsp cinnamon

1/2 c. apple juice concentrate

FILLING:

1 can canned pumpkin
1/2 c. water
1/2 tsp cinnamon
1/4 tsp ginger

2 1/2 tsp vanilla extract
1 env. unflavored gelatin
1/2 c. apple juice concentrate
2 egg whites

Combine crust ingredients and press into standard pie plate. Combine filling ingredients, except for gelatin, apple juice, and egg whites. Sprinkle gelatin over apple juice concentrate and let stand for 2 minutes. Heat gently until dissolved and stir into pumpkin filling mixture. Chill for 30 minutes. Beat egg whites stiffly and fold into pumpkin mixture. Mound into pie pan and chill until firm.

SUMMER FRUIT PIE

CRUST:

1 1/2 c. Grave Nuts cereal or
   Nutty Rice cereal

1/3 c. apple juice
   concentrate
1 tsp cinnamon

Mix above ingredients in a 9 inch pie pan. Press to form shell. Bake in 350 degree oven for 10 minutes.

FILLING:

1 (8 oz.) can pineapple slices
   (juice pack)
1 env. unflavored gelatin
Unsweetened pineapple juice

2 sm. bananas

2 c. sliced strawberries
2 kiwi fruit, peeled and sliced

For Glaze: Drain pineapple slices, reserving juice. Cut pineapple into small pieces and set aside. Add enough unsweetened pineapple juice to the reserved juice to make 1 3/4 cup total liquid.

In a small saucepan, stir together pineapple liquid and gelatin. Let stand 5 minutes. Cook and stir over low heat until gelatin dissolves. Cover and chill to the consistency of unbeaten egg whites (partially set).

Slice bananas. Arrange evenly over cooled crust, then top with 2/3 cup of the glaze. Arrange strawberry slices over glaze. Stir together pineapple pieces and remaining glaze, then spoon over strawberries. Chill for 2 to 4 hours or until set. Just before serving, arrange kiwi fruit on pie. Makes 8 servings.

APRICOT COBBLER

2 3/4 c. mashed fresh apricots, pitted   1/3 c. oatmeal
    but not peeled (20 to 25 sm. apricots)   1/3 c. dates
1 c. apple juice   1/2 tsp cinnamon
1 tsp cinnamon   1 c. pitted dates

Spread apricots evenly in the bottom of a 6 x 10 inch baking dish. Pour apple juice in a blender and add dates. Puree, then add 1 teaspoon cinnamon. Pour over apricots. Make topping by grinding oatmeal, dates, and 1/2 teaspoon cinnamon in blender.

CHERRY COBBLER

CRUST:
1 1/2 c. Grape Nuts   1 tsp cinnamon
1/3 c. apple juice concentrate

Mix above ingredients into 9 inch pie pan. Press to form shell.
FILLING:
3 c. frozen cherries   2 tsp water
3 tsp cornstarch   1 c. walnuts, chopped

Place cherries, water, and cornstarch in a saucepan. Mix well to dilute cornstarch. Bring to a boil, reduce flame to low, and simmer for 3 to 5 minutes. Stir to prevent lumping and sticking. Remove from flame and allow to cool. Add walnuts. Pour over crust in pie pan. Bake at 375 degrees for about 15 minutes. Serves 6.

PEACH COBBLER

1 c. pineapple juice   3 c. mashed fresh peaches
1/2 c. pitted dates   1 Tbsp almonds
1 tsp vanilla   1/2 c. pitted dates
1 tsp cinnamon   1/3 c. oatmeal
1 tsp tapioca

Blend first 5 ingredients. In a non-stick baking dish, layer peaches; pour juice mixture over. Grind remaining ingredients as topping and spoon over top. Bake at 350 degrees for 45 minutes. Serves 6 to 8.

BLUEBERRY - APPLE CRISP

1 c. Grape Nuts or Nuggets	1/4 c. Butter Buds
1 c. toasted oat cereal	1/4 to 1/3 c. apple juice concentrate

FILLING:

3 apples, cored and sliced (or 1 can water packed apples)	1/2 c. apple juice concentrate
	1/4 c. cornstarch
1 c. blueberries	

Combine crust ingredients and set aside. Combine filling ingredients in a bowl. Pour filling ingredients in baking pan; sprinkle with crust ingredients. Bake at 350 degrees for 30 minutes or until bubbly.

APPLE CRISP

5 lg.. Pippin apples	2 Tbsp whole wheat pastry flour
Juice of 1/2 lemon	
1 Tbsp cinnamon	3/4 c. dark raisins

TOPPING:

1 1/2 c. rolled oats or cereal flakes	3/4 c. honey or apple juice concentrate
3/4 c. whole wheat pastry flour	
1 Tbsp cinnamon	

Core and slice apples in thin pieces. Place in a 9 x 13 inch baking dish. Sprinkle with lemon juice, cinnamon and flour. Mix well, making sure the apples are evenly coated. Sprinkle raisins over apples. In a separate bowl, combine oats, 3/4 cup flour, and cinnamon. Mix in honey. Drop topping evenly over the apple mixture. Cover with foil and bake at 350 degrees for 25 minutes. Uncover and bake 15 minutes more or until browned.

In glass baking dish, sprayed with non-stick spray, spread fruit evenly. Then sprinkle and continue layering all ingredients in order. Blend apple juice and vanilla together and pour evenly over all. Bake at 350 degrees for 20 minutes.

PEACH OR PEAR CRISP

1 lg. can peaches or pears, totally
   drained in colander
1/2 c. raisins
1/4 to 1/2 c. chopped walnuts or pecans
1/4 c. unsweetened coconut,
   shredded (optional)

1/2 tsp cinnamon
1/2 c. old fashioned oats
1/2 c. Grape Nuts or Perky's
   Nutty Rice cereal
6 oz. apple juice
1/2 tsp vanilla extract

In glass baking dish, sprayed with non-stick spray, spread fruit evenly, then sprinkle and continue layering all ingredients in order. Blend apple juice and vanilla and pour evenly over all. Bake at 350 degrees for 20 minutes.

TAHINI CUSTARD

3 apples
1/2 c. raisins
2 c. apple juice
2 to 3 Tbsp Erewhon Sesame Tahini

Pinch of Instead of Salt
5 Tbsp Erewhon Agar Flakes
2 c. spring water

Wash, cored, and slice apples. Place in a pot with the liquids, tahini, salt, and agar. Mix well. Bring to a boil reduce heat to low and simmer 2-3 minutes. Chill in a shallow bowl until almost hardened. Place cooled mixture in a blender and blend until smooth and creamy. Place custard back in serving bowl and chill once more before serving.

LEMON CUSTARD

2 c. pear or apple juice
2 c. natural lemonade
2 bars agar-agar (or 3 Tbsp
   agar flakes)
Pinch of sea salt
1 tsp . vanilla

1 c. lemon non-dairy frozen
   dessert
1 pt. berries (raspberries,
   strawberries, or
   blueberries) (optional)

Combine juice and lemonade in a saucepan. Rinse agar bars; tear into 1 inch pieces and add to saucepan (or measure flakes and sprinkle on juice). Stir until agar softens. Bring mixture to a light boil; lower heat and simmer for 10 minutes until agar dissolves. Add salt and vanilla. Add frozen dessert; stir to dissolve and pour into shallow, heat-proof dish. Place dish in refrigerator for 30 minutes until custard is set. Serve as is or with berries. Serves 6.

Variation: For extra creaminess, place chilled custard in a blender and whip for 30 seconds immediately before serving. Per serving: 138 calories, 1 g protein, 2 g fat, 32 g carbohydrates, 0 cholesterol, 9 mg sodium.

BROWN RICE PUDDING

1 c. cooked brown rice
2 egg whites
2 c. rice or nut milk

1/2 tsp vanilla extract
1/2 c. raisins
1/2 tsp cinnamon

In blender, mix milk, vanilla, egg whites, and cinnamon. Spray 8 x 10 inch class baking dish with non-stick spray. In a separate bowl, mix together brown rice, raisins, and the blender mixture. Pour entire recipe into the baking dish; sprinkle with additional cinnamon and bake at 350 degrees for 35 to 40 minutes. Serve warm or cold.

DATE NUT BREAD PUDDING

1 1/3 c. fresh whole grain bread crumbs
1/4 c. wheat germ
1 c. chopped dates

1/4 c. chopped almonds and
    sunflower seeds
2/3 c. orange juice

Combine all dry ingredients. Add juice until mixture is moist but not soggy. Line a 9 inch pie pan with waxed paper and press mixture into pan. Cover loosely with wax paper, foil or plastic wrap, and chill for several hours. To serve lift wax paper with pudding from pan and slice into very thin wedges. This dessert is very rich so serve small portions.

SWEET QUINOA PUDDING

2 c. cooked quinoa*
1 c. apple juice concentrate
1/2 c. raisins
1 c. chopped water chestnuts

1 1/2 tsp vanilla extract
Grated zest of 1 lemon
Pinch of ground cinnamon
1 kiwi fruit for garnish

In a medium saucepan, combine quinoa, apple juice concentrate, raisins, water chestnuts, vanilla, lemon zest, and cinnamon. Cover pan and bring to a boil, then reduce heat and simmer for 15 minutes. Slice kiwi fruit. Divide pudding among 5 dessert dishes and top with kiwi fruit slices. Makes 5 servings. *(Quinoa -pronounced Keen-wa- has the texture of whole cereal grains but, like buckwheat, is actually the fruit of an annual herb. It's available in most large health food stores and in some supermarkets.)

To prepare 2 cups of cooked quinoa: Thoroughly rinse 1/2 cup quinoa and drain. Combine quinoa with 1/2 cup water in a saucepan and bring to a boil. Cover pan, reduce heat to medium-low, and simmer for 10 to 15 minutes or until water is completely absorbed and grain is translucent.

PINEAPPLE BARS

CRUST:

1/2 c. almonds ground fine	1/4 c. water
1/4 c. whole wheat flour	1 c. granola crumbs

Mix together with a fork in bottom of 9 x 13 inch pan. Press against bottom. Bake 5 to 10 minutes at 350 degrees.

FILLING:

1 1/2 c. apple juice	2 Tbsp cornstarch
1 c. dates	1 tsp vanilla
2 1/2 c. crushed pineapple	Coconut for topping

Blend water and dates in blender until smooth. Mix together with other ingredients; pour over crust and sprinkle with coconut, then bake at 350 degrees for 15 minutes or until coconut is light brown. Cool well before cutting into desired squares.

CHAROSES Jewish Passover Ceremonial Food

6 med. apples, chopped very fine	1/2 c. chopped nuts
1/2 c. raisins	1/4 c. sweet wine
1/2 tsp cinnamon	

Make from apples, raisins, and sweet wine to resemble the mortar used in laying the bricks for the pyramids. It also symbolizes the sweetness of freedom. Mix and serve.

ORANGE PILLOWS, TART

5 peeled, baked potatoes (about 2 1/2 c.)	3 bananas
12 oz. frozen orange juice concentrate	1 tsp almond extract

Preheat oven to 375 degrees. Beat the above list of ingredients together until smooth:

Beat 6 egg whites into stiff peaks. Fold into above mixture. Drop by heaping spoonfuls onto ungreased cookie sheet. Bake 15 minutes. Remove from oven and let sit 5 minutes before removing from cookie sheet. Makes 90 pillows, 17 calories each. *To make sweet, replace orange juice " with apple juice " and the almond " with vanilla ".*

SWEET POTATO APPLE CASSEROLE

1 1/4 lbs. sweet potatoes
1 lb. apples
1 c. apple juice

2 Tbsp cornstarch
4 Tbsp water
Cinnamon

Cook (either bake or steam) sweet potatoes until tender. Peel and slice. Layer in a non-stick casserole. Core and slice apples. Lay apple slices on top of sweet potatoes. Heat apple juice to boiling point. Combine cornstarch and water; add to juice, cooking until sauce is clear and thickened. Spoon sauce over apples; sprinkle with cinnamon. Bake at 350 degrees for 30 to 45 minutes. Serves 6.

SWEET POTATOES WITH ORANGE

4 lg. sweet potatoes
1/2 c. orange juice
2 crushed pineapple

Grated zest of 1/2 orange
Pinch of grated nutmeg
Pinch of white pepper

1. Place potatoes in a large pot of water; bring to a boil and cook for 30 to 40 minutes or until tender. Set aside to cool slightly.
2. When potatoes are cool enough to handle, peel them and place in a bowl. Mash with the orange juice, crushed pineapple, orange zest, nutmeg, and pepper.
3. Return mashed potatoes to the pot and reheat over medium heat. If not serving immediately, cover bowl and refrigerate mashed potatoes until 1 hour before serving. Transfer to an oven-proof dish. Cover and reheat in a 350 degree oven for 25 minutes or until hot. Makes 5 servings.

YAM SOUFFLE

2 c. cooked, mashed yams
4 to 5 egg whites

1 Tbsp cinnamon
1 Tbsp grated orange peel

Beat the egg whites to soft peak stage. Fold egg whites, cinnamon and orange peel into the yams. Divide into 4 individual soufflé dishes and bake at 350 degrees for 25 minutes. Serve immediately. Serves 4.

GLAZED YAMS

1 lb. yams   1/4 c. fresh orange juice
1/3 c. unsweetened pineapple   1 tsp cornstarch juice

1. Bring a large saucepan of water to a boil. Add yams and cook for about 15 minutes or until barely tender. Drain and set aside to cool slightly.
2. When yams are cool enough to handle, peel and cut into 3/4 inch slices. Place in a single layer in a baking dish.
3. Preheat oven to 350 degrees. In a small bowl, combine pineapple and orange juices with cornstarch and stir until cornstarch is dissolved. Pour the mixture over yams and bake for 45 minutes. Makes 8 servings.

BANANA - PINEAPPLE ICE CREAM - Fast Weight Loss

4 lg. bananas, cut into chunks   4 oz. crushed pineapple,
1 tsp vanilla   frozen and unsweetened
                                   (or any fruit you desire)

Cut bananas into slices. Lay on cookie sheet and freeze. Pour pineapple into a bowl and freeze. Place the frozen fruit and vanilla in a blender. Blend, stopping the motor to stir frequently until the mixture is smooth. Serve at once. Serves 2.

CHOCOLATE BANANA ICE CREAM

1 c. apple juice concentrate   2 Tbsp tahini
1 c. apple juice   2 Tbsp maple syrup
3 Tbsp brown rice flour   4 ripe bananas
1/2 c. carob powder

Combine juice and concentrate in a saucepan. Blend in rice flour and carob powder. Bring to a boil, stirring constantly. Pour into blender or food processor and blend with remaining ingredients. Chill well and freeze. Remove from freezer and blend in food processor until smooth. Serves 8.

PUMPKIN ICE CREAM

1 pkg. unflavored gelatin	1/2 tsp nutmeg
1/4 c. hot water	1/2 tsp ginger
1 c. frozen orange juice concentrate	1/2 tsp cinnamon
1 lb. can pumpkin	1/2 c. rice, nut, or soy milk

Dissolve gelatin in hot water. Place orange juice, pumpkin, and spices in blender, then add rice milk. Put in shallow freezer trays and freeze. Stir often to break up ice crystals. Serves 4 to 6.

ROCKY BANANA CREAM

10 med. ripe bananas 2 c. chopped, dried apricots

Blend bananas in blender until smooth. Fold in apricots. Turn mixture into a freezer container Stir once when semi frozen, then freeze overnight to harden. Serve with slices of fresh fruit. Fresh strawberries, blueberries, or raspberries can be substituted for apricots. Serves 6.

APRICOT SORBET

1 lb. California fresh apricots	1 c. water
(about 2 1/2 c.), peeled and sliced	1/2 c. apple juice concentrate
2 tsp finely chopped, candied ginger	2 Tbsp fresh lemon juice
(optional)	2 Tbsp rum or orange juice

Plunge whole apricots into a pan of boiling water, about 30 - 60 seconds. Remove to ice water. Peel and puree apricots. Stir in lemon juice. Add rum and ginger, as desired; set aside. Cook water and sugar over low heat, stirring occasionally. When sugar dissolves, bring to full boil over medium high heat; simmer about 5 minutes. Remove syrup from stove; chill. Combine syrup and apricot mixture. Freeze in ice cream maker according to manufacturer's instructions. Best served fresh. Makes 1 quart (8 servings).

STRAWBERRY SORBET

4 c. ripe strawberries, washed and	Juice of 2 oranges
hulled plus 8 whole strawberries	1 Tbsp lemon juice
for garnish	1 c. apple juice concentrate

1. Place 4 cups of strawberries in a food processor or blender and process until pureed.
2. Transfer puree to a large bowl, add apple juice concentrate, orange and lemon juices; mix well.
3. Freeze, let soften in refrigerator and serve.
4. Scoop sorbet into dessert dishes and garnish each serving with a whole strawberry. Makes 8 servings.

WATERMELON SORBET - Fast Weight Loss

1 sm. watermelon   Finely chopped mint
3 egg whites

Scoop out watermelon; puree in blender and pour in ice cream trays and freeze. Remove from freezer and scoop out mixture and fold through egg whites until well combined. Refreeze until ready to serve. Remove from freezer to soften slightly before serving. Garnish with fresh mint. Serves 6.

PINEAPPLE BANANA SHERBET

1/2 c. orange juice   1 Tbsp fresh lime juice
1 lg. ripe banana   2 Tbsp honey
1 lg. ripe pineapple, peeled, cored,   2 Tbsp fresh mint, plus
    and coarsely chopped   additional for garnish

Blend orange juice and mint together in a blender until mint is very finely chopped or liquified. Blend in remaining ingredients, except garnish, and puree until smooth. Pour into ice trays or a baking dish and freeze until just beginning to set. Remove from freezer again and repeat once more when just beginning to set. Pack into a container and freeze. If frozen solid; let soften in refrigerator 1 hour before serving . Serve garnished with fresh mint. Serves 4.

PINEAPPLE SHERBET - Fast Weight Loss

1 pineapple (sweet and ripe)   Fresh mint sprigs
1 pt. fresh strawberries, sliced

Blend pineapple until smooth in blender. Pour into a freezer container and freeze semi-hard. Then stir well and fold in sliced strawberries. Freeze overnight. When serving, garnish with fresh mint. Serves 4.

BLUEBERRY HONEYDEW ICE - Fast Weight Loss

4 c. honeydew melon   2 c. frozen blueberries

Combine the ingredients in blender and puree until smooth. Pour into a bowl or shallow pan. Place in freezer. Stir or beat the mixture every 15 minutes to break up ice crystals. Ready to serve in about 2 hours. Serves 8.

For a variation: Blend 4 cups honeydew melon or cantaloupe with 2 cups orange juice, juice of 1 lemon, 2 cups crushed ice. Garnish with mint leaves.

PEACH FROST

3 c. fresh peaches   3 c. fresh orange juice

Blend peaches, then blend with orange juice. Pour mixture in shallow freezer trays. Freeze until solid. Cut frozen mixture into strips and put through food grinder and blender. Serves 6.

PINEAPPLE - COCONUT TOFU DESSERT

1 c. tofu, whipped in blender   4 Tbsp frozen apple juice
1 c. diced fresh pineapple   concentrate
1 c. grated fresh coconut   1 tsp vanilla

Combine all ingredients. Chill. Spoon into dessert dishes and garnish with kiwi fruit slices and fresh strawberries. Serves 4.

APRICOT MOUSSE

1 1/2 c. dried apricots   1 1/3 c. orange juice
1 1/2 c. agar agar   Generous squeeze lemon juice
2 Tbsp undiluted soy milk or rice milk

Wash the apricots, then cover them with boiling water and leave to soak overnight. Add lemon juice and cook the apricots gently 10 to 20 minutes or until tender. Set aside to cool; drain well, then mash or puree. Put the orange juice in a saucepan and bring gently to a boil. Whisk in the agar and continue heating and whisking a few minutes. Combine the apricot puree with the orange juice, mixing well. Stir in enough soy milk to give the mixture a creamy color. Divide among 4 glasses and leave to coo, then chill well before serving. Top with chopped nuts, if desired. Serves 4.

BANANA MOUSSE

6 very ripe bananas   2 Tbsp carob powder
1 1/2 c. unsweetened applesauce   1/4 tsp vanilla extract

Blend the applesauce and the bananas in a food processor using the steel blade. (Cut the bananas into quarters and add them to the blending applesauce one piece at a time.) Add carob powder and vanilla extract. Continue to blend until the mixture is smooth and all of the bananas have been blended with no chunks remaining. Spoon into individual dessert cups. Refrigerate for 30 minutes before serving. Serves 4.

FROZEN CHERRY MOUSSE

1 container Amazake rice milk   1 Tbsp apple juice concentrate
   (plain or almond)   1 egg white
1/2 c. frozen cherries   1/2 tsp almond extract
1/2 pkg. gelatin, softened in hot water

Pour rice milk in a bowl and place in freezer. In food processor or blender, whip egg white with sweetener. Add frozen rice milk, cherries, gelatin, and almond extract. Whip 1 minute. Transfer to serving dish. Freeze 1 hour before serving.

APPLESAUCE SOUFFLE

1 1/4 c. unsweetened applesauce   2 tsp raisins
1/2 tsp cinnamon   3 egg whites

Preheat oven to 350 degrees. Blend applesauce and cinnamon. Spoon 1 tablespoon of applesauce into bottom of each of 4 (6 ounce) cups. Top with raisins. Beat egg whites until stiff but not dry. Fold half into remaining applesauce and blend well. Fold remaining whites into applesauce very gently. Spoon into cups and sprinkle tops with cinnamon. Bake about 15 to 20 minutes until puffed and brown. Serve immediately. Serves 4.

BAKED APPLE

1/2 c. cranberry juice   1 tsp apple juice concentrate
1 baking apple   Pinch of cinnamon
1/2 c. red wine   1Tbsp raisins

Core apple and stand it bottom down in a baking dish. Sprinkle with sweetener and cinnamon, making sure some gets inside the apple. Stuff raisins into the center of the apple. Pour juice and wine into baking dish around apple. Bake, uncovered, at 350 degrees for 20 to 25 minutes or until skin splits and the apple is tender.

BAKED BANANAS NEW ORLEANS

2 bananas peeled
1/2 tsp nutmeg or mace
1 tsp cinnamon
3 Tbsp Grand Marnier or other
orange liqueur (optional)

1 tsp Butter Buds
3 Tbsp apple juice concentrate
1/2 c. orange juice
3 Tbsp rum (dark preferred)

Place bananas in small baking dish (cut in half, if desired). Dot with Butter Buds and sprinkle with apple juice concentrate, cinnamon and nutmeg or mace. Pour orange juice over all. Bake lightly covered 15 minutes at 375 degrees or microwave approximately 4 minutes.

To serve, place bananas in dessert dishes. In medium ladle or dish pour the liqueur and rum. Heat slowly over flame (while stove burner will do, a candle is more dramatic). Tip ladle slightly into fire or light with a match. Pour flaming liquid over the individual dishes. Serves 2.

BANANA AMBROSIA

1 lg. ripe yellow banana
1/4 c. pineapple or orange juice
1 lg. ripe papaya
1/4 c. vanilla rice dream or
strawberry sorbet

1/2 tsp vanilla extract
1/2 tsp coconut extract
Pinch of powdered ginger
1 Tbsp sesame seeds or
sesame tahini

Peel and mash banana with fork. Place in bowl and add juice. Cut papaya in half; scoop out and discard seeds. Scoop out papaya meat with spoon and add with rice dream or sorbet to bowl. Mix in seasonings. Stir until well mixed.

FLAMING PINEAPPLE - Easy Weight Loss - Microwave

1 pineapple, halved lengthwise
1 c. strawberries, sliced
1 c. melon balls

1/2 c. blueberries
1/4 c. light rum

Remove fruit in chunks from each pineapple half, leaving a 1/2 inch thick shell. Cut pineapple in cubes. In a large bowl, combine pineapple, strawberries, melon balls, and blueberries. Fill pineapple halves with fruit mixture. Cover with wax paper. Microwave on full power for 4 minutes. In a 1 cup glass measure, microwave rum on full power for 25 seconds. Pour over fruit mixture, carefully ignite. Makes 10 servings.

FRUIT AMBROSIA - Fast Weight Loss

2 oranges, sectioned and cut
2 c. fresh pineapple, diced
2 bananas, sliced
2 nectarines, sliced

2 baskets fresh strawberries
1/2 c. shredded coconut
1/4 c. lemon juice

Peel the fruit, cut it up, and toss very lightly in a bowl. Add the coconut and the lemon juice. Cover and chill. 8 servings.

FRUIT KABOBS - Fast Weight Loss

2 Spanish blood oranges, sm.
  navel oranges, or mandarins
12 kumquats or seedless grapes
2 thick slices fresh pineapple
1 lg. ripe kiwi fruit

12 strawberries or pitted
  cherries
Watermelon, honeydew, or,
  cantaloupe cut into 12
  (1 inch) cubes

Cut fruit into bite sized slices, cubes, or wedges. Spear fruit on thin skewers. Stand spears in bowl or bucket of crushed ice or use a hollowed out pineapple or watermelon filled with ice, to support the skewers. 12 servings, 1: skewer each. 40 calories per serving. 2 mg sodium.

FRUIT COMPOTE

2 Tbsp water
1 Tbsp honey
1 1/2 Tbsp lime juice
1 tsp grated lime rind
Fresh mint

1 c. cantaloupe balls
1/2 c. seedless green grapes,
  halved
1 kiwi fruit, peeled and
  coarsely chopped

Combine honey and water in a small non-aluminum saucepan. Simmer over low heat until honey dissolves, stirring occasionally. Remove from heat and let cool. Add lime juice and rind. Combine fruit in a medium bowl; add lime syrup, tossing gently. Cover and chill 2 hours. Garnish with mint. Serves 2.

GLAZED PEARS

4 to 6 ripe pears, cut in half   Pinch of Instead of Salt
1 c. apple juice   1/2 tsp grated fresh ginger
1 Tbsp Erewhon Kuzu

Place pears in a baking dish, facing up. Pour juice over the pears, cover the baking dish, and cook in a 350-400 degree oven until soft. When done, drain the liquid from the pears into a small pot; add the kuzu dissolved in a little cold water and stir thoroughly. After 30 minutes add the salt and ginger to the pot. Stir occasionally and cook until the mixture thickens and becomes transparent, usually only several minutes. Pour topping over the pears and bake for 15 minutes more until glazed. Be careful pears don't burn.

SUMMER FRUIT PARFAITS

1/2 c. sorbet or rice dream   2 c. seedless grapes
2 peaches, sliced   1/2 c. blueberries
1 Tbsp lemon juice

Toss peaches with lemon juice. In 4 wine glasses, layer grapes, peaches, and blueberries. Drizzle with sorbet or frozen rice dream. Serves 4.

MONKEYS IN A BLANKET

1 slice whole grain bread   Cinnamon
1/2 banana   Honey
1/2 Tbsp Butter Buds

Preheat oven to 400 degrees. Roll bread flat with a rolling pin and trim crust. Spread with a thin layer of honey. Place banana on half of bread and wrap jelly roll fashion. Prepare Butter Buds. Allow 1 tablespoon for each whole banana. Roll bread-covered banana in Butter Buds sprinkle with cinnamon and bake for 15 minutes until crust is crisp and banana is hot and creamy.

WHIPPED CREAM SUBSTITUTE

1 c. cashews   1 tsp vanilla
2 c. water   1 Tbsp honey
2 tsp cornstarch   1 tsp apple juice concentrate

Put cashews, water, and cornstarch in a blender. Blend about 1 minute until smooth. Place in saucepan; add the rest of the ingredients. Cook over medium heat until thickened, stirring constantly. Use as a topping on desserts.

WHIPPED TOFU CREAM

1 (8 oz.) container soft tofu, drained   1 tsp lemon rind
1/4 c. maple syrup   1 tsp lemon juice
2 tsp vanilla extract

Place all ingredients in blender and whip for 5 minutes. Stir 4 or 5 times, then whip again for 5 minutes until creamy. Serves 4 to 6.

VANILLA FRUIT CREAM

1 c. millet   2 c. water

Bring water to a boil; add millet and cook for 30 to 40 minutes.
1 c. raw cashew pieces, washed   1/4 c. honey
1 c. water   4 Tbsp vanilla
1 tsp salt

Blend cashews in water until smooth. Blend in other ingredients and add millet until smooth. Refrigerate unused portions. Goes great on fruit or bread. *Recipe by Country Life Restaurant.*

CHERRY SOUP

2 pkgs. frozen and pitted sweet   8 Tbsp apple juice concentrate
    dark cherries   5 c. water
1/4 c. white wine

Place the cherries in a large pot along with the apple juice concentrate and water. Bring to a boil and simmer for about 15 to 20 minutes. Remove cherry (save the water) and puree them. Return pureed cherries to water and add the white wine. Serves 6.

Main Dishes: Italian

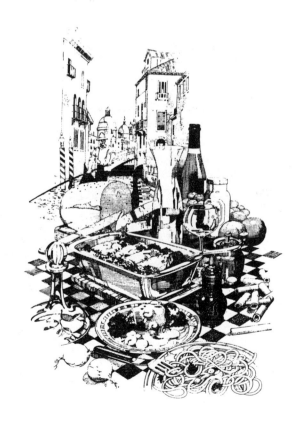

How to Look Great & Feel Sexy

EGGPLANT ITALIAN

1 eggplant sliced 1/2 - 1 in. thick
(do not peel)
1 jar Johnson's spaghetti sauce (no oil)

1 tsp garlic powder
Italian bread crumbs
Mushrooms

Place some of the eggplant in the bottom of baking dish. Cover with some of the spaghetti sauce and sprinkle some of the garlic powder and mushrooms over sauce. Continue this layering process until pan is full. Sprinkle a coating of Italian bread crumbs on top. Bake in oven at 350 degrees for about 1 hour or until eggplant is tender.

FETTUCINE WITH TOMATOES & WILD MUSHROOMS

1/2 c. Butter Buds
1/4 c. minced shallots
6 oz. fresh mushrooms, chopped
6 tomatoes, sliced

White pepper to taste
1 lb. whole wheat fettuccine
2-3 green onions, sliced

Place Butter Buds in skillet; add shallots and stir 1 minute over medium heat. Add mushrooms and tomatoes and stir 3 minutes. Season with pepper.
Cook fettuccine in a large pot of boiling water until just tender. Drain well. Transfer to a large bowl. Add mushrooms and tomatoes. Garnish with green onion and serve.

HOMEMADE MARINARA SAUCE - Fast Weight Loss

5 tomatoes, chopped
2 (15 oz.) cans tomato sauce
1 can tomato paste
1 onion, chopped
3 cloves garlic, minced
1 sm. bell pepper, diced
12 mushrooms, sliced
2 carrots, sliced

2 sm. zucchini, sliced
2 bay leaves
1 tsp black pepper
1/2 Tbsp basil
1/2 Tbsp oregano
1/4 tsp sage
1 Tbsp soy sauce
1/4 c. red cooking wine

Add all the ingredients together (except for the dry herbs) into a large pot on the stove. Simmer for about 2 hours. Add the dry herbs and simmer for another 1 to 2 hours. Use sauce on spaghetti, in lasagna, or with any other Italian dishes.

BAKED VEGETABLE ITALIANO - Fast Weight Loss

1 lg. eggplant, peeled and diced
1 (9 oz.) pkg. French cut green beans
1 (16 oz.) can tomatoes, mashed

1 zucchini, sliced into rounds
1 clove garlic, minced
2 tsp oregano

Combine vegetables in casserole dish. Stir in seasonings. Bake at 375 degrees for 30 to 40 minutes. Serves 6.

ITALIAN EGGPLANT CASSEROLE

4 oz. whole wheat spaghetti,
  broken into 2 in. pieces
1 lg. eggplant, peeled and cut
  into 1/2 in. cubes (6 c.)
1 med. onion, chopped
1 med. carrot, chopped
1 (4 1/2 oz.) can sodium reduced
  tomatoes

1 (6 oz.) can sodium reduced
  tomato paste
2 cloves garlic, minced
1 1/2 tsp dried oregano,
  crushed
1 tsp dried basil, crushed
1/2 tsp pepper
1 sm. zucchini, chopped

Cook spaghetti according to directions; drain. Meanwhile in a steamer basket, place eggplant, onion, carrot, and zucchini. In a Dutch oven, place filled basket over, but not touching, boiling water. Cover and reduce heat. Steam for 5 to 7 minutes or until vegetables are crisp tender; remove from Dutch oven.

In a large mixing bowl, stir together steamed vegetables, undrained tomatoes, paste, garlic, basil, oregano, and pepper. Spread 2 cups tomato mixture on the bottom of a 12 x 7 1/2 x 2 inch baking dish. Top with cooked spaghetti; sprinkle with Parmesan cheese if desired. Spoon remaining tomato mixture over top; sprinkle with a dash more Parmesan. Bake, uncovered, in a 350 degree oven for 30 to 35 minutes or until bubbly. Serves 6.

ITALIANO ZUCCHINI - Fast Weight Loss

1/2 c. onions, chopped
1/2 c. green bell peppers, chopped
3 celery stalks, chopped
1 clove garlic, minced
5 tomatoes, chopped

1 lg. zucchini, sliced into
  spears
1 tsp Italian seasoning
Parsley sprigs
Non-stick spray for sautéing

Place onions, pepper, and celery in a pan (spray with non-stick spray) with garlic and sauté. Add remaining ingredients and cook, covered until zucchini is done. Remove cover and evaporate tomato water. Serve with sprigs of parsley. Serves 4.

ITALIAN POTATO CASSEROLE - FAST WEIGHT LOSS

5 lg. potatoes
1 lg. onion, sliced
4 c. fresh green beans
1 (28 oz.) can pureed tomatoes

2 cloves garlic, pressed
2 tsp Italian seasoning
Freshly ground pepper

Chop potatoes into large chunks and place in large casserole dish with onion and green beans. Mix pureed tomatoes with garlic and seasoning; pour over vegetables. Add ground pepper if desired. Bake at 350 degrees for approximately 1 1/2 hours. Check potatoes with a fork for softness. Makes 4 to 6 servings.

LASAGNA

SAUCE:

1/2 med. onion, chopped
1 stalk celery, chopped
1 carrot, grated
1/2 green pepper, chopped
1/2 c. fresh mushrooms, chopped
1 (28 oz.) can crushed tomatoes with
    added puree (Progresso)

1/2 tsp basil
1 tsp oregano
1/2 tsp thyme
1/2 tsp marjoram
1/2 tsp onion powder
2 Tbsp fresh parsley

Sauté onion in 1/2 cup water. Add celery, carrots, green peppers, and mushrooms and cook 5 minutes. Add herbs and onion powder. Then add the tomatoes. Simmer 10 to 15 minutes.

LASAGNA:

Whole wheat or whole grain lasagna
    noodles ((9-10, 12 in.) strips), cooked
1 med. zucchini, sliced thin
1/2 - 3/4 c. frozen green peas

1/2 sm. eggplant, peeled and
cut in half or quarters,
sliced thin

Spread a little sauce on the bottom of a shallow rectangular baking dish, 8 x 11 1/2 inches. Cover with a third of the noodles. Spread one half of the zucchini, eggplant, and peas over the noodles. Then spread with some (1/3) sauce. Repeat these layers. Cover with remaining noodles and sauce. Cover and bake for 45 minutes at 350 degrees. Remove the cover and bake for 10 to 15 minutes.

LENTIL SPROUT LASAGNA

1 (8 oz.) pkg. whole wheat lasagna
noodles
1 lg. eggplant, peeled and sliced thin

1 recipe lentil sprout filling
1(32 oz.) jar spaghetti sauce
(meatless and sugarless)

Place sliced eggplant under broiler a few minutes, turning once. In baking dish, alternate layers, beginning with whole wheat lasagna noodles, then eggplant, lentil sprout filling, and spaghetti sauce. Repeat once more. Heat in low heat oven (250 to 300 degrees) for 30 to 35 minutes or until warm. Makes large 9 x 13 inch casserole.

LENTIL SPROUT FILLING:

3 c. lentil sprouts (1/2 c. dry lentils,
sprouted for 3 days)

1 c. spaghetti sauce (meatless
and sugarless such as
Ragu Natural or other
brands found in health
food stores)

Place lentil sprouts and spaghetti sauce in food processor with grinding blades. Mix lightly to resemble a meat filling.

SPINACH LASAGNA

8 oz. uncooked lasagna noodles
1 eggplant, thinly sliced into rounds
1 lg. bunch fresh spinach, stems
removed
1 tsp oregano

1 1/2 c. fresh mushrooms,
sliced
1 onion, chopped
1 c. spaghetti sauce (no oil)

Cook noodles, remove from water immediately, and separate. Spray 9 x 14 inch baking dish with non-stick cooking spray. Layer first with noodles, then with eggplant. Spread 4 tablespoons of sauce over this. Layer again with noodles and top with remaining sauce, mushrooms, and onion. Sprinkle with Parmesan, if desired. Cover with foil and bake at 350 degrees for 45 minutes. Cut into squares after allowing to cool. To serve, layer 2 squares together for thickness. Serves 4.

PASTA

4 oz. Vegeroni
2 c. broccoli flowerettes
1/2 c. spaghetti sauce (no oil)

1 tsp sesame seed
1/8 tsp garlic powder
1/8 tsp pepper

In a large saucepan, cook broccoli and pasta in boiling water for 6 minutes or until tender; drain. Add the rest of the ingredients and serve. 4 servings

PASTA WITH SAUCE

4 med. size zucchini
1/3 c. low-sodium chicken stock, defatted
1 Tbsp low-sodium soy sauce
1 lg. red bell pepper, seeded and thinly sliced
2 Tbsp balsamic vinegar or mild red wine vinegar
8 oz. whole wheat pasta such as fusilli or rotelle

1 (28 oz.) can unsalted peeled plum tomatoes, drained, seeded and coarsely chopped
1 Tbsp chopped fresh rosemary or 1 1/2 tsp dried rosemary
1/2 med. size onion, thinly sliced

Cut each zucchini crosswise into 4 equal pieces. Then cut each piece lengthwise into 6 to 8 wedges; set aside. Bring a large pot of water to a boil.

For the sauce, heat 3 tablespoons stock and the soy sauce in a large non-stick skillet over medium heat. Add onion. Reduce heat to medium low, cover pan, and cook for 3 minutes or more until onion is limp and slightly caramelized. Add bell pepper and cook, covered, for 2 minutes. Add zucchini and remaining stock and cook, covered, for 5 to 6 minutes more.

In a large pot bring 2 cups water to a boil and add pasta. Bring back to a boil, turn heat off, cover pot with a lid, and let sit for 20 minutes until al dente. While pasta is cooking, add tomatoes and rosemary to sauce and cook, uncovered, over low heat for 2 minutes. Stir in vinegar and cook for 2 minutes more. Drain pasta and transfer to a large serving dish. Pour sauce over pasta and serve immediately. Makes 8 servings.

PASTA LA MER

2 c. cooked whole wheat or vegetable shell macaroni
1 c. cooked wheat meat*
1/4 c. chopped celery
1/4 c. frozen green peas (or fresh)
1/4 c. diced green bell or red bell pepper

1 Tbsp vinegar
1 tsp low sodium Dijon mustard
Juice from 1 lemon
1 c. bean sprouts
1/4 c. chopped green onions

*Seitan wheat meat is available ready made at certain health food stores. Toss all ingredients together in bowl. Chill before serving. Serves 4.

PASTA PRIMAVERA

1/2 c. peas
1/2 c diced carrots
1/2 c. diced zucchini
1 c. broccoli flowerettes, broken in
   sm. pieces
1 lg. onion diced (1 c.)

1/4 lb. spinach pasta shells
   (2c.), cooked
6 c. water (to boil pasta)
2 tsp cornstarch
1 c. chicken stock

Steam the vegetables until crisp-tender and set aside. Bring the water to a boil. Add the pasta, return to a boil and cook 8 to 10 minutes or until it has a slight resiliency (al dente). While the pasta is cooking, combine the chicken stock and cornstarch and stir until the cornstarch is completely dissolved. Bring to a boil. Reduce the heat and simmer stirring constantly, until thickened; set aside. Drain the pasta thoroughly and put it in a large bowl. Pour the thickened chicken stock over the pasta and toss thoroughly. Add the steamed vegetables and again toss thoroughly. Divide into 4 servings (1 3/4 cups each).

SPAGHETTI

6 oz. dry whole wheat spaghetti

SAUCE:

4 oz. tofu or Seitan's wheat meat
2 c. tomato sauce
1/2 lb. mushrooms, thinly sliced
1/2 c. celery, thinly sliced

1 clove garlic, pressed
1/2 tsp basil
2 Tbsp chopped parsley
1 Tbsp chopped chives

Place tofu or wheat meat in a medium size saucepan. Using a fork, mash tofu into small chunks resembling cottage cheese. Add tomato sauce, mushrooms, celery, garlic, and basil. Heat and stir until sauce is hot and mushrooms are cooked, about 5 to 10 minutes. Remove from heat and stir in parsley and chives. Keep warm.

To cook spaghetti, boil water, add spaghetti, bring back to a boil, turn off heat, cover pan with lid, and let sit for 20 minutes. Drain thoroughly and return to saucepan. Pour tomato sauce over and mix gently to coat spaghetti Garnish with parsley sprigs.

SPAGHETTI SQUASH - Fast Weight Loss

1/2 spaghetti squash	1/4 tsp pepper
1 c. Ragu Garden Style spaghetti	1/8 tsp basil leaves
sauce with extra tomatoes and	1 c. grated zucchini
garlic or spaghetti sauce	Dash of garlic powder
(no oil, no meat)	

Cut squash in half lengthwise and clean out seeds. Place squash, cut side down, in a pot with 2 inches of water. Cover and boil for 20 minutes. If you are using a microwave, place squash, cut side up, in a dish with 1/4 cup water. Cover with a clear wrap and cook 7 to 8 minutes. Run fork over inside of cooked squash to get spaghetti-like strands.

Scoop out spaghetti from 1/2 cooked squash. Add the other ingredients. Mix well and spoon back into empty squash. Sprinkle on 2 tablespoons grated Parmesan cheese and bake at 350 degrees for 20 minutes.

This exciting squash will separate into spaghetti-like lengths and have the texture of firm, cooked spaghetti. It has only 66 calories in an 8 ounce serving.

SPAGHETTI SAUCE, TOMATO - LESS - Fast Weight Loss

1/2 c. beets	1 green pepper, diced
4 stalks celery, sliced	1 c. warm water
4 carrots, sliced	

Dice the beets. Steam the beets, celery, carrots, green pepper, and warm water for 20 minutes or until tender.

Heat a pan and sauté:

3 cloves garlic, minced	1/4 c. water
2 lg. onions, chopped	Pam spray

Add to vegetables and mash or puree in blender. Dissolve:

3 Tbsp dark miso	1/2 c. warm water

Add to vegetables with:

1/2 c. warm water	1 tsp oregano
2 Tbsp tamari	1 tsp basil
2 Tbsp mirin *	Pinch of cayenne

Simmer sauce 5 minutes. Serve over whole wheat spaghetti or buckwheat noodles. Per serving: 130 calories, 4 gm protein, 14 gm carbohydrates, and 2 gm fat.

*Mirin is a sauce found in the macrobiotic section of a health food store.

BROILED RED PEPPER AND EGGPLANT ANTIPASTO

1 round sm. firm purple eggplant or
4 to 5 Japanese eggplants
1/2 tsp granulated garlic

2 Tbsp minced sweet basil
1 lg. red bell pepper (in season
mid-spring to late fall)

With sharp knife, cut eggplant into very thin sheets. Cut into 2 inch strips lengthwise, if using round eggplant. Seed and cut red pepper into quarters. Prepare baking sheet by lightly spraying with Pam (or use nonstick cookware). Place eggplant and peppers close together on baking sheet and sprinkle with spices. Place in broiler fairly close to flame. Broil until browned and tender. Eggplant will become moist as broiled. This also is good cooked on a barbecue grill. Serves 4 to 5 as side dish or appetizer.

WHOLE WHEAT CRUST PIZZA

1 pkg. active dry yeast
1 1/2c. warm water
2 tsp dry basil
2 tsp oregano
1/4 c. oat bran
1 1/2 c. whole wheat flour
1 1/2 c. all-purpose flour
All-purpose flour for kneading
1/2 green or red bell pepper,
    seeded and thinly sliced
1 c. diced Liteline cheese(optional)

1 (15 oz.) can tomato paste
2 zucchini, thinly sliced
1 lg. red onion
4 green onions including
    tops, thinly sliced
1 can sliced ripe olives
1 (14 oz.) can artichoke hearts,
    drained and quartered
4 Tbsp grated Parmesan cheese
1/2 c. red wine

In a large bowl, dissolve yeast in water. Add 1 teaspoon basil, 1 teaspoon oregano, oat bran, and all-purpose flour. Beat until smooth (about 5 minutes) using an electric mixer. Using a wooden spoon, beat in whole wheat flour until dough holds together. Turn onto a lightly floured board and knead until dough is smooth and elastic, about 5 minutes. Turn over in a greased bowl, cover, and let rise in a warm place until dough has doubled in size (about 45 minutes). Meanwhile, prepare tomato sauce

Tomato Sauce: In a frying pan, sauté the onion. Stir in tomato sauce, tomato paste, red wine, 1 teaspoon oregano, and 1 teaspoon basil. Simmer, uncovered, for 10 minutes.

Punch down dough and divide in half. Roll out each half to form a 14 inch circle, then transfer each circle onto a greased 14 inch pizza pan. 1 at a time, bake on next to bottom rack of a 450 degree oven for about 7 minutes or until bottom of crust just starts to brown. During baking, watch carefully and prick any bubbles that form. Remove from oven and set aside.

To assemble pizza, spread tomato sauce over crust. Arrange zucchini, bell pepper, green onions, olives, and artichoke quarters over sauce. Sprinkle Liteline cheese and Parmesan cheese over the top (optional). Bake in a 450 degree oven for 12 to 15 minutes or until cheese melts. Cut hot pizzas in wedges to serve. Makes 2 pizzas, each serves 6.

WHOLE WHEAT VEGETARIAN PIZZA

1 pkg. active dry yeast
1 1/2 c. warm water
2 tsp dry basil
2 tsp oregano
1/4 c. oat bran
1 1/2 c. whole wheat flour
1 1/2 c. all-purpose flour
All-purpose flour for kneading
1 (14 oz.) can artichoke hearts, drained and quartered

1 lg. red onion
1 (15 oz.) can tomato sauce
1 (6 oz.) can tomato paste
2 zucchini, thinly sliced
1/2 green or red bell pepper, seeded and thinly sliced
4 green onions (including tops), thinly sliced
1 can sliced ripe olives
1/2 c. red wine

In a large bowl, dissolve yeast in water. Add 1 teaspoon basil and 1 teaspoon oregano, oat bran and all-purpose flour. Beat until smooth (about 5 minutes, using an electric mixer). Using a wooden spoon, beat in whole wheat flour until dough holds together. Turn out onto a lightly floured board and knead until dough is smooth and elastic, about 5 minutes. Turn over in a greased bowl; cover and let rise in a warm place until dough has doubled in size, about 45 minutes. Meanwhile, prepare tomato sauce.

PITA & VEGETABLE PIZZAS

Vegetable cooking spray (Pam)
1/2 c. chopped onion
1 clove garlic, minced
4 c. seeded and chopped tomatoes (about 3 lbs. whole tomatoes)
1 med. yellow or green bell pepper, finely chopped
3 oz. fresh mushrooms, thinly sliced

1 sm. zucchini, thinly sliced
3 (6 in.) whole wheat pita bread rounds
2 tsp dried whole oregano
1/4 tsp pepper
2 Tbsp minced fresh basil leaves
3 Tbsp red wine vinegar

Coat a large, heavy pan with cooking spray. Sauté onion and garlic until tender. Stir in tomatoes, vinegar, basil, oregano, and pepper. Bring to a boil, reduce heat, and simmer, uncovered, 20 minutes or until sauce is reduced. Set aside. Cut slit around edge of each bread round; carefully split apart. Place split rounds on baking sheet; toast at 450 degrees for 5 minutes or until dry and beginning to brown. Spread 1/4 cup tomato sauce mixture evenly over each toasted rounds. Bake at 450 degrees for about 10 minutes until vegetables are tender. Serves 6.

How to Look Great & Feel Sexy

Main Dishes:
Mexican

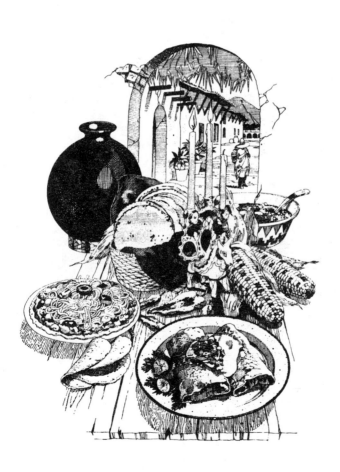

BURRITOS

Whole wheat Chapati
Vegetarian refried beans
Sliced black olives

Chopped tomatoes, carrots,
celery, green onions,
avocado, lettuce,
sprouts, etc.

Heat refried beans in 350 degree oven for 20 minutes. Spread onto chapati and sprinkle in vegetables. Yum. Favorite kids' treat.

BAKED BURRITOS WITH SPICY SAUCE

SAUCE:

1 onion, chopped
2 cloves garlic, pressed
1/2 c. water
1/3 c. chopped canned green chilies
2 Tbsp chili powder
1 tsp cumin

1/2 tsp ground coriander
1/2 tsp cayenne
1 (8) oz. can tomato sauce
1 (6) oz. can tomato paste
3 1/2 c water

FILLING:

1 onion, chopped
1 green pepper, chopped
3/4 lb. mushrooms, chopped
1/2 c. water
1 1/2 c. corn kernels

3 1/2 c. chopped zucchini
2 tsp chili powder
1 tsp ground cumin
12 to 15 whole wheat tortillas

To make Sauce: Sauté onion and garlic in 1/2 cup water for 5 minutes. Add green chilies and spices. Stir and sauté a few more minutes. Add remaining ingredients. Mix well and simmer for 15 minutes; set aside.

To make Filling: Sauté onion, green peppers, and mushrooms in water for 5 minutes. Add corn, zucchini, and spices. Sauté 10 minutes more; set aside.

To assemble Burritos: Spread 1 cup of sauce on bottom of a baking dish. Place 1/3 to 1/2 cup filling down the center of each tortilla. Roll up tortillas and place, seam side down, in baking dish. Pour remaining sauce over burritos. Cover and bake at 350 degrees for 30 minutes. Serves 8 to 10.

GUACAMOLE - Fat Free Ole'

1 can Anderson's Split Pea Soup
1 lg. tomato, chopped
1/4 med. onion, minced
1/4 tsp garlic powder

1 Tbsp salsa
1/2 c. shredded lettuce
1/4 c. shredded cabbage

Blend all ingredients. Excellent on veggie tacos, tostadas, or dip with chips.

BEAN DIP

1 (1 lb.) can kidney beans, well
   drained
1 (4 oz.) can diced green chilies,
   drained
2 to 3 Tbsp lime or lemon juice
1/8 tsp crushed red chili or
   1/2 tsp hot pepper sauce
2 tsp Worcestershire sauce

2 cloves garlic
4 green onion tops, thinly
   sliced
12 corn or whole wheat
   tortillas
1 lg. tomato, coarsely
   chopped

Drain beans thoroughly. Put all ingredients, except green onions, in a blender or food processor. Blend for 1 to 2 minutes until smooth. Turn mixture into serving bowl and sprinkle with green onions. Serve immediately or chill. Makes 1 1/2 cups. 6 servings, 1/4 cup each. 48 calories per serving, 104 mg sodium.

Toasted Tortilla Chips: Use 12 corn tortillas or whole wheat flour tortillas (chapatis).

Preheat oven to 400 degrees. Cut each tortilla into 6 pie shaped wedges. Spread half of the tortilla chips on a baking sheet. Bake in the preheated oven for 10 minutes. Remove from the oven, turn each tortilla chip over and return them to the oven for 3 more minutes. Remove from the baking sheet and let cool. Repeat with remaining tortilla chips.

CORN TORTILLAS

2 c. masa harina
1 1/4 c. warm water

Mix masa flour with enough warm water to make dough hold together well. Using your hands, shape dough into a smooth ball. Divide dough into 12 equal pieces, then roll each into a ball.

Use 2 cloths which have been dipped in water and wrung dry. Flatten a ball of dough slightly and place between the cloths. Roll with rolling pin until cake is about 6 inches in diameter. Carefully pull back cloths, trim tortilla to a round shape, and sandwich it between 2 squares of waxed paper.

Peel off top piece of waxed paper carefully. Turn over tortilla, paper side up, onto a preheated, ungreased medium-hot griddle, or into a heavy frying pan over medium heat. As tortilla becomes warm, you will be able to peel off remaining paper.

Bake for about 1 1/2 to 2 minutes, turning frequently, until tortilla looks dry. Makes 1 dozen.

CHILI BEANS I

1 (14 oz.) can kidney beans
1 c. frozen corn

2 c. salsa, Pace Picante mild
or your favorite

Blend all ingredients in a medium-sized saucepan. Heat to a boil, reduce heat, cover, and cook for 6 to 10 minutes until corn kernels are heated through. Each serving: 0 mg cholesterol and 169 calories. Serves 4. *If you are in a hurry, try this recipe. It is easy, delicious and an excellent source of soluble fiber.*

CHILI BEANS II

1 (29 oz.) can pinto beans
1 (27 oz.) kidney beans
1 (15 oz.) black eyed peas
1 (20 oz.) tomato sauce
3 lg. tomatoes, chopped
1 onion, chopped
3 cloves garlic

1 med. green pepper
1 1/2 Tbsp chili powder
1 1/2 Tbsp cumin
1 1/2 Tbsp oregano
1 1/2 Tbsp paprika
1 Tbsp soy sauce

Add all ingredients together in large pot. Simmer for about 1 hour or until all ingredients are soft.

CHILI RANCH STYLE

8 oz. dry pinto beans
2 cloves garlic, minced
2 onions, chopped
4 oz. can green chilies, drained
and chopped

2 jalapeno peppers, diced
28 oz. can tomatoes with
liquid
1 tsp oregano
Dash of Tabasco

Soak beans overnight. Cook about 1 hour until tender. Cook onions and garlic in small amount of water until tender. Add to beans with remaining ingredients and bring to a boil. Simmer 1 hour or until sauce reduces. Serves 4.

CHILI BEAN STUFFED PEPPERS

4 green bell peppers
2 c. cooked kidney beans
3 c. cooked brown rice
1 c. corn

2 tsp chili powder
2 Tbsp chill salsa
1 c. tomato sauce

Wash peppers and cut off tops. Remove and discard seeds and pulp. Place in pot with cold water to cover, then bring to a boil; reduce heat and simmer or 5 minutes. Drain, then mix together remaining ingredients. Fill peppers with mixture, place into small baking dish and top with a mixture of salsa and tomato sauce. Cover and bake at 350 degrees for 45 minutes. Uncover and bake another 15 minutes more. Serves 4.

CHILI PIE

FILLING:

2 (15 oz.) cans kidney beans, drained
1 onion, chopped fine
1 green bell pepper, chopped fine
6 oz. tomato paste
1/4 c. water

2 tsp chili powder
1 Tbsp low sodium soy sauce
1 c. canned corn, drained
1/2 c. red wine vinegar

Sauté onions and pepper in small amount of water; add remaining ingredients and heat through.

CRUST:

3/4 c. cornmeal
1/4 c. whole wheat flour

1/2 c. water
1 egg white

Let water and egg white sit until they are at room temperature, then mix together. Preheat oven to 375 degrees; combine egg white and water with dry ingredients. Form a ball with dough and place into pie pan sprayed with non-stick spray. Flatten dough with fingers and form into shape of pie crust. Add filling and bake for 35 to 40 minutes or until crust is light brown. Serves 6 to 8.

CHILES RELLENOS

1 (7 oz.) can California green chilies
1 sliced zucchini
1/2 c. whole wheat flour
8 egg whites
Butter Buds
Sliced green onion tops

Drain canned chilies and cut a slit down side of each; gently remove seeds and pith. Stuff each chile with a slice of zucchini, about 1/2 inch wide, 1/2 inch thick, and 1 inch shorter than the chile. Slightly lap cut edges to hold filling inside. Roll each chile in flour to coat all over; gently shake off excess.

Beat egg whites until they form soft peaks. Prepare 1 package Butter Buds and place in frying pan or omelet pan. Over medium heat, take about 1/2 cup of egg whites and place in frying pan. Quickly lay a stuffed chile in center of mound and spoon about 1/3 cup egg whites over top to encase chile. Cook for 2 to 3 minutes; gently turn and cook for 2 to 3 minutes longer. If you like, top with hot salsa and green onion tops. Serve immediately. Makes 3 to 4 servings.

ENCHILADAS

Leftover or available beans,
  vegetables, sprouts, potatoes
6 corn tortillas or desired quantity
Las Palmas green enchilada
  sauce (lg. can) or
  favorite sauce

Wrap corn tortillas in napkin and place in microwave for 2 minutes or until soft.

One by one, fill tortillas with desired filling and form enchilada; place each one in a Pyrex baking dish. (Enchilada can be large or small depending on filling.) Pour desired sauce over enchiladas and return to microwave for heating or heat in oven at 250 degrees for 30 minutes.

ENCHILADA PIE

1 (16 oz.) pkg. dried pinto beans
1 (16 oz.) pkg. dried lentils
2 pkgs. corn tortillas
3 (10 oz.) cans Rosarita enchilada sauce
1 (29 oz.) can tomato sauce
1 (29 oz.) can tomato puree
4 Tbsp onion flakes
1/2 tsp cayenne pepper
1 sm. can Ortega green
  chilies (mild)

Soak pinto beans overnight. Cook several hours until tender. Add lentils the last 3/4 hour of cooking. Layer all ingredients in a large baking pan; start with sauce and end with sauce. Bake at 350 degrees for 1 1/2 hours.

ENCHILADA BEAN CASSEROLE

6 c. enchilada sauce
  (see recipe below), or use
  Rosarita Enchilada Sauce
12 corn tortillas
3 c. brown rice

4 c. cooked and mashed
  pinto beans or Rosarita
  Vegetarian Refried beans
3/4 c. chopped black olives
1 1/2 c. chopped green onions

Spread 2 cups of sauce over the bottom of an oblong baking dish. Set aside. Place 1/2 cup beans and some rice, onions, and olives in the center of each tortilla. Repeat until all ingredients are used. Roll up tortillas and place, seam side down, in baking dish. Pour remaining sauce over the rolled tortillas. Cover and bake at 350 degrees for 30 minutes. Serves 6 to 8.

ENCHILADA SAUCE:

3 c. tomato sauce
3 c. water
1/2 tsp garlic powder

1/2 tsp onion powder
3 Tbsp chili powder
5 Tbsp cornstarch

Combine all ingredients in a saucepan. Cook, stirring constantly, until mixture boils an thickens. Makes 6 cups.

MEXICAN PASTA BAKE

1 med. onion, chopped
1 clove garlic, chopped
1/4 tsp cayenne
1 Tbsp chili powder
1 qt. undrained canned tomatoes
1 tsp oregano
1/2 tsp cumin

1 c. uncooked whole wheat
  elbow macaroni
1 1/2 c. corn kernels
3 c. cooked pinto beans
1/3 c. sliced olives
1 c. (5) broken corn tortillas
1 c. sliced Lifetime cheese

Sauté onion and garlic for 3 minutes to soften. Add cayenne and chili powder and cook briefly. Add tomatoes, oregano, and cumin; bring to a boil. Add pasta and corn and simmer, uncovered for 15 minutes until pasta is just tender. Stir in beans and olives. Preheat oven to 325 degrees. Transfer bean mixture to a shallow 2 quart casserole. Bake for 10 minutes to melt cheese. If casserole is assembled in advance of baking and chilled, increase baking time to approx. 20 minutes or until heated through. Serves 6.

How to Look Great & Feel Sexy

PEPPERS AND CORN - Fast Weight Loss

2 c. canned corn
1 can green chilies, chopped
2 green peppers, chopped

2 onions, chopped
4 lg. tomatoes, chopped
1/8 tsp cayenne pepper

Combine all ingredients in a non-stick skillet, adding 1/4 cup water to sauté until vegetables are tender. Serve over brown rice. Serves 6.

POLENTA PIE

CRUST:

1 c. cornmeal
1/2 tsp sage
1/4 tsp cumin

1/2 tsp chili powder
4 c. cold water

FILLING:

1 onion, chopped
1 clove garlic, pressed
1/2 lb. mushrooms, sliced
1 eggplant, diced
2 c. tomato sauce

6 oz. tomato paste
1 bay leaf
1/2 tsp basil
1 tsp oregano

Combine cornmeal, sage, cumin, and chili powder in a saucepan. Stir in the cold water. Cook, stirring constantly until very thick. Pour into a non-stick oblong baking dish. Bake at 425 degrees for 30 minutes. Remove from oven and let cool for 30 minutes. In the meantime sauté onion, garlic, mushrooms, and eggplant in 1/2 cup water for 10 minutes. Add remaining ingredients and simmer 20 minutes. Spoon this mixture over the cornmeal crust. Bake at 350 degrees for 30 minutes. Serves 3 to 4.

SPANISH RICE

1/2 c. celery, chopped
1 med. onion, thinly sliced
1/2 med. green pepper, chopped
2 Tbsp Ortega Taco Sauce (mild)
    or Pace Picante (mild)

1 c. brown rice, uncooked
3 (8 oz.) cans tomato sauce
3/4 c. hot water
1 Tbsp garlic powder
Dash of oregano and paprika

Heat water in skillet. Add the onions, green peppers, celery, and rice. Stir over high heat until lightly browned. Add the tomato sauce and the remaining ingredients. Bring to a boil. Cover tightly and simmer 25 minutes.

SPANISH RICE & VEGETABLES

2 heads cauliflower, separated
   into flowerettes
2 lg. bell peppers, diced
4 lg. stalks celery, diced
3 Tbsp (or to taste) chili powder

4 Tbsp onion flakes
1 (46 oz.) can tomato juice
1 clove minced garlic
Salt to taste

Place all ingredients in a large pot. Bring to a boil. Simmer over low heat until cauliflower becomes tender. Mash with a potato masher until the cauliflower breaks into small rice-like pieces. Continue to simmer until mixture is the consistency of Spanish rice.

TAMALE PIE

CORN MEAL CRUST:

2 1/2 c. cold water
1/2 tsp chili powder

1 1/4 c. yellow cornmeal

Combine all ingredients in a saucepan over medium heat. Cook until quite thick and stiff, about 10 minutes, stirring frequently. Set aside 3/4 cup. Line sides and bottom of 1 1/2 quart casserole with the rest of the mixture.

TAMALE PIE FILLING:

1 3/4 c. Dennison's chili beans
1/2 c. chopped green pepper

1/2 c. drained, sliced ripe
   olives (2 1/4 oz. can)

Combine all ingredients in a saucepan over medium heat. Heat until hot. Pour into casserole. Top with rounded tablespoons of remaining crust. Bake in a moderate oven (350 degrees) for about 25 minutes.

TAMALES PRONTO

2 c. masa harina
1 1/4 c. chicken broth
2 c. cooked corn
1/2 c. pitted olives, chopped

1/2 c. canned green chili salsa
1 med. onion, chopped
Foil

Cut 30 pieces of foil, each 6 inch square. Stir together masa flour and chicken broth to make a thick paste. Place about 1 1/2 tablespoons of the paste on each foil square and spread in center of foil in a 3 inch square.

Mix together corn, olives, onion, and salsa. Place about 1 1/2 tablespoons of filling down center of each masa square. Fold foil edges together so mesa edges meet, then seal all sides.

Arrange tamales in a kettle with a rack placed on the bottom, so that the tamales are not in the water. Add about 1 inch of water, cover, and steam about 45 minutes. About 6 servings.

TOFU TACOS

1 onion, diced	2 Tbsp flour
1 green bell pepper, diced	2 Tbsp tomato puree
1 tsp paprika	Dash of Tabasco
Water for sautéing	6 taco shells
1 lb. firm or tofu, cut into chunks	

In a large frying pan, sauté onion, bell pepper, and paprika in a small amount of water for 3 to 5 minutes. Crumble tofu into small pieces and add to pan; sauté for several minutes. Add 2 tablespoons of water and tomato puree. Cook until mixture is heated thoroughly. Remove from heat. Stuff taco shells with mixer. Serves 6.

BEAN TACO

2 wheat flour or corn tortillas	Sliced black olives
Vegetarian refried beans, heated	Sliced green onions
Salsa	Chopped tomatoes

Lightly brown tortillas in a 400 degree oven on both sides. Top tortillas with remaining ingredients in the order listed (tomatoes may either be added after or baked with other ingredients).

SOFT VEGGIE TACOS

Have ready:

2 c. cooked brown rice	1 cucumber, thinly sliced
2 c. chopped Bibb or Boston lettuce	1 sm. can black olives, chopped
10 tortillas (yellow or blue corn)	1 chopped tomato

ADDITIONAL OPTIONS:

1/2 c. grated jicama	1/4 c. grated carrots
1/2 c. grated zucchini	1/2 c. sprouted sunflower seeds

Sprinkle rice with a dash of tamari; mix with chopped olives. Warm tortillas in microwave or on stove, one at a time, and fill with a few slices of cucumber, some rice, lettuce, veggies, tomatoes, and top with taco sauce. Yield: 10 tacos. Per taco: 119 calories, 3 gm carbohydrates, 3 gm fat. *An easy to fix lunch for little ones at home.*

TOSTADAS

12 corn tortillas
2 c. Pinto beans (or Del Monte burrito
   filling or Rosarita Vegetarian beans)
1/4 head lettuce, shredded

1/2 onion
Salsa (your favorite)
Garlic powder as desired
2 tomatoes, diced

Soak pinto beans overnight in water, then cook several hours. Add water as needed. Cook beans about 4 hours until tender. Add garlic powder. Mash or blend the beans. Place corn tortillas on cookie sheet and bake at 400 degrees until hard and crispy, about 10 minutes. Spread beans on top of tortillas, then add lettuce, tomatoes, onions, and salsa.

SALSA - Fast Weight Loss - Yield 2 Cups

4 fresh, red ripe med. sized tomatoes
1/4 c. diced onion
1/4 c. fresh lemon juice
2 Tbsp fresh cilantro, minced
1 clove galic minced

3 whole mild green chilies,
   diced or fresh green chili
   pepper (jalapeno or
   serrano) to your taste

With food processor, cut tomatoes in 4 parts and place in processor with remaining ingredients. Chop, using an on-off motion (pulse) until desired consistency. By hand, mince all ingredients and combine in a bowl. Chill 1 hour before serving. Makes 2 cups.

SALSA FRESCA - Fast Weight Loss

4 med. tomatoes, minced
1/2 sm. onion, minced
8 sprigs cilantro, minced
1/3 c. red wine vinegar

2 serrano or jalapeno
   peppers, diced
1/2 c. water

Mix all ingredients and serve or chill first and serve. Best when served very fresh but will keep for 2 days in refrigerator. Yield: 2 cups.

SANTA FE SALSA - Fast Weight Loss

1 c. finely chopped tomato
1/2 c. finely chopped purple onion
1 (4 oz.) can chopped green chilies,
   drained

1 lg. clove garlic, minced
1/8 tsp Mrs. Dash Extra
   Spicy seasoning

Mix all ingredients and serve. Yield: About 2 cups.

SALSA VERDE GREEN I - Fast Weight Loss

1/2 lb. fresh tomatillos: (Mexican
    green tomato)
4 to 6 cloves garlic

1 c. fresh cilantro leaves
1 Tbsp fresh green chile
    or pickled jalapeno pepper

Remove brown husks from tomatillos. Wash thoroughly and cut into chunks. Place all ingredients in a blender or food processor and chop finely but do not liquefy. Makes 1 cup. Serving size: 1 tablespoon. 7 calories, 3 mg. sodium.

SALSA VERDE GREEN II - Fast Weight Loss

1 lb. tomatillos
1 chopped onion
1 chopped green onion

2 tsp minced jalapeno
1 c. chicken stock
Salt and pepper to taste

Sauté onion in large skillet until soft. Cook tomatillos in boiling, salted water for 2 to 3 minutes, then puree in blender. Add green onions to skillet just before regular onions are ready. Combine all ingredients in a saucepan and simmer for 20 minutes. Serve at room temperature.

How to Look Great & Feel Sexy

Main Dishes:
Oriental

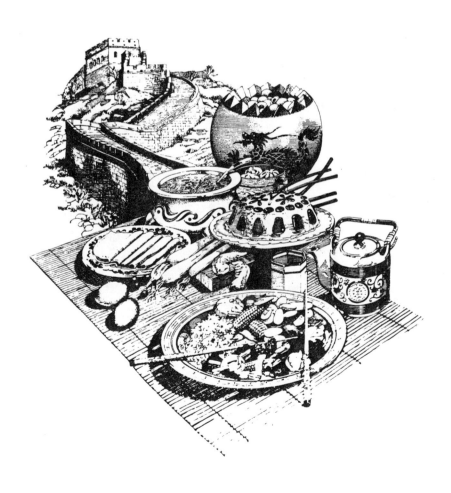

How to Look Great & Feel Sexy

BEAN SPROUTS IN STOCK - Fast Weight Loss

1 lb. (8 c.) bean sprouts
2 shallots, finely chopped
1 clove garlic, finely chopped

4 Tbsp vegetable stock
Freshly ground pepper

SAUCE:

1 Tbsp low-salt soy sauce
3 Tbsp vegetable stock

1 tsp corn flour

Stir fry bean sprouts, shallots, and garlic in a non-stick frying pan for 2 minutes with 3 tablespoons of vegetable stock.
Mix sauce ingredients. Add to frying pan and simmer for 1 minute. Season with pepper and serve.

BROCCOLI WITH WATER CHESTNUTS - Fast Weight Loss

2 1/2 c. broccoli, roughly chopped
3 Tbsp bean sprouts
2 cloves garlic, finely chopped
2 tsp finely chopped fresh ginger
1/2 c. water chestnuts,
   thinly sliced

8 Tbsp basic Chinese
   vegetable stock
2 Tbsp bamboo shoots,
   thinly sliced
1 Tbsp low-salt soy sauce
1 tsp corn flour

Stir fry broccoli, bean sprouts, garlic, and ginger in a non-stick frying pan for 3 minutes with 3 Tbsp of stock. Add chestnuts and bamboo shoots and toss for 1 minute.
Mix soy sauce. Chinese wine or sherry with corn flour and remaining vegetable stock. Add to frying pan. Simmer for 1 minute and serve.

CHINESE BROCCOLI, CAULIFLOWER, & ALMONDS

2 Tbsp soy sauce
2 cloves garlic, minced
4 Tbsp dry sherry
1/2 c. chopped almonds

3 c. broccoli, cut into bite
   sized pieces
3 c. cauliflower, cut into bite
   sized pieces

Sauté garlic in a large skillet or wok, using water in place of oil. Add the sherry and soy sauce. Turn the heat to moderate and add the broccoli and cauliflower. Stir quickly to coat the veggies with the liquid. Stir fry just until the pieces are well distributed. Serve as soon as possible. 4 servings. Top with almonds.

CHINESE EGGPLANT - Fast Weight Loss

4 med. long eggplants
4 cloves garlic, crushed
1 thumb-size piece ginger root
2 stalks green onions

3 Tbsp low-sodium soy sauce
1/4 tsp crushed red chili
   pepper(optional)

Cut eggplant into 1/4 x 1 inch pieces. Cook in a small amount of boiling water until almost done, 5 to 8 minutes. Drain. Serves 6.

CHINESE SPICY VEGETABLES - Fast Weight Loss

VEGETABLES:

1 onion, cut in half and sliced
1 c. celery, sliced
1 1/2 c. chopped broccoli
1/2 c. Chinese peas

1 c. bean sprouts
1/2 lb. mushrooms, thinly
   sliced
2 c. chopped Chinese cabbage

SAUCE:

4 Tbsp low-sodium soy sauce
2 Tbsp cider vinegar
2 cloves garlic, crushed
3 Tbsp chopped fresh coriander
1/4 tsp crushed red pepper

1 1/2 Tbsp cornstarch or
   arrow root
1/4 tsp grated fresh ginger
   root

Mix sauce ingredients together. Set aside. Sauté onions and celery in a small amount of water for 5 minutes. Add broccoli and Chinese cabbage; cook and stir for 5 more minutes. Add mushrooms. Cook and stir until soft, 5 minutes. Add bean sprouts. Stir in sauce. Heat through. Use to fill pita bread. 4 servings

GREEN PEPPERS AND CHINESE MUSHROOMS

3 lg. green peppers, diced
8 Chinese mushrooms, soaked in hot
   water for 30 minutes, remove
   stems, and cut them into quarters
4 Tbsp vegetable stock

1 Tbsp low-salt soy sauce
1 tsp corn flour
Freshly ground pepper
3 cloves garlic, chopped

Stir fry mushrooms, garlic, and green peppers with stock in non-stick frying pan for 3 minutes. Mix soy sauce and corn flour. Add to frying pan and simmer for 2 minutes. Season with pepper. Serve hot. *This is a Fast Weight Loss Recipe.*

MIXED VEGETABLES - Fast Weight Loss

1 1/2 c. snow peas, stems and
 strings removed
1 1/4 c. Chinese cabbage,
 roughly chopped
6 dried Chinese mushrooms, soaked
 in hot water for 30 minutes, discard
 stems, and cut into quarters
1 c. basic Chinese vegetable stock
1 3/4 c. bean sprouts

2 shallots, finely diced
1 tsp corn flour
1 Tbsp toasted sesame seeds
Freshly ground pepper
1 med. carrot, cut into
 thin slices
1 sm. red or green pepper,
 seeded and cut into strips

Stir fry mangetout (snow peas), cabbage mushrooms, carrots, and pepper strips in a non-stick frying pan with half the vegetable stock for 2 minutes. Add bean sprouts and shallots. Toss for 30 seconds. Mix remaining stock with corn flour. Add to frying pan and simmer for 2 minutes. Sprinkle with sesame seeds. Season with pepper and serve.

PUMPKIN TREAT

1 c. water
3 c. pumpkin, diced
1 clove garlic, chopped
1 Tbsp fresh ginger, chopped
3 tsp toasted sesame seeds

1 Tbsp low-salt soy sauce
Freshly ground pepper
1 tsp corn flour, mixed with
 1 Tbsp cold water

Bring water to the boil and stir fry pumpkin for 15 minutes with garlic clove and ginger. Add soy sauce and pepper; simmer for another 2 minutes. Thicken with corn flour mix. Simmer for 1 minute. Sprinkle with sesame seeds and serve.

RED COOKED CABBAGE - Fast Weight Loss

1 Chinese cabbage, roughly chopped
2 Tbsp finely chopped fresh ginger
1 clove garlic, finely chopped
1 shallot, finely chopped

1 red chili, finely chopped
1 1/2 c. stock vegetable
2 Tbsp low-salt soy sauce
1 Tbsp fresh orange juice

Stir fry cabbage, ginger, garlic, shallots, and chili in half the stock for 3 minutes. Reduce heat. Add remaining stock, soy sauce, and orange juice. Simmer for another 5 minutes and serve.

SPINACH AND BAMBOO SHOOTS - Fast Weight Loss

1 lb. spinach, roughly chopped
2 Tbsp canned bamboo shoots,
    thinly sliced
2 tsp finely chopped fresh ginger

4 Tbsp vegetable stock
1 Tbsp low-salt soy sauce
1 tsp corn flour
1 clove garlic, finely chopped

Add spinach, bamboo shoots, ginger, and garlic to wok or non-stick frying pan. Stir fry for 2 minutes with 3 tablespoons of stock.

Mix soy sauce and corn flour. Add to wok and simmer until sauce thickens, about 1 minute. Serve hot.

VEGETABLES ORIENTAL - Fast Weight Loss

2 c. sliced celery
1 c onion, sliced
1 c sliced mushrooms
1 lb. broccoli, sliced
1/2 c. sliced water chestnuts
Water for sautéing

1 c. water
1 1/2 tsp low-sodium soy
    sauce
3 Tbsp cornstarch, dissolved
    in 3 Tbsp water

Stir-fry vegetables in a small amount of water for about 5 minutes. Add 1 cup water and soy sauce; bring to a boil. Add cornstarch to vegetable mixture and combine thoroughly. Cook until sauce thickens. Serves 8.

STIR - FRY - Fast Weight Loss

1/2 c. chicken stock
1/2 sm. onion, chopped
1 clove garlic, minced
4 carrots, sliced or grated
4 celery stalks, chopped
1/2 head cabbage

1/4 green pepper, diced
4 c. bean sprouts
12 lg. mushrooms, chopped
1 bunch scallions, chopped
1 can water chestnuts, sliced

Heat the stock. Add onion and garlic. Stir fry 1 to 2 minutes. Add the carrots and celery. Stir them quickly to seal in their juices. When these are about half done, add in cabbage and green pepper. When these veggies are nearly cooked, add in bean sprouts, mushrooms, scallions, and water chestnuts. Stir continuously, until all the veggies are tender crisp.

SAUCE FOR STIR - FRY VEGETABLES:

1 clove garlic, minced	1/2 tsp ginger
1 1/2 c. chicken stock	2 1/2 Tbsp cornstarch
3 Tbsp soy sauce	

Sauté the garlic over low heat. Pour stock over the garlic and add the soy sauce, sherry, and ginger. Turn the heat to medium. Dissolve the cornstarch in a little cold water. Add the cornstarch. Let the sauce boil slowly until it has thickened, stirring almost continuously. Pour this over the stir fry veggies when they are done and serve over brown rice.

ZUCCHINI AND GARLIC - Fast Weight Loss

1 lb.(2 2/3 c.)zucchini, cut into thin slices	3 Tbsp basic Chinese vegetable stock
2 cloves garlic, finely chopped	1 Tbsp low-salt soy sauce
2 tsp finely chopped fresh ginger	1 tsp corn flour
1 shallot, finely chopped	Freshly ground pepper

Stir fry zucchini, garlic, ginger, and shallot in non-stick frying pan with the vegetable stock for 3 minutes. Mix soy sauce and corn flour. Add to frying pan. Simmer for 2 minutes. Season with pepper and serve.

CARROT SALAD

4 c. grated carrots	1 fresh red chili, chopped
1 c. chopped fresh coriander	1 Tbsp toasted sesame seeds
1/2 c. shallots, sliced	3/4 c. fresh orange juice
2 tsp vinegar	1/4 c. fresh bean sprouts

Combine all ingredients. Marinate for 30 minutes before serving.

CHINESE FRUIT SALAD

1 c. watermelon balls	1 Tbsp finely chopped fresh ginger
1 c. honeydew melon balls	1/4 clove crushed garlic
2 c. diced fresh pineapple or canned unsweetened pieces	1 c. fresh orange juice
1 c. kiwi fruit circles	1 c. unsweetened pineapple juice
2 c. fresh lychees	1 c. diced apple
1 c. sliced fresh mango	

Combine all ingredients, except garnish. Chill before serving.

CHINESE SALAD - RAW

4 c. shredded Chinese cabbage
2 c. diced water chestnuts
1 sm. white onion, finely chopped
2 shallots, sliced
2 c. carrots, grated

2 c. bean sprouts
1 Tbsp toasted sesame seeds
1 c. fresh orange juice
1 Tbsp low-salt soy sauce

Combine all ingredients and serve.

COLD NOODLE SALAD

5 c. cooked whole wheat or rice
   noodles
1 c. carrots, grated
1/2 c. diced shallots
1/2 c. finely shredded red cabbage
1 clove garlic, chopped

1 tsp finely chopped fresh
   ginger
1 Tbsp low-salt soy sauce
1/4 c. fresh lemon juice
2 tsp toasted sesame seeds

Combine all ingredients and serve.

CUCUMBER SALAD

3 med. cucumbers
1 clove garlic, chopped
1 tsp finely chopped fresh ginger
2 tsp freshly ground
Szechuan or black pepper

1 Tbsp toasted sesame seeds
1 Tbsp low-salt soy sauce
1/2 c. fresh orange juice
2 tsp vinegar

Peel cucumbers and slice into thin discs. Mix with other ingredients, except sesame seeds. Marinate for 30 minutes before serving. Toss in sesame seeds and serve.

EGGPPLANT SALAD

2 med. eggplants
3/4 c. basic Chinese vegetable stock
   or water
2 cloves garlic, chopped

2 tsp finely chopped fresh
   ginger
1 Tbsp chopped fresh
   coriander

Cut eggplants in half lengthwise, then into thin strips. Bring stock to the boil and stir fry eggplant strips with garlic and ginger for 2 minutes. Drain and allow to cool. Garnish with fresh coriander and serve.

PICKLED VEGETABLES - Side Dish

2 cucumbers, thinly sliced
2 carrots, cut into thin strips
1 c. cauliflower flowerettes
4 sticks celery, diced
1 clove garlic, chopped

1/2 tsp finely chopped fresh
  ginger
1 c. fresh orange juice
2 Tbsp vinegar
Freshly ground pepper

Place cucumber, carrots, cauliflower, and celery in a serving bowl. Mix together remaining ingredients and pour over vegetables. Combine well and marinate for 1 hour before serving.

SPROUTS AND FRESH VEGGIES

4 c. mixed sprouts (bean,
  alfalfa, mung)
3 shallots, diced
3 carrots, grated
2 1/2 c. red cabbage, finely shredded
1 tsp chopped fresh ginger
Freshly ground pepper

2 cloves garlic, chopped
1 Tbsp toasted sesame seeds
1 Tbsp low-salt soy sauce
2 Tbsp fresh lemon juice
1 c. basic Chinese vegetable
  stock

Toss and stir all ingredients together, except lemon juice. Sprinkle with lemon juice just before serving.

NAM PRIK (THAI)

1/2 c. shredded green apple
2 Tbsp chopped canned green chilies
2 tsp apple juice concentrate
1/2 tsp anchovy paste

1 tsp grated lime peel
2 Tbsp lime juice
2 Tbsp green onion

Choose an assortment of vegetables, i.e. carrot sticks, cucumber rounds, green pepper strips, whole green onions - and arrange on a tray around the chili sauce.

Combine all ingredients in a small dish. 1/2 cup servings.

CHINESE NOODLES

8 dried Chinese mushrooms, soaked
for 30 minutes in hot water,
discard stems, and finely slice
1/4 c. bean curd, diced
2 c. bean sprouts
1 c. sliced shallots
2 fresh red chilies, chopped

2 1/2 c. fresh rice noodles,
cut into thin strips
1 green pepper, finely sliced
1 red pepper, finely sliced
5 Tbsp basic Chinese
vegetable stock

SAUCE:

1 tsp corn flour
2 cloves garlic, chopped
2 tsp chopped fresh ginger
2 tsp sesame seeds
Freshly ground pepper
1 Tbsp low-salt soy sauce

1 Tbsp mild-medium hot
curry powder
3 Tbsp basic Chinese
vegetable stock
1 Tbsp fresh orange juice
1 Tbsp dry sherry

Mix sauce ingredients in a bowl. Bring a large saucepan of water to the boil. Plunge in noodles for 30 seconds. Remove and drain. Stir fry bean curd in a hot wok or non-stick frying pan for 1 minute with 2 tablespoons of vegetable stock. Remove bean curd from wok and set aside. Stir fry bean sprouts, shallots, mushrooms, peppers, and chilies for 2 minutes in wok with 3 tablespoons of vegetable stock. Return bean curd and noodles to wok. Add sauce and toss over low heat for 2 minutes. Serve hot.

FRIED NOODLES

Spring water
1 (8 oz.) pkg. Erewhon Soba or
Udon noodles
2 c. shredded cabbage

1/2 c. sliced scallions
1 to 2 Tbsp Kikkoman Lite
Soy Sauce

Cook the noodles according to directions on package. Use non-stick frying pan and add the cabbage. Put the cooked noodles on top of the cabbage; cover the pan and cook over low heat for 5 to 7 minutes or until the noodles are warm. Add the soy sauce and mix the noodles and vegetables well. Do not stir the ingredients together until this time; they should be left to cook peacefully until the very end. Cook for several minutes longer and add the scallions at the very end. Serve hot or cold.

Variation: Many combinations of vegetables may be used, including carrots and onions, scallions and mushrooms and cabbage and Seitan wheat meat. Hard root vegetables take longer to cook and they should be sautéed in the frying pan before the noodles are added. Add the soft vegetables just before sprinkling on the soy sauce.

ORIENTAL NOODLES

1 pkg. brown rice ramen
1 lb. broccoli
1 clove garlic, minced
1 onion, chopped
3/4 c. chicken broth
2 carrots, sliced

1 red or green bell pepper,
   sliced
1/4 lb. mushrooms, sliced
1 lb. tofu, drained and cut
   into cubes
2 stalks celery, chopped

Cut off broccoli flowerettes; peel off and discard tough outside layer of stalks, then cut stalks into 1/4 inch thick slices. Slice large broccoli flowerettes in half or thirds lengthwise. Cook noodles, according to package directions; drain well.

Place other ingredients in wok. Stir fry on high heat for 5 to 6 minutes until veggies are crisp-tender. Serve over noodles. 4 servings.

RICE NOODLES AND GREEN PEPPERS IN BLACK BEAN SAUCE

1 Tbsp black beans soaked in cold
   water for 15 minutes to remove
   excess salt, drain and mash
3 c. fresh rice noodles, cut into strips
1 Tbsp finely chopped fresh ginger
2 shallots, finely chopped
2 Tbsp dry sherry
2 med. green peppers,
   seeded and cut strips

3 Tbsp basic Chinese
   vegetable stock
3 Tbsp basic Chinese
   vegetable stock
2 tsp corn flour
3 cloves garlic, finely chopped

Stir fry garlic, black beans, shallots, ginger, and green peppers in a non-stick frying pan with 3 tablespoons of stock for 3 minutes. Bring a large saucepan of water to the boil. Plunge rice noodles in for 1 minute. Remove and drain. Mix 2 tablespoons vegetable stock, corn flower, and sherry. Add to frying pan. Add rice noodles and stir over low for heat for 2 minutes. Serve hot.

RICE NOODLES WITH LETTUCE AND MUSHROOMS

1 sm. lettuce, roughly chopped
6 dried Chinese mushrooms,
  soaked in hot water
  for 30 minutes, discard
  stems, and cut into quarters
2 tsp corn flour
3 cloves garlic, finely chopped
1 Tbsp finely chopped fresh ginger

3 c. fresh rice noodles, cut
  into strips
1 Tbsp low-salt soy sauce
Freshly ground pepper
1 shallot, finely chopped
1 c. basic Chinese vegetable
  stock
2 Tbsp dry sherry

Stir fry lettuce, mushrooms, garlic, ginger, and shallots with half the stock in a non-stick frying pan for 3 minutes. Bring a large saucepan of water to the boil. Plunge in noodles for 1 minute. Remove and drain. Mix soy sauce, corn flower, and sherry with remaining stock and add to frying pan. Stir in rice noodles. Season with pepper and simmer for 2 minutes. Serve hot.

SZECHUAN -SPICY NOODLES

6 Tbsp lite soy sauce
6 Tbsp rice vinegar
2 Tbsp finely chopped scallions
6 tsp Szechuan sauce
1 tsp chili powder

1/2 lb. fresh Chinese noodles
2 Tbsp finely chopped
  roasted cashews
1 tsp minced garlic

In a small bowl, combine soy sauce, vinegar, garlic, scallion, chili powder, and Szechuan sauce (from the oriental section at the supermarket) set aside.

In a large pot, bring 6 to 8 cups of water to a boil over a moderate flame. Drop in noodles and loosen them with chop sticks or a fork. When the noodles and water come to a boil, add 1 cup cold water. Cook noodles until the water comes to a boil again; remove noodles from heat and drain.

Pour the spicy sauce into a large serving bowl and put the cooked noodles on top of the sauce. Mix the noodles and the sauce together; sprinkle chopped cashews on top and serve at once. Serves 4.

ORIENTAL VEGETABLES AND RICE

2 Tbsp water
1/2 c. green onions, chopped
1 c. celery, chopped
1/2 lb. mushrooms, chopped
2 c. broccoli
1 c. unsweetened pineapple chunks
  (save juice)

1 c. frozen peas, defrosted
1 can water chestnuts,
  drained and sliced
2 Tbsp cornstarch
1/2 tsp ground ginger
4 Tbsp soy sauce (low sodium)
1/2 c. chicken stock (defatted)

Heat 2 Tbsp water in non-stick skillet. Add onions and sauté. Add celery and mushrooms; heat over low flame, stirring constantly, for 5 minutes. Add chestnuts and pineapple. Separately, combine cornstarch, ginger, soy sauce, pineapple juice (chunks), and stock. Mix well to remove lumps. Add to mixture. Add defrosted peas. Cook until mixture thickens, stirring constantly. Serve over a bed of brown rice. Serves 4 to 6.

VEGETABLE AND RICE

3 c. cooked brown rice
1 Tbsp ginger, finely chopped
3 shallots, chopped
3 cloves garlic, finely chopped
3 Tbsp basic Chinese vegetable stock

2 c. broccoli, chopped
1 c. bean sprouts
1 green pepper, seeded and
  cut into strips
Freshly ground pepper

Stir fry garlic, ginger, and shallots in non-stick frying pan for 1 minute with 1 Tbsp of stock. Add green pepper, broccoli, and sprouts to pan and stir fry for 3 minutes w/ 2 Tbsp of stock. Add rice to pan and stir fry over medium heat until heated through. Season w/ pepper and serve hot. If you like spicy rice, add a diced red or green chili.

WILD RICE & VEGGIES

2 1/2 c. plus 3 Tbsp low-sodium
chicken stock, defatted
1/2 c. wild rice
1/2 c. long-grain brown rice
1 Tbsp low-sodium soy sauce
1 Tbsp salt-free Dijon style mustard
1 1/2 c. sliced fresh mushrooms

1/2 c. fresh or frozen peas or
snow peas
1 c. sliced water chestnuts
1/2 c. diced red bell pepper
1 scallion or shallot, chopped
1 clove garlic, minced
Chopped fresh parsley

Place 2 1/2 cups stock in a medium size saucepan and bring to a boil over high heat. Add wild rice and brown rice; do not stir. When stock returns to a boil, cover pan. Reduce heat to medium low and simmer for 45 minutes or until rice is tender and liquid is absorbed. Remove pan from heat and let stand, covered, for 10 to 15 minutes.

Meanwhile, heat soy sauce, mustard, and remaining stock in a medium size non-stick skillet over medium heat. Add mushrooms, peas, water chestnuts, bell pepper, scallion, and garlic; cook, stirring constantly, for 10 minutes or until vegetables are crisp-tender.

Add rice to vegetables; stir well to combine and divide among 8 plates. Sprinkle with parsley and serve. Makes 8 servings.

CHINESE FRIED RICE WITHOUT OIL

1/2 c. chicken broth
3 Tbsp sesame seeds
1 c. thinly sliced carrots
1 onion, sliced
2 cloves garlic, minced
1 green pepper, cut into strips
1 c. zucchini, sliced

1 c. mushrooms, sliced
2 c. bean sprouts
1 c. cooked brown rice
1 tsp ginger
1/4 c. soy sauce
3 Tbsp cilantro, chopped

Heat chicken broth in wok. Add carrots and stir fry for 1 minute over high heat. Mix in onion, garlic, and green pepper; stir fry for 1 more minute. Add zucchini and mushrooms; stir fry until all vegetables are tender-crisp (about 2 more minutes). Mix in bean sprouts and rice and cook until heated through.

In a small bowl, mix ginger with soy; blend into rice mixture. Serve immediately, sprinkled with cilantro and sesame seeds. 4 servings.

ORIENTAL STIR- FRY WITH BROWN RICE

Parsley Patch oriental blend
(no salt, no MSG, no sugar)
1 (16 oz.) pkg. frozen vegetables
orient

1 (14 oz.) pkg. fresh chop
suey mix
1 (6 oz.) pkg. frozen Chinese
pea pods

Spray a non-stick pan; stir fry the above ingredients in a large skillet over medium heat until lightly brown. Add about 1 cup cooked brown rice; stir in and blend well. Sprinkle with Oriental Blend seasoning to taste.

ORIENTAL RICE

2 tsp minced ginger
2 lg. cloves garlic, minced
1/2 c. defatted chicken stock
3 Tbsp reduced sodium soy sauce
3 c. sliced mushrooms
2 c. sliced bok choy

1 c. diced bell pepper
1 c. diced carrots
1 1/4 c. sliced water chestnuts
4 c. cooked brown rice
1 c. chopped green onions
1 1/2 tsp sesame seeds, toasted

1. Sauté ginger and garlic in 1/4 cup chicken stock and soy sauce.
2. Add mushrooms, bok choy, bell pepper, carrots, water chestnuts, and rice. Cook until vegetables are tender, adding more chicken stock as needed.
3. Add green onion and sesame seeds. Makes 10 servings. Each 1 cup serving contains 120 calories, 7% fat, 173 mg sodium, and 0 mg cholesterol.

MEE KROB

1 lb. rice vermicelli
1 lg. onion, finely chopped
4 cloves garlic, finely chopped
6 dried Chinese mushrooms,
   soaked and finely sliced
2 sm. fresh chilies, seeded and sliced
3 Tbsp soy sauce
2 Tbsp rice vinegar

4 egg whites
5 Tbsp apple juice concentrate
Handful of bean sprouts
6 green onions, finely chopped
4 Tbsp fresh coriander,
   chopped
Juice of 2 limes

Boil the noodles in water until tender. Sauté the onions and garlic in a little water. Add the mushrooms and chilies. Reduce heat. In a separate bowl, mix the egg whites, soy sauce, lime juice, vinegar, and apple juice concentrate. Add this to mixture and simmer until it becomes thicker. Add the bean sprouts, noodles, green onion, and coriander. Heat the combination through.

EGG FOO YONG

1 c. vegetable stock
6 dried mushrooms, soaked for
   30 minutes in hot water,
   discard stems, and slice
7 egg whites

1 c. fresh bean sprouts
1 c. bamboo shoots, sliced
2 Tbsp low-salt soy sauce
12 water chestnuts, chopped
2 shallots, finely sliced

Only egg whites are used in this recipe
Bring stock to the boil and add all ingredients except egg whites. Stir fry in stock for 5 minutes. Swirl through egg whites; simmer for 2 minutes and serve.

CHOP SUEY - Microwave

2 c. wheat meat
1 c. chopped onion
1 tsp instant beef bouillon
1 c. boiling water
2 Tbsp cornstarch
1/4 c. soy sauce

1/4 tsp ginger
1 (4 oz.) can sliced mushrooms
1 (8 oz.) can bamboo shoots
1 (8 oz.) can water chestnuts
1 (16 oz.) can bean sprouts

Place wheat meat and onion in 2 quart casserole. Cook on full power for 3 minutes; drain. Combine bouillon and boiling water. Gradually stir into cornstarch. Add soy sauce and ginger. Pour over wheat meat. Cook on full power for 6 minutes. Add remaining ingredients. Cook on full power for 3 minutes. Serve over rice.

RAW CHOP SUEY

2 med. heads bok choy
2 lg. heads napa
2 c. broccoli flowerettes
1/4 c. minced parsley
1/4 c. chopped watercress
4 Tbsp lime juice
3 Tbsp soy sauce or tamari

3 sheets nori, crumbled
3 c. red bell pepper strips
4 stalks celery, trimmed and
   chopped
1 1/2 c. mung bean sprouts
Cherry tomatoes for garnish
1 c. sliced mushrooms (optional)

Cut off and discard the base ends of each head of bok choy and napa. Shred bok choy and napa in a food processor, using the medium shredding disk; place in large bowl. Add broccoli, parsley, and watercress; set aside.

Puree lime juice, soy sauce or tamari, and nori in a food processor, using the metal "S" blade. Add to bok choy mixture. Stir in remaining ingredients except cherry tomatoes and mix well. Place in a serving bowl and top with a circle of cherry tomatoes. Serves 4.

Per serving: 217 calories, 20 g protein, 2 g fat, 37 g carbohydrates, 0 cholesterol, 87 mg sodium.

CHOW MEIN I

3 onions, chopped
1 c. sliced mushrooms
3 c. cooked celery
2 c. chicken broth
2 tsp soy sauce

2 tsp cornstarch
1 c. mung bean sprouts
4 c. cooked brown rice
Water

Put a little water in a skillet and sauté the onions until cooked. Add the mushrooms and celery; cook a little more. Stir in the broth and soy sauce; bring to a boil. Mix the arrow root with a little water until smooth and pour into the onion mixture. Add the sprouts. Serve over brown rice. 4 servings.

CHOW MEIN II

4 c. fresh rice noodles
4 Tbsp basic Chinese vegetable stock
1 c. bean sprouts
5 dried Chinese mushrooms soaked
   in hot water for 30 minutes,
   discard stems, and slice

1 c. bamboo shoots
3 cloves garlic, chopped
1 c. sliced carrots
1 c. broccoli flowerettes
10 snow peas, trimmed

SAUCE:

2 tsp corn flour
1/2 c. basic Chinese vegetable stock
1 Tbsp diced shallots
1 tsp chopped fresh ginger

Freshly ground pepper
1 Tbsp low-salt soy sauce
1 Tbsp dry sherry

Drop noodles into boiling water. Reduce heat. Simmer for 1 minute and drain. Stir fry remaining ingredients in a non-stick frying pan or wok for 3 minutes with 4 tablespoons of stock. Return drained noodles to frying pan. Mix sauce ingredients. Pour sauce over chow mein and toss for 3 minutes over low heat. Serve hot.

NORI MAKI SUSHI

1 c. short grain brown rice
2 c. water
4 sheets dried nori

1/2 tsp Instead of Salt
2 to 4 Tbsp rice vinegar
2 tsp honey

FILLING INGREDIENTS: Choose 3 for each roll.

Grated raw carrot or jicama
Cooked chopped spinach
Strips of scallion bell pepper, celery,
  omelette (no yolk), lightly steamed
  asparagus, carrot or green beans
Avocado

Pickled umeboshi plum
  (use just a bit)
Chopped watercress
Mushrooms
Toasted sesame seeds

CONDIMENTS:

Shoyu, sweet and hot mustard

Pickled ginger

The outside wrapper nori, is made from seaweed. It has best flavor when freshly toasted and eaten soon after.

If you want to include mushrooms, shiitakes are traditional, but normal ones work too, sautéed and cut in strips. If you do come upon some dried shiitakes soak several in water, then simmer in 2 teaspoons each shoyu and sherry. Chop fine or cut into strips.

Cook rice, uncovered, in boiling water for 5 minutes, then cover and reduce heat to low. Simmer for 45 minutes.

While the rice is cooking, select and prepare your choice of fillings. You'll be making 4 rolls, it's fun to vary the fillings in each. Combine about 3 of the suggested ingredients in each.

Unless the nori sheets you have are pre-toasted, wave each one over a flame (a gas burner is ideal), holding it with tongs or fingertips, so that each sheet changes color and texture slightly, becoming light and coarser.

Dissolve Instead of Salt in rice vinegar in a small saucepan and add honey; heat gently to liquefy. When the rice is cooked, turn it out onto a large platter or baking dish with sides. Pour the vinegar mixture over it, stirring as you do, and fanning the steam away, a folded newspaper works nicely. When the rice has cooled to room temperature, it is ready.

For rolling the sushi, a traditional bamboo mat is great, but not essential; a big cloth napkin works fine, just a little bigger than the nori sheets. Place the mat or cloth flat in front of you and put the first sheet of nori on it. Moisten your fingers with water or vinegar and spread 1/4 of the seasoned rice on the meat, covering it except for an inch or 2 at the top, which you'll use to seal the roll.

The rice should be not quite 1/2 inch thick. Across the middle, parallel to the top, form an indentation and place the filling materials there, forming a thin line from one end to the other. For example: A strip of omelette, a line of chopped watercress, and strips of red bell pepper. Aim for beauty and harmony too.

Grasping the nearest side of the mat, roll it up and away from you toward the top, pressing the whole thing together tightly and pushing the filling ingredients into place if necessary. Dampen the remaining "flap" of nori and seal the roll by pressing the flap along the length of the roll. Place the roll on a cutting board and slice It with a very sharp knife into 1 inch segments. Arrange, cut side up, and serve. Makes about 6 servings.

SUKIYAKI - Microwave

1/2 lb. wheat meat	3 stalks celery, sliced
1 (8 oz.) can bamboo shoots	3 Tbsp apple juice
1 (8 oz.) can water chestnuts	concentrate
1 (16oz.) can bean sprouts	1/3 c. soy sauce
1/2 lb. fresh mushrooms, sliced	1/2 c. beef bouillon
1 med. onion, sliced	

Slice wheat meat into very thin pieces. Place in 2 quart casserole. Cook on full power for 4 minutes. Add vegetables to skillet. Combine apple juice concentrate soy sauce, and bouillon. Pour over vegetables. Cook on full power for 6 minutes.

SWEET & SOUR STIR - FRIED VEGETABLES WITH TOFU

1/2 lb. tofu or seitan wheat meat	1 Tbsp fresh ginger, finely
1 1/2 c. chicken stock	chopped
3 c. of any combination of these	Fresh vegetables
or other vegetables:	2 cloves garlic, minced

HIGH DENSE:

Carrots	Green beans
Cauliflower	Sweet potato

MEDIUM DENSE:

Snow peas	Red peppers
Broccoli	

SLIGHTLY DENSE:

Water Chestnuts	Bean sprouts

SAUCE:

1/2 c. chicken stock (salt free and defatted)
1/4 c. vinegar
1/4 c. apple juice concentrate

1/4 tsp garlic powder
1/4 tsp ginger
1 Tbsp cornstarch

Cut tofu into bite sized pieces and marinate at least 1/2 hour in the sauce before adding the cornstarch to it. Prepare vegetables in bite sized pieces. Preheat wok or large skillet over medium heat. Pour in 1/2 cup stock; add fresh ginger and minced garlic. Sauté until stock evaporates and herbs are browned. Deglaze pan by adding 1/3 cup more stock, then turn up fire to high temperature. Start adding vegetables, beginning with the High Dense. Solid, firm vegetables, such as carrots, are the most dense and require the longest cooking time. Cook the most dense vegetables until they are slightly tender (2 minutes), then clear a space in the center of the wok and add the vegetables that are Medium Dense and so on. Repeat until all the vegetables are done, adding stock as needed to keep vegetables from scorching.

When they are done, clear a space in the center of the wok and add tofu. Clear space again. Add cornstarch to the sauce mixture and pour sauce into the center of the wok. Cook stirring continuously, until the sauce thickens. Fold the vegetables and tofu into the sauce and serve. Vegetables cooked over a high heat come out best. Overcooked vegetables lose their color, so be careful not to overcook!

STUFFED STEAMED PEPPERS IN MUSTARD SAUCE

6 sm. green or red peppers, cut tops
off and remove seeds

STUFFING:

1 1/2 c. cooked brown rice
1 shallot, finely chopped
1 Tbsp finely chopped fresh ginger
2 cloves garlic, finely chopped

Freshly ground pepper
6 Tbsp vegetable stock
1 tsp corn flour
3 1/2 c. bean sprouts

MUSTARD SAUCE:

1 Tbsp low-salt soy sauce
1 Tbsp vinegar

2 tsp Dijon mustard
3 Tbsp vegetable stock

Mix stuffing ingredients together, except bean sprouts. Allow to stand for 15 minutes. Stir fry stuffing mixture in hot wok or frying pan for 3 minutes. Add bean sprouts and stir fry for 2 minutes. Allow to cool. Stuff the peppers with the filling. Transfer stuffed peppers to steamer and steam vigorously on a plate for 10 minutes. Remove peppers from the plate. Mix mustard sauce ingredients with liquid on the plate. Pour over stuffed pepper and serve.

SWEET AND SOUR LENTILS WITH BROWN RICE

1/2 c. dry lentils	1 tsp arrow root or cornstarch
3 c. water	1 sm. onion, sliced
2 Tbsp vinegar	Cooking spray (Pam)
2 Tbsp honey	4 to 5 stalks celery,
1/2 tsp grated fresh ginger or	diagonally sliced
1 tsp ground ginger	1 Tbsp soy sauce
1/2 c. water	

To cook lentils, bring water to a boil, then reduce heat and cook about 25 minutes or until tender. Do not overcook Drain and set aside.

To make sweet and sour sauce: Combine next 4 ingredients and 1/2 cup water in a small saucepan. Bring to a boil. Put arrow root or cornstarch in a small glass and add a little water. Mix thoroughly and add to boiling water to thicken it. Sauté onion in large frying pan lightly sprayed with Pam. When onion is soft, add pieces of celery and cook 5 minutes more over medium heat. Drain cooked lentils and add to frying pan; mix well. Pour sweet and sour sauce into pan and cook for 5 minutes. Serve over a bed of brown rice.

SWEET AND SOUR SOYBEANS

1 onion, chopped	1 1/2 Tbsp cornstarch
2 carrots, sliced	1 1/2 Tbsp soy sauce
1 clove garlic, minced	1/3 c. chicken broth
1 green pepper, chopped	1/2 c. apple juice concentrate
2 tomatoes, sliced	1/2 c. wine vinegar
2 1/2 c. cooked soy beans	1 1/2 Tbsp sherry
3/4 c. canned pineapple chunks	

Sauté onion, carrots, and garlic. Add green pepper and cook about 1 minute longer. Add pineapple, tomatoes, and soy beans and cook for 2 more minutes.

In a bowl, combine cornstarch, soy sauce, apple juice concentrate, chicken broth, wine vinegar, and sherry. Pour on top of beans and cook until sauce bubbles and thickens. 6 servings.

LYCHEES STUFFED

1 1/4 c. currants
1/4 c. toasted sesame seeds
1 c. finely chopped dried apricots
1 Tbsp sweet cherry

20 fresh or canned lychees
(remove lychee stones
from fresh ones, rinse
canned lychees to remove
excess sugar)

Blend together currants sesame seeds, dried apricots, and sherry. Stuff mixture into lychees. Chill and serve.

PEARS AND CINNAMON

6 fresh pears, with stems on
1 c. unsweetened apple juice
1 c. dry sherry
1 c. water

2 sm. pieces cinnamon stick
1 Tbsp finely chopped fresh
ginger

Combine all ingredients in saucepan. Stand pears upright. Cover and simmer for 20 minutes and serve.

SOY LEMON SAUCE

1/3 c. whole wheat flour
1 Tbsp Butter Buds (liquid)
2 1/2 c. water
2 Tbsp lemon juice

2 Tbsp low-sodium soy sauce
1/2 tsp thyme
1 tsp basil
1/4 tsp pepper

Toast the flour in a non-stick pan. Add the spices. Then add the liquids gradually while stirring. Simmer 5 to 10 minutes.

SWEET AND HOT CHILI SAUCE - SAUS PRIK

1 1/2 c. seedless golden raisins
5 Tbsp white vinegar
3 tsp red chili flakes
8 cloves garlic
1 tsp Instead of Salt
2 fresh red chili peppers,
    seeded and sliced

1 c. whole canned tomatoes
(with juice)
12 oz. Red Plum jam
9 oz. pineapple juice
4 Tbsp apple juice concentrate

Place the first 7 ingredients in a food processor blender and blend to an even consistency. This will take several minutes and require stopping occasionally to scrape down the sides. Place the remaining ingredients in a saucepan over medium heat. Pour the blended ingredients in the saucepan. While stirring, let this mixture come to a boil. Reduce heat to simmer and cook for 20 more minutes. Store in air-tight, sterilized jars. It will keep for at least 2 months, refrigerated. Yield: 3 1/2 cups, approximately.

Saus Prik is my attempt to re-create the marvelous, hot sauce served in so many Thai restaurants . Similar sauces may be purchased bottled and labeled "All Purpose Sauce". They are also sweet-hot and garlicky but lack the personality of homemade. It is interesting to experiment and find your own application. This recipe yields 3 1/2 cups and will noticeably become more spicy with age.

SAUCE II FOR STIR- FRY VEGETABLES

1 clove garlic, minced	1/2 tsp ginger
1 1/2 c. chicken stock	2 1/2 Tbsp cornstarch
3 Tbsp soy sauce	1/2 c. dry sherry

Heat garlic and chicken broth. Add soy sauce, ginger, and sherry. Dissolve the cornstarch in a little cold water. Add the cornstarch to broth. Let the sauce boil slowly until it has thickened, stirring continuously. Pour this over the stir-fry veggies and serve over brown rice.

Sweet and sour stir fry: Follow the instructions for basic stir fry, but include 2 medium ripe tomatoes and 2 cups of diced pineapple, preferably fresh, when you add the bean sprouts, mushrooms, scallions, and water chestnuts. For the sauce substitute 1 1/2 cups pineapple juice for the 1 1/2 cups stock and add 2 tablespoons honey and, 1/4 cup white vinegar.

SWEET AND SOUR SAUCE III

1 (12 oz.) can vegetable juice	1 tsp corn flour or 2 Tbsp
1/2 c. unsweetened pineapple juice	tomato paste
1/2 c. unsweetened pineapple	1/2 c. red bell pepper
2 Tbsp wine vinegar	1/2 c. green bell pepper
1/2 tsp black pepper	

Combine all ingredients, stirring frequently, and bring to a boil. Boil gently until sauce thickens; garnish with parsley or chives.

How to Look Great & Feel Sexy

Main Dishes:
Casseroles, Stews,
Veggies, Etc.

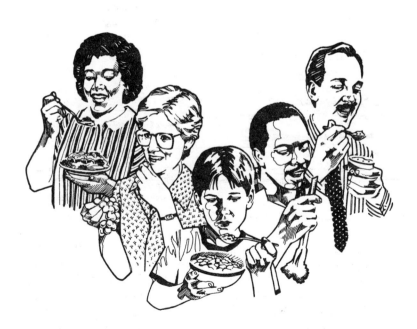

How to Look Great & Feel Sexy

BARBECUED LENTIL BURGERS

1 c. lentils
3 c. water
1 onion, chopped fine
1 clove garlic, crushed
2 stalks celery, finely chopped

1 carrot, grated
1/2 c. bulgur wheat
3 Tbsp ketchup or tomato sauce
2 tsp chili powder

Place lentils and water in a medium saucepan and bring to a boil. Add onion, garlic, celery, and carrot. Reduce heat, cover, and simmer for 30 minutes. Add remaining ingredients. Cook an additional 15 minutes. Remove from heat and let cool. Shape into patties and cook on a non-stick griddle until browned (about 15 minutes). Serve on whole wheat buns with a variety of condiments. Makes 10.

ELEANOR'S OAT BURGERS

1 diced onion
1 tsp garlic powder
2 dice cloves garlic

1 tsp crushed oregano
1 tsp sweet basil

In a small amount of water, sauté (approximately 3 minutes): the above ingredients that are listed.

Add 4 1/2 cups water and 1/3 cup "green" label Kikkoman Milder Soy Sauce. Bring to a boil and add 4 1/2 cups old fashioned "Quaker" oats.

Lower heat and cook 5 minutes. Cover and let set until cooled enough to form patties with wet hands. Bake in 350 degree oven for 15 minutes on each side. Makes 15 medium patties.

MUSHROOM BURGERS

2 onions, chopped
3/4 lb. mushrooms, chopped
3 cloves garlic, crushed
2 lbs. tofu
3 c. rolled oats
Whole wheat buns and any
   garnish you wish
2 Tbsp low-sodium soy sauce

4 Tbsp vegetarian
   Worcestershire sauce
1/2 tsp black pepper
1 tsp paprika
1 tsp lemon juice
1 (10 oz.) pkg. frozen,
   chopped spinach
   thawed and pressed

Sauté onions, mushrooms, and garlic in a small amount of water until they are softened and water is absorbed. Mash tofu in a large bowl. Add oats; spinach (make sure all excess water is removed), seasonings and lemon juice. Mix well. Stir in onion-mushroom mixture. Shape into patties and place on non-stick cookie sheet. Bake at 350 degrees for 20 minutes; turn over, then cook an additional 10 minutes. Makes 15 to 18 medium size burgers.

KASHA HAMBURGERS

1 c. toasted whole buckwheat groats	2 tsp soy sauce
2 c. water to cook buckwheat	2 tsp garlic sauce
8 Tbsp onion flakes	1/2 tsp black pepper
2/3 c. chopped mushrooms	6 Tbsp potato flour
12 oz. wheat meat	3 egg whites

Bring the water to a boil. Add buckwheat; cover and cool on a low heat 10 minutes. Don't overcook. At the same time, brown the wheat meat in a skillet. Mix in cooked buckwheat and the rest of the ingredients; mold the mixture into hamburger patties on a cookie sheet. Bake in a 400 degree oven for 20 minutes or cook individually in the microwave on high for 2 minutes apiece. Delicious served with the tasty sauce below:

SAUCE:

2 (15 oz.) cans tomato sauce	1/2 tsp ginger
1 (10 oz.) can enchilada sauce	1/2 tsp garlic powder
1/4 c. prepared mustard	1/2 tsp onion powder

Combine all sauce ingredients in a saucepan. Heat to blend flavors. Serve hot over Kasha hamburgers or other grain dishes.

NATURE'S BURGER LOAF OR PATTIES

In large saucepan, add:

1 can beef consommé	2 c. water
2 med. finely chopped onions	1 tsp tarragon dry leaves,
Lots of chopped parsley	ground to powder form

Bring to boil and cook 10 minutes. Turn off heat and add:

1 box Nature's Burger meatless mix	1 c. whole grain flour
(with brown rice as main	
ingredient)	

Let stand 15 minutes. When cool enough, form into patties. Cook in a non-stick skillet about 5 minutes on each side.

Variation: Pour into shallow baking dish. Top with 1 can tomato sauce and bake at 350 degrees for 30 minutes.

ORIENTAL GARBONZO BURGERS

1 lb. Falafal	1/2 tsp coriander
1/4 c. oat bran	1 Tbsp low-sodium soy sauce
1/2 tsp ginger	

Mix all ingredients together in large bowl. Form into 4 patties and cook in non-stick skillet (use non-stick spray) until browned. Serves 4.

VEGETABLE BURGERS

2 c. shredded carrot	1/2 tsp ground ginger
1 c. cooked brown rice	1/4 tsp pepper
1/2 c. chopped onion	1/2 tsp ground coriander
1/2 c. chopped almonds	4 egg whites
1/2 c. fine dry bread crumbs	2 Tbsp soy sauce
1 Tbsp parsley, chopped	Non-stick spray coating

In a large bowl, stir together carrot, rice, onion, almonds, bread crumbs, parsley, ginger, coriander, and 1/4 teaspoon pepper. Stir together egg whites and soy sauce; add to rice mixture and mix well. Cover and chill. Shape rice mixture into 6 patties. Spray a baking sheet with non-stick spray coating. Place patties on baking sheet. Broil 3 to 4 inches from heat for 3 to 5 minutes on each side. 6 servings.

RED - BEAN PATTIES

4 c. cooked red or pink beans, drained	Tabasco to taste
4 green onions, sliced thin	1/2 tsp thyme
1/2 red bell pepper, chopped	1/4 tsp garlic powder
1/2 c. chopped fresh parsley	About 1/2 c. apple fiber
1/4 tsp cayenne	

In a food processor or blender, combine beans, onions, red pepper, parsley, cayenne, Tabasco, thyme, garlic powder, and 1/4 cup of the apple fiber. Process until smooth.

Place remaining apple fiber in a shallow bowl. Dipping your hands in the apple fiber, shape the bean puree into patties about 2 1/2 inch diameter and 3/4 inch thick.

Spray a skillet with Pam or Baker's Joy and heat. Cook patties for 5 minutes on each side. Serve the patties like burgers on whole bread buns with onions, lettuce, tomatoes, ketchup, barbecue sauce, or mustard. Makes 12 (2 1/2 inch) patties. 1 patty = 1 serving, 84 calories, .4 grams fat, 0 cholesterol, 100 milligrams sodium.

SUNRISE PATTIES

12 egg whites
8 oz. tofu
1 celery stalk, chopped
1 green onion, chopped
1/2 c. zucchini, shredded

1/8 lb. mushrooms, sliced
1/4 lb. bean sprouts
Pepper
1 tsp soy sauce
1 tsp sherry

Crumble tofu into a large bowl; add sherry and soy sauce. Let stand 5 minutes. Add the rest of the ingredients.

Heat a griddle or large frying pan over medium heat; spray with Pam. Spoon mixture, about 1/4 cup for each patty, onto griddle. From the bowl, spoon about 2 more Tbsp's of only the liquid egg over each patty and distribute evenly over vegetables. Cook until egg is set and bottoms of patties are golden brown. Turn and cook other side. 5 servings.

LENTIL SPROUT SLOPPY JOES

3 c. lentil sprouts (1/2 c. dry lentils,
   sprouted for 3 days)
1 c. spaghetti sauce (no oil)

1/2 c. sliced onions
10 whole wheat
   hamburger buns

In processor, grind lentil sprouts with spaghetti sauce (no oil, meatless, sugarless) to make a thin mixture. Heat and serve over warmed, whole wheat hamburger buns. May top with chopped onion, if desired. *Mitzi Narrarnore.*

WHEAT MEAT CHILI A LA NICK

6 oz. wheat meat
Celery tops
1 onion, sliced
Poultry seasoning to taste
1 c. chopped onions
1/2 c. chopped celery
1/3 c. chopped green pepper
3 cloves garlic, minced
1 1/2 c. broth from cooking turkey
1 (28 oz.) can tomato sauce
1 (15 oz.) can tomato sauce

2 Tbsp tomato paste
1 Tbsp onion powder
2 Tbsp chili powder
2 tsp cumin
1 tsp garlic powder
1 tsp oregano
1 Tbsp soy sauce
Dash of cayenne pepper
1 1/2 c. cooked pinto beans
1 c. cooked kidney beans

Place the wheat meat in a non-stick baking dish with 1 1/2 cups water. Add the celery tops and sliced onion; sprinkle with poultry seasoning. Sauté the chopped onion, celery, green pepper, and garlic in 1/2 cup of the water. Add the remaining ingredients, except the wheat meat and beans. Simmer the sauce, uncovered, for 45 minutes, stirring occasionally.

Meanwhile, dice the wheat meat. Add 1 cup of the diced wheat meat and all the beans to the chili. Cook and stir about 5 minutes more.

WHEAT MEAT VEVESTEAKS

2 1/2 lb. pkg. 100% stone ground
   whole wheat flour
1 lg. onion
2 bay leaves

Soy sauce to taste
Spike seasoning
Water

Pour regular temperature water over the flour and mix until it is like bread dough. Let stand in refrigerator for 2 hours. Wash it slowly until all starch is out; keep changing the water. Takes about 20 minutes. Will become stretchy like meat. Cut in pieces and flatten out. Have kettle boiling water with soy sauce, onion, bay leaves, and spike ready; drop the pieces in and cook until tender. Roll in flour and yeast; brown in non-stick skillet, no oil. Make gravy with broth. *Dale Shinkle*

ZUCCHINI AND WHEAT MEAT DELIGHT - Microwave

1 c. wheat meat
4 c. zucchini, sliced
1 onion, sliced
1 clove garlic, minced
2 Tbsp whole wheat flour

2 tsp instant chicken bouillon
1/4 tsp thyme
2 tomatoes, cut in wedges
1 c. seasoned salad croutons

Cut wheat meat into bite sized pieces. Place in 2 quart casserole. Add zucchini, onion, garlic, flour, bouillon, and thyme. Mix well. Cook at full power for 8 minutes. Add tomatoes. Cook on full power for 2 minutes. Garnish with croutons. 4 servings.

BEAN & VEGETABLE LOAF

8 oz. dried white northern beans
4 c. water
1 Tbsp low-sodium soy sauce
3 cloves garlic, minced
1 bouquet garnish (4 sprigs parsley,
   1 tsp thyme, 1 bay leaf, 1/2 tsp
   crushed red pepper)
5 lg. Swiss chard leaves, stems removed

1/4 lb. fresh whole string beans
1/4 lb. fresh whole okra
1/4 lb. fresh sm. whole carrots
5 artichoke hearts
1/2 c. egg whites (4 to 5 lg.
   eggs), slightly beaten

Cook beans in water and soy sauce with bouquet garnish for 1 1/2 hours. Drain and puree beans in blender. Mix pureed beans with slightly beaten egg whites and garlic. Blanch Swiss chard leaves, string beans, and okra for 3 minutes in boiling water and refresh in cold water. Line a non-stick 6 cup loaf pan with overlapping Swiss chard leaves. Spread a 1/4 layer of bean puree, then a layer of vegetables. Continue alternating bean paste and vegetables.

The first layer should be okra, then artichokes, then carrots, then string beans, end with beaten paste. Cover with foil and place in a baking pan with 1 inch hot water.

Bake in a preheated oven at 350 degrees for 30 to 45 minutes or until mixture is firm. Serve hot with a tomato sauce or cold with a vinaigrette dressing (no oil). Serves 8 to 10.

GARBANZO MEATLOAF

1 pkg. Falafal
2 egg whites
1/2 c. oat bran
1/2 sm. onion, chopped fine
1 clove garlic, minced
1/2 tsp pepper

1/2 tsp sage
1/2 tsp marjoram
2 Tbsp ketchup
2 Tbsp Worcestershire sauce
1/2 tsp Dijon mustard

Combine all ingredients; mix well in a large bowl. Form loaf and place in non-stick loaf pan and bake at 350 degrees for 1 hour or until done. Serves 4.

LEGUME LOAF

3/4 c. whole grain bread crumbs
1/4 c. oat bran
1 egg white
1/2 c. onion, chopped fine
1/2 to 3/4 c. carrots, grated
1 stalk celery, chopped fine
1/4 tsp thyme
1 tsp basil
1/2 tsp savory

2 c. garbanzos, cooked &
  mashed or chopped in a
  food processor or lentils
  and black-eyed peas,
  mashed or chopped
  or a combination
2 Tbsp fresh parsley
  or 2 tsp dried parsley

Combine the bread crumbs and oat bran. Add the egg white and mix. (If the mixture is not moist, add a little water.) Add the other ingredients. Put the mixture in a loaf pan or casserole dish, non-stick or sprayed with Pam. Bake for 1 hour at 350 degrees. Serve with a tomato sauce or Soy Lemon Sauce.

NUT LOAF

2 c. finely ground mixture of seeds
and nuts, such as sunflower seed,
kernels almonds, walnuts, and
cashews
1 onion, chopped
3 celery stalks, chopped
3/4 c. wheat germ

3 cloves garlic, chopped
1 c. cooked brown rice
1/8 tsp dried rosemary
1/4 tsp dried sage
1 tsp caraway seeds
2 egg whites, lightly beaten
1 Tbsp soy sauce

Preheat the oven to 350 degrees. Mix all ingredients together in a large bowl until well blended.

Turn into a 9 x 3 x 5 inch pan sprayed with Pam and bake for 40 minutes. Serve like a meatloaf. For leftovers, cold nut loaf can be served with crackers. 6 servings.

VEGETABLE LOAF

1/2 c. Butter Buds
1 c. chopped onion
1 c. minced celery
1 c. grated raw carrots
1 c. finely ground English walnuts
1 tsp poultry seasoning

1 c. dry whole wheat
bread crumbs
4 egg whites
1 c. chicken broth
1 can tomato sauce

Cook onion in Butter Buds until tender. Add vegetables, nuts, crumbs, and seasonings. Sauté. Mix egg whites and chicken broth. Combine both mixtures and turn into a loaf pan, sprayed with Pam. Bake at 350 degrees for 40 minutes. Serve with tomato sauce. Serves 4.

VEGELOAF

2 c. canned green beans
1 c. liquid reserved from
canned beans
4 slices whole wheat bread
(crumbs equal 2 c.)
3/4 c. brown rice, cooked

1/4 c. spaghetti sauce
(no oil, no meat)
2 cloves garlic minced
1/4 c. cooked mushrooms,
chopped
1 egg white

Blend green beans and liquid in blender. Add remaining ingredients, except bread crumbs and blend. Pour mixture into a bowl over crumbs and mix well. Pour into a non-stick loaf pan (use non-stick spray). Bake at 300 degrees for 45 minutes. Serves 4.

ARTICHOKE & PINTO BEAN CASSEROLE

2(1 lb.) cans pinto or pink beans
1 (1 lb.) can artichoke hearts,
  drained and chopped

1/8 tsp each cayenne and
  ground cloves
1/2 tsp ground cumin

Preheat oven to 350 degrees. Empty 1 can of beans and liquid into a 9 inch square baking pan. Drain and rinse the other can of beans, then roughly chop the beans. Add chopped beans and artichokes to the whole beans. Add spices and chili sauce; mix together well. Set pan in oven, uncovered, and bake for 30 minutes. Serving size: 1/4 recipe, 259 calories, 72 grams fat, 0 cholesterol, 80.2 milligrams sodium.

CARROT CASSEROLE

1 c. carrot, peeled and shredded
1 c. potato, peeled and shredded
3/4 c. sweet potato, peeled and
  shredded
3 Tbsp chopped onion

1 1/2 c. cooked brown rice
1 tsp Mrs. Dash extra spicy
  seasoning
1/3 c. rice milk
1 Tbsp low sodium soy sauce

Preheat oven to 350 degrees, then bring 1 cup water to a boil and add vegetables; cook 5 minutes. Add 1/2 cup water to vegetables and add remaining ingredients; mix well. Pour into non-stick casserole dish (use non-stick spray) and bake for 30 minutes. Serves 4 to 6.

CORN ZUCCHINI CASSEROLE

2 (10 oz.) pkgs. kernel corn, defrosted
6 sm. zucchini, cut in 1/2 inch slices
4 ripe tomatoes, cut in 1/4 inch slices
2 onions, thinly sliced
2 cloves garlic, crushed

1 tsp red pepper, crushed
Juice of 1/2 lemon
4 low sodium bouillon cubes,
  melted

Place first 6 ingredients in a covered casserole. Sprinkle with lemon juice and mix together gently. Pour cubes over vegetables. Cover and bake in a preheated oven at 325 degrees for 45 minutes.

CREOLE CASSEROLE

1 med. size eggplant, peeled and
thickly sliced
2 1/2 c. tomato puree
2 c. water
1 1/2 c. thinly sliced mushrooms
1 1/2 c. coarsely chopped onions

1 c. green chili salsa
1 tsp Italian seasoning
1/2 tsp garlic powder
3 c. fresh or frozen okra, cut
into lg. pieces
1/3 c. whole wheat flour

1. Soak eggplant in cold water to cover for 30 minutes. Meanwhile, combine tomato puree, water, mushrooms, onions, salsa, Italian seasoning, and garlic powder in a large saucepan; bring to a boil. Reduce heat and simmer, uncovered, for 20 minutes. Add okra and cook for another 5 minutes; set aside.
2. Preheat oven to 350 degrees. Pat eggplant slices dry with paper towels. Dredge eggplant slices in flour. Place them on a baking sheet and bake for 10 minutes or until browned. Increase oven temperature to 375 degrees.
3. Line a 9 x 11 inch baking dish with eggplant slices and pour okra mixture over them. Bake for 30 minutes. Makes 8 servings.

EGGPLANT & PEPPER CAPONATA - Fast Weight Loss

1 sm. eggplant
1 red pepper or 1 (4 oz.) jar pimento
peppers or roasted peppers
1/4 c. salt free tomato paste
2 cloves garlic, minced
1/4 c. onion, finely chopped

1 stalk celery, finely chopped
2 Tbsp sweet basil
1 Tbsp Butter Buds
1/4 tsp cayenne pepper or
crushed red pepper
1/4 Tbsp red wine vinegar

With sharp knife, pierce whole eggplant several times and place half whole into baking dish. Cut red pepper in half; discard seeds. Place in pan with eggplant. Place in broiler, several inches away from fire, and broil 10 minutes or until eggplant and peppers are soft and charred on one side. May also be baked in 450 degree oven. Turn and broil or bake an additional 10 minutes until soft and charred.

In bowl or food processor, place the remaining ingredients, the eggplant, and peppers and any liquid from cooking. Process or mash with a fork until ingredients are blended but still chunky. Chill 1 hour before serving. Serve as a vegetable dip or on bread or crackers. Makes 2 cups (approximately).

GARDEN CASSEROLE - Fast Weight Loss

4 potatoes, peeled and sliced
1 zucchini, sliced
1 onion, sliced
2 carrots, sliced
2 tomatoes, cut in chunks

1 c. chicken broth
1/4 tsp pepper
1 tsp summer savory
Nutri Grain wheat flakes

Spread potatoes over the bottom of a 2 quart casserole. Separate the onion into rings and place them over the potatoes. Top these with the zucchini, then the carrots and then the tomatoes. Mix the broth, pepper and savory together. Pour over the casserole; cover and bake at 375 degrees for 1 hour. Sprinkle the wheat flakes over the top. Return to the oven and bake for another 15 minutes. Serves 4.

LENTIL CASSEROLE

1 c. lentils
2 c. water
1 c. chopped tomatoes
1 green pepper, chopped

1 clove garlic, minced
1 tsp chili powder
Dash of cayenne pepper

Bring lentils and water to a boil in saucepan. Reduce heat and simmer for 1 to 1 1/2 hours until tender. Add tomatoes, onion, garlic, chili powder, and cayenne. Place in a baking dish and bake, covered, for 20 minutes at 350 degrees. Serves 4 to 6.

RICE CASSEROLE OR STUFFING

2 c. brown rice
2 cloves garlic, minced
1 c. sliced celery
3 Tbsp chopped fresh basil or
   1Tbsp dried

1/2 c. chopped parsley or
   1 to 2 Tbsp dried
1 c. chopped onion
5 c. defatted chicken broth
1/2 c. pine nuts

Sauté rice in a skillet in a little chicken broth. Add onion and garlic. Sauté a little longer. Stir in chicken broth and celery. Bring to a boil. Reduce heat, cover, and simmer 40 minutes or until rice is tender. Toast pine nuts on a cookie sheet in the oven. Watch carefully as they burn easily. For a casserole, add pine nuts, basil, and parsley when casserole is about half done. For stuffing, add pine nuts, basil, and parsley when rice is done.

SPICY VEGERONI

1 (8 oz.) Vegeroni
1/4 lb. wheat meat
2 (16 oz.) cans tomato sauce
1 can Rosarita enchilada sauce
3 Tbsp raisins

1 onion, chopped
1/2 c. celery, chopped
1 tsp garlic powder
Liteline cheese (optional)

Cook Vegeroni and cook wheat meat. Directions on box. Then to wheat meat add tomato sauce, enchilada sauce, raisins, onion, celery, garlic powder, Vegeroni and Liteline cheese (optional).

SWEET PEA NOODLE CASSEROLE

8 oz. Seitan wheat meat
1 jar sweet peas, drained

1 can kidney beans, drained
1 pkg. whole wheat noodles

Bring 4 cups of water to boil; add noodles. Set aside from heat; let set for 20 minutes. Rinse and drain. In a large mixing bowl, combine all ingredients. Mix and pour into casserole dish. Bake at 400 degrees for 15 minutes.

SQUASH CASSEROLE

6 to 8 med. yellow squash, sliced
1 lg. onion chopped
3 stalks celery, diced
1/2 green bell pepper, diced

2 Tbsp water
1 (13 oz.) lite soy milk
1/2 c. unsalted matzo crumbs
1/4 tsp white pepper

Preheat oven to 350 degrees. Boil squash until tender, not mushy, and mash. Sauté onion, celery, and green pepper in 2 tablespoons water in a non-stick pan. Add to squash along with milk, matzo crumbs, and white pepper; mix well. Pour into a non-stick pan and sprinkle top with more matzo crumbs. Bake at 350 degrees for about 45 minutes. Serves 6 to 8.

VEGERONI CASSEROLE

1 1/2 lbs. vegeroni, cooked
2 onions, chopped
2 cloves garlic, minced
1 c. chopped carrot
1 c. chopped celery

1 c. chopped green pepper
1 lb. chopped mushrooms
1/2 tsp black pepper
5 c. tomato sauce

Pour vegeroni into baking dish sprayed with non-stick cooking spray. Combine remaining ingredients and pour over noodles. Bake, covered, in preheated 300 degree oven for 30 minutes. Bake, uncovered, for 10 minutes more. Serves 4 to 6.

VEG - RICE CASSEROLE

1 (20) oz. bag frozen corn
1 (20) oz. bag frozen peas
1 (20) oz. bag frozen broccoli
1 (24) oz. bag stew vegetables
   (carrots, onions, celery,
   and potatoes)

3 c. cooked brown rice
3 c. cream of mushroom soup
   (Hain Natural brand)
2 tsp garlic powder
2 Tbsp chopped onion (instant)

Place all ingredients in oblong baking dish and bake at 350 degrees for about 1 hour.

ZUCCHINI CASSEROLE - Fast Weight Loss

4 c. sliced zucchini
1 onion, thinly sliced
1 (4 oz.) jar chopped pimento

1 1/2 tsp oregano
1 tsp basil
1 (15 to 16 oz.) can tomato sauce

Slice the zucchini about 1/4 inch thick. Lay in the bottom of a medium sized oblong baking dish. Separate onion into rings and lay over zucchini. Next, spoon the pimento over the top of the onions and zucchini. Sprinkle herbs over this, then pour the tomato sauce over it all. Cover baking dish with foil and bake at 375 degrees for 30 minutes. Serves 6.

ARMENIAN STEW

1/4 c. dried garbanzo beans
1 1/2 c. dried apricots
5 c. chicken broth

1 c. lentils
3 red onions, sliced
2 Tbsp malt syrup

Soak the garbanzo beans overnight. Soak the dried apricots for 1 hour. In a large pan, bring the soaked apricots and their water to a boil. Add the soaked, drained garbanzo beans and 1 cup chicken broth. Bring to a boil; cook for 30 minutes. Add the lentils, onion, and 4 cups chicken broth to the pot. Bring to a boil. Lower heat, cover, and cook about 2 hours until garbanzos are tender. Add 2 tablespoons malt syrup and mix well. Serve over brown rice. Serves 8.

BARLEY STEW

1/3 c. each: Pinto beans, red beans, lentils, split peas, and black eyed peas
1/2 c. pearled barley
6 c. fresh water

1 (24 oz.) can V-8 juice Instead of Salt (Health Valley)
1 chopped onion
Any favorite vegetables
Garlic powder

Soak beans overnight, covering with 2 inches of water. Drain off and rinse next morning. Simmer in a large pot soaked beans, water, V-8 juice, garlic powder, and Instead of Salt. Simmer, covered, over a very low heat for 6 hours, then add onion and barley. Simmer 45 minutes, then add any vegetables. Simmer 30 more minutes. Serves 10.

BLACK - EYED PEA STEW

2 c. black-eyed peas, dry
1/2 c. onions
2 lg. tomatoes
1 tsp garlic powder

Dash of cinnamon
Salt (optional)
6 c. water
1/4 c. soy sauce

Soak black-eyed peas overnight. Cook black-eyed peas for 2 hours until tender soft. Add onions, tomatoes, soy sauce, garlic, and cinnamon. Simmer for 15 to 30 minutes to desired tenderness.

RAW "BARBECUED" STEW

VEGETABLES:

1 c. fresh corn kernels
1/2 lg. red bell pepper, diced
1/2 lg. green bell pepper, diced
1/4 c. chopped parsley
1 c. broccoli flowerettes

3 stalks celery, trimmed and chopped
1 c. sliced mushrooms
1 c. cubed zucchini

SAUCE:

1/4 med. onion, chopped
6 med. tomatoes, chopped
1 sm. clove garlic, pressed

2 tsp soy sauce or tamari
1/3 c. minced cilantro
1/4 tsp chili powder

GARNISH:

1 c. peeled and shredded banana squash   1 c. mixed salad greens

In a large bowl, combine vegetable ingredients. Set aside. Puree sauce ingredients in a food processor, using a metal "S" blade. Add puree to vegetable mixture and stir to combine. Arrange salad greens on 4 plates. Top with stew and garnish with banana squash. Serves 4. Per serving: 167 calories, 9 g protein, 1 g fat 35 g carbohydrates, 0 cholesterol, 255 mg sodium.

STEW - Fast Weight Loss

1 pressure cooker
4 potatoes, peeled and cubed
4 carrots, peeled and sliced
3 celery stalks, sliced

2 zucchini, sliced
6 oz. wheat meat (brand
   name, Seitan)
Dash of pepper

Combine all ingredients and 1 1/2 cups fresh water into pressure cooker. Put the lid and regulator on the pressure cooker and once the regulator starts rocking, cook for 10 minutes.

STEW FOR YOU

1 c. garbanzo beans, dry
1 c. kidney beans, dry
1 onion, sliced
1 clove garlic, crushed
1 tsp curry powder
3 carrots sliced

2 zucchini, sliced
2/c. whole wheat pasta, cooked
1/2 c. bulgur
2 c. fresh spinach, chopped
1 Tbsp lemon juice

Place beans in a large pot with 2 quarts water. Soak overnight or bring to a boil; cook for 2 minutes. Turn off heat and let rest for 1 hour. Then add onion, garlic and curry powder. Bring to a boil, reduce heat, and cook for 2 hours. When beans are almost tender, add carrots and zucchini. Cook for 30 minutes more, then add pasta and bulgur. Cook an additional 5 minutes. Serve immediately. Serves 6.

SUMMER STEW - Fast Weight Loss

2 onions, sliced
2 cloves garlic, crushed
6 sm. zucchini, sliced 1/2 inch thick
4 sm. yellow crookneck squash,
   sliced 1/2" thick
1 green pepper, coarsely chopped
2 c. snow peas, trimmed and left whole

3 c. tomato chunks
2 c. corn kernels
1 tsp basil
1 1/2 tsp dill weed
1 1/2 tsp paprika
3 Tbsp low-sodium soy sauce

Sauté onions and garlic in 1/2 cup water in a large saucepan. Cook until soft, about 5 minutes. Add both kinds of summer squash, green pepper, snow peas, and tomatoes; plus another 1/2 cup water. Cover and simmer over medium heat for 15 to 20 minutes. Stir occasionally. Add corn and seasonings. Simmer an additional 10 minutes. Mix 1 tablespoon cornstarch or arrow root in 1/4 cup cold water. Gradually add to stew while stirring. Cook and stir until thickened. Serve hot. Serves 6 to 8.

How to Look Great & Feel Sexy

SUCCOTASH

5 c. peeled, diced potatoes	2 c. diced fresh tomatoes
3 c. low sodium chicken stock, defatted	1 lg. clove garlic, minced
1 c. coarsely chopped onions	1 Tbsp low-sodium soy sauce
2 1/2 c. frozen corn kernels	1/2 tsp dried thyme
2 1/2 c. frozen baby lima beans	1/2 tsp poultry seasoning

1. Place potatoes, stock, and onions in a large pot. Bring to a boil and cook until potatoes are barely tender and almost all of the stock has been absorbed. If potatoes are cooked before all stock is absorbed, puree 1/3 of the vegetables and stock in a food processor or blender and return it to the pot; this will thicken the mixture.
2. Stir in corn, lima beans, tomatoes, garlic, soy sauce, thyme, and poultry seasoning, and cook for another 10 minutes or until frozen vegetables are heated through and flavors are well blended. Makes 10 servings.

BROWN GRAVY - NO OIL

7 Tbsp whole wheat flour	1 tsp minced dried onion
1/4 tsp onion powder	1 Tbsp salt-reduced tamari
1/8 tsp garlic powder	2 c. cold water

Combine flour and water. Stir until well blended. Cook over low heat until thickened, about 10 minutes. Add remaining ingredients. Continue to cook over low heat for 10 minutes, stirring occasionally. Great over vegetables, rice, or casserole dishes or stews. Makes 2 cups.

FAT - FREE GRAVY

6 Tbsp whole wheat flour	1/2 tsp poultry seasoning
2 1/2 c. defatted chicken broth	Pepper

In a saucepan, whisk flour, stock, and poultry seasoning until smooth. Cook, stirring constantly, over medium heat until gravy is thickened (about 10 minutes). Season with pepper. Great on mashed potatoes.

MUSHROOM GRAVY - Fast Weight Loss

1/2 c. onion, chopped
1 c. cooked mushroom pieces
1 Tbsp arrow root
1/2 tsp black pepper
1 c. water

1 Tbsp vegetable broth
  seasoning
Dash of Tabasco
1 Tbsp white wine

In a small saucepan, sauté onion in small amount of water. Dissolve broth seasoning and arrow root into cup of water. Add mushrooms to the onions. Cook gently until thickened, then add remaining ingredients. Serves 4. Use on vegetables, casseroles, or stews.

STUFFED ACORN SQUASH

1 sm. acorn squash, trimmed
  and halved
1 tart apple, sliced
1/2 tsp Butter Buds

1 Tbsp chopped pecans
1 Tbsp raisins halved
1/2 tsp cinnamon
1/3 c. apple juice concentrate

Preheat oven to 375 degrees. Place squash halves, cut side down, in a baking pan; add 1/2 inch of water. Cover pan. Bake 35 minutes or until tender. Sauté apple slices in Butter Buds in a non-stick skillet until soft. Add nuts, sauté 1 minute more. Add raisins and apple juice concentrate. Simmer until juice thickens, about 3 minutes. Add cinnamon.

Remove seeds and fiber from cooked squash. Scoop out flesh and add to apple mixture. Stir well; place back in squash shells. Return to oven, about 12 to 15 minutes. Serves 2.

AZUKI BEANS AND SQUASH

1 c. azuki beans
1 strip Erewhon Kombu 6 to 8
  inches long - seaweed
Spring water

1 c. buttercup squash or any
  squash, cubed but not peeled
Instead of Salt to taste

This makes a nice sweet dish for the autumn.
Wash the beans; cover them with water and soak for 6 to 8 hours. Put the kombu in the bottom of a pot and cover with the squash. Next, add the azuki beans. Add water to just cover the squash layer. Do not cover the beans at the beginning. Place the bean mixture over low heat and bring to a boil slowly. Cover after about 10 to 15 minutes. Cook until the beans are 70 to 80 percent done, about 1 hour or more. The water will evaporate as the beans expand, so add cold water occasionally to cover to keep the water level constant and make the beans soft. When the beans are 70 to 80 percent done, add the Instead of

Salt and cook until done and most of the liquid has evaporated another 15 to 30 minutes. Transfer to a serving bowl and serve.

Variation: This dish may also be pressure cooked. First pressure, cook the kombu and beans for 15 to 20 minutes. Bring down the pressure, uncover, and add the squash. Continue to cook without pressure until the beans are 70 to 80 percent done. This makes for a less bitter taste. Then season and continue to cook until done. If you add the squash at the beginning of pressure cooking, it will melt too much.

BAKED BUTTERNUT SQUASH AND ONIONS - Fast Weight Loss

3 c. butternut squash, cut into lg. chunks	1 strip Erewhon Kombu, about 6 inches long
2 c. spring water	1 c. onions, sliced
1 to 3 Tbsp Kikkoman lite soy sauce	2 to 3 Tbsp Erewhon Kuzu

Put the sliced squash in a baking dish. Add a few drops of water to squash to keep it moist. Cover baking dish and bake in preheated 350 degree oven for about 35 to 40 minutes or until it is almost done. Pour the water into a pot and add the onions and kombu. Bring to a boil. Reduce to simmer for about 15 minutes. Reduce the heat to very low. Remove the kombu from the pot.

BELL PEPPERS STUFFED WITH BARLEY

1 c. pearled barley	2 Tbsp chopped fresh mint or
6 med. green or red bell peppers	2 tsp dried
1/4 c. chopped onions	3/4 tsp ground cinnamon
1/2 c. raisins	2 Tbsp lemon juice
Pepper	

Cook barley in 6 to 8 cups boiling water for 30 minutes; it should be tender but still have some bite to it. Drain and reserve for later.

Preheat oven to 350 degrees.

Cut 1/2 inch slice off stem end of each bell pepper. Discard stem but chop up what pepper remains and reserve for later. Empty peppers of seeds and ribs.

Spray a large skillet with Pam or Baker's Joy; add onions and reserved chopped peppers. Stir fry for a couple of minutes. Add 1/2 cup water to the skillet, cover, and simmer over low heat for 10 minutes or until vegetables are tender.

Add to the skillet the cooked barley, raisins, mint, cinnamon, and lemon juice. Stir around for a minute or so and remove from heat. Season to taste with pepper.

Scoop the barley mixture into the hollowed-out pepper cases. Fit the peppers into a baking pan so that the peppers touch and help support each bother. Add about an inch of water to the pan. Cover and bake for 45 minutes to 1 hour or until tender. Makes 6 stuffed peppers. Serving size: 1/4 recipe - 193 calories, 77 grams fat, 0 cholesterol, 6 milligrams sodium.

BELL PEPPERS STUFFED WITH MUSHROOMS

3 lg. green peppers
1 1/2 c. tomatoes
1 c. fresh mushrooms
1 1/2 c. cooked lentils, seasoned with
herbs and drained

1 c. cooked brown rice
1/2 c. diced celery and onion
Dash of garlic powder
Dash of Mrs. Dash

Cut green peppers in half lengthwise. Parboil about 4 minutes. Sauté 1/2 cup diced celery and 1/3 cup diced onion in Teflon skillet (use Pam spray) until soft. Mix onion and celery with rest of ingredients. Season with a bit of black pepper. Stuff mix in green peppers. Bake 30 to 35 minutes in 350 degree oven or until green pepper as tender. Serve hot. Serves 6.

BELL PEPPERS STUFFED WITH RICE ITALIAN STYLE

2 lg. bell peppers
1 1/2 c. tomato sauce
2 c. cooked brown rice

2 Tbsp chopped parsley
1/2 tsp Italian seasoning

Cut peppers in half lengthwise; remove seeds and membranes. Steam pepper halves until cooked crisp-tender; set aside. Combine 1/2 cup tomato sauce with cooked brown rice, 1 tablespoon chopped parsley, and 1/2 teaspoon seasoning. Heat over moderate heat, stirring gently until well blended. Add a little water if need to prevent sticking. Spoon remaining tomato sauce into bottom of a 9 inch pie pan. Place pepper halves on top of sauce, then fill with rice mixture. Bake at 350 degrees until hot. Sprinkle with chopped parsley and serve. Serves 4.

FALAFELS

4 c. cooked garbanzos
4 egg whites
1 c. chopped onions
2 tsp parsley
1/2 tsp garlic powder

1/4 tsp basil
1/4 tsp pepper
3/4 c. matzo meal
1/4 c. potato pancake mix
1/2 c. water

Put garbanzos and water in a blender. Blend until smooth. Mix the garbanzos egg whites, onions, and spices in a large bowl. Add matzo meal and pancake mix. Form into small balls. Bake on a non-stick pan at 350 degrees for 15 to 20 minutes. Serve in pita bread with tomatoes, lettuce, onions, etc.

MACARONI NO - CHEESE

3 to 4 c. butternut squash, peeled
   and cubed
2 Tbsp tahini
2 Tbsp light miso
About 3 c. water
Pinch of salt and white pepper(optional)
2 c. elbow or spiral noodles

Water for boiling
1 c. or more fresh or frozen
   green peas,
   steamed (optional)
1/3 c. dry bread crumbs
1 to 2 tsp no-oil Italian dressing

Place squash in a pot; add water almost to cover. Cover pot and bring to a boil. Lower heat and simmer until squash is very soft, about 15 to 20 minutes. Drain. Place squash in blender or food processor. Add tahini, miso, and salt and pepper if desired. Puree until smooth.

Add noodles to a large pot of boiling water and cook until al dente. Drain and rinse. Combine noodles with puree and add peas, if desired. Place mixture in an oiled 9 inch square baking dish.

Preheat oven to 350 degrees. In a small bowl, mix bread crumbs with no oil Italian dressing. Sprinkle evenly over macaroni mixture. Bake for 20 minutes. Serve hot. Serves 6. Per serving: 184 calories, 6 g protein, 6 g fat, 29 g carbohydrates, 0 cholesterol, 283 mg sodium.

WHOLE WHEAT ALMOND NOODLES

Cook and drain 1 pound whole wheat noodles. Stir in 3/4 cup sliced, toasted blanched almonds. Put in serving dish and top with 1/4 cup toasted, whole wheat bread crumbs and an additional 1/4 cup sliced toasted blanched almonds. 4 servings.

LUNCH/SANDWICHES

Whole wheat pita bread stuffed with any kind of leftover. Warmed, rolled tortilla filled with California green chili.

Whole wheat bread, mustard, lettuce, and tomato sandwich.

Pita bread pizza - pita bread, covered first with spaghetti or tomato sauce and then with garlic powder, oregano, caraway seeds, and Lifetime cheese. Warmed in the oven or microwave.

Bread, mustard, ketchup lettuce, and tomato sprouts.

Bread, tomato, green chili, and cilantro.

SPECIAL SANDWICH

1 slice whole wheat toast	2 slices avocado
1 sliced red onion (raw)	2 slices tomato

Place onion, avocado, and tomato on top of whole wheat toast. Good substitute for a BLT sandwich.

HERBED WHEAT PILAF

1 3/4 c. vegetable stock	2 green onions, sliced
1 sm. carrot	1 bay leaf
1 med. stalk celery	1 c. raw bulgur wheat
1/2 green pepper	1 tsp vegetables seasoning
1/4 c. chopped mushrooms	

Dice carrot, celery, green pepper, and onions. Place small amount of liquid in a heavy pot with a close fitting lid. Add all the vegetables and the bay leaf; stir over medium heat for several minutes. Pour in stock; bring to a boil and simmer for 5 minutes, covered. Add wheat and seasoning and bring to a fast boil again. Cook, covered, over very low heat for 15 minutes. If too moist, uncover and simmer another few minutes until the liquid diminishes.

For special occasions, add 1 cup garden peas towards the end of the cooking time. Pilaf can be made with just about any grain. Try millet cracked wheat, rice or triticale in this dish, or a partial substitution of barley for any of these.

BROWN RICE

2 c. chicken stock	1 c. brown rice

Bring stock to a boil. Stir in rice and bring back to boil. Turn flame low, cover pot tightly, and cook for 40 minutes w/o lifting the lid. Add rice to vegetables, beans or soup.

BROWN RICE MUSHROOM RING

1 c. brown rice, cooked   1 Tbsp grated onion
1/2 lb. mushrooms, sliced   2 Tbsp parsley, chopped

Combine all ingredients, then spoon into a 1 quart ring mold (use non- stick spray) and set in a pan of hot water. Bake in a preheated 350 degree oven for 30 minutes. Turn out into a platter. Serves 4 to 6.

BROWN RICE WITH ZUCCHINI

1/4 c. Butter Buds   1 onion, chopped
2 zucchini, sliced   3 c. chicken broth
1/3 c. Molly McButter   Pepper to taste
     (optional) (cheese flavor)

Place Butter Buds and zucchini in saucepan and cook over medium heat, about 3 minutes, until zucchini begins to soften. Transfer to a bowl. Place broth and onion in saucepan; cook until tender (about 6 minutes). Add rice and cover; cook until liquid is absorbed, about 40 minutes. Season with pepper. Add zucchini and cheese flavor; mix well. 2 servings.

CORN AND BROWN RICE STIR - FRY

1 lg. can corn, drained   2 Tbsp soy sauce (low sodium)
1/4 c. water   1/2 c. chopped green onion
4 c. brown rice

Place corn in skillet sprayed with non-stick coating. Sauté for 4 to 5 minutes. Add water, rice, and soy sauce. Continue cooking, stirring frequently until liquid has evaporated. Remove from heat and add green onion. Serves 4.

CRUNCHY RICE AND PEAS

1 c. leftover rice, cooked and chilled   Garlic powder and salt
3/4 c. frozen peas   1/2 c. chicken broth
4 oz. can water chestnuts, sliced

Add peas, water chestnuts, and seasonings; stir fry over high heat with chicken broth. Toss in rice and heat thoroughly. Makes 2 servings. 1 cup serving provides 151 calories, 85% carbohydrates, 14% protein, and 1% fat.

CURRIED LENTILS AND BROWN RICE

2 c. lentils, cooked
2 c. brown rice, cooked
2 tsp curry

1 tsp garlic powder
1/2 tsp parsley
Water

Add the ingredients together with enough water to cover. Simmer for about 15 minutes. It's ready to eat.

FRUIT - RICE STUFFING

3/4 c. Butter Buds
1 1/2 c. chopped onion
1 1/2 c. chopped celery
1/2 c. chopped parsley
7 c. cooked brown rice
1 tsp marjoram
1/2 c. chopped nuts
1/2 tsp thyme

1/2 tsp sage
Salt and pepper
3 egg whites, lightly beaten
3/4 c. turkey stock or chicken
bouillon
6 oz. mixed dried fruit
1/2 c. raisins

Sauté onions, celery, and parsley in Butter Buds. Remove from heat and combine with rice in large bowl. Stir in marjoram, thyme, and sage. Season to taste with salt and pepper. Add egg whites, stock, fruit, and nuts. Mix well. Makes enough stuffing for a 10 to 12 pound turkey or 6 side dishes.

INDIAN SPICE RICE

2 c. cooked brown rice
1 c. chopped onion
1 1/2 c. chopped celery
1 c. frozen green peas, thawed
    and rinsed to separate

2 Tbsp chopped mint leaves
1 Tbsp onion powder
1 tsp curry powder
1/2 c. orange juice

Sauté onion and celery in non-stick pan (use non-stick spray) for about 3 to 5 minutes on low heat. Add orange juice and continue cooling until liquid is almost evaporated. Stir in mint leaves, onion, and curry. powder, and blend to combine flavors. Stir in the rice and peas and heat through. Serves 4 to 5.

NICK'S SPICY BROWN RICE & NOODLES

2 c. brown rice
1/4 c. lentils
1/2 c. whole wheat noodles
1 clove garlic, minced

Onion powder
6 c. chicken broth
1/2 c. Pace Picante Chili
   Salsa(med. or mild)

Mix all ingredients, except chili salsa and cook in a large, covered pan for 40 minutes. Add the chili salsa; cover pan again and let sit for 20 minutes without heat. Ready to eat.

QUICK BROWN RICE - Microwave

1 1/4 c. chicken broth
1 c. brown rice

1/2 c. green bell pepper, diced
1/2 c. chopped onions

Place chicken broth in a 2 quart microwave dish. Cover tightly. Microwave on high for 4 minutes. Stir in rice, bell pepper, and green onions. Recover. Adjust power level to medium. Microwave 10 to 15 minutes or until rice is tender and water is absorbed. Fluff with a fork. 6 servings.

RAINBOW RICE

2 c. cooked brown rice
1 onion chopped
1 green bell pepper, finely chopped
2 c. whole kernel corn
1 (4 oz.) jar pimento, chopped

1 tsp oregano
1/2 tsp paprika
1/2 tsp soy sauce (low-sodium)
1 c. green peas

In a large skillet, sauté onion and green pepper (use non-stick spray) until vegetables are crisp-tender. Add next 5 ingredients, cooking for another 5 minutes, then add green peas and rice and heat through for about 5 minutes until done. Serves 4 to 6.

RED BEANS AND RICE, CAJUN STYLE

1/2 lb. dry red beans (kidney beans)
7 c. vegetable stock
1 lg. yellow onion, chopped
1 lg. green pepper, chopped
1 1/2 c. chopped celery
Salt to taste (optional)

2 bay leaves
1 Tbsp Cajun seasoning
4 c. hot cooked rice
Freshly ground pepper
2 cloves garlic, minced

This is a hearty dish. Serves 8.

Cover beans with cold water and soak overnight. Drain the beans. In a large soup pot, heat vegetable stock. Add the beans, onion, green pepper celery, garlic, bay leaves, and Cajun seasoning. Bring to a boil, reduce heat, cover, and simmer for 1 hour.

Continue cooking the beans until they become tender. Watch the pot carefully to prevent scorching of beans. Add more water to the pot as needed. When beans are tender, remove bay leaves, salt to taste, and serve by ladling a portion of red beans over 1/2 cup hot cooked rice in a large bowl. Pepper to taste. Each serving: 281 calories.

RICE PILAF WITH ALMONDS

1/2 c. Butter Buds
1/4 c. minced onion
1/2 c. chopped blanched almonds

1 c. raw brown rice
Pepper to taste
2 c. hot chicken broth

Heat Butter Buds in saucepan. Add onion and sauté until onion is transparent. Do not let it brown. Add almonds and sauté for 1 to 2 minutes or until barely golden. Add rice and sauté until rice is transparent, stirring constantly. Add hot broth all at once, mixture will sizzle. Cover tightly. Simmer on low heat for 30 to 40 minutes or until rice is tender. Season with pepper. 4 servings.

SAFFRON RICE

1/2 tsp crushed saffron threads
3 Tbsp water
1 Tbsp Butter Buds
1/3 c. currants or raisins
1/4 c. shelled, chopped pistachios
    or pine nuts

3 c. chicken stock or water
1 Tbsp Veg-It
Lg. pinch of cinnamon
1 1/2 c. long grain brown or
    basmati rice

Dissolve the saffron in water. Melt the Butter Buds in a medium large saucepan and add the currants, nuts, and rice. Stir over low heat for several minutes, then add the stock or water and dissolved saffron. Stir once, raise the heat, and bring to a boil, then lower heat, cover, and simmer for 35 minutes or until steamed. Serves 6 to 8.

STUFFED ARTICHOKES

4 whole fresh artichokes
1/4 c. lemon juice
2 pepper corns
4 whole cloves
2 slices toasted whole wheat bread

1 c. chopped mushrooms
1 onion, diced
2 Tbsp chopped parsley
1/2 tsp garlic powder

Cut stem from artichokes and trim points from leaves. In a skillet, roll artichokes in lemon juice then place in a pan upright. Add about an inch of water and place peppercorns and garlic in the water. Crumble toast as fine as possible and add rest of ingredients. With a spoon, sprinkle this mixture among the leaves, use small amounts in each place. Cover and cook over a low heat for 30 minutes or until done. Serves 4.

BAKED ASPARAGUS

3 Tbsp bread crumbs
1/2 c. Butter Buds
1/2 c. chicken broth, defatted

Dash of nutmeg
1 lb. asparagus, boiled

In a small saucepan, simmer bread crumbs, Butter Buds, chicken broth, and nutmeg for about 5 minutes. Arrange cooked asparagus in a casserole dish. Pour sauce over asparagus. Bake at 350 degrees for 30 minutes. Serves 3.

BAKED BEANS

1 c. finely chopped celery
2 c. cooked pinto beans
1 med. chopped onion
1/2 c. spaghetti sauce (no oil or salt)

1/4 c. water
1 Tbsp unfiltered apple juice
1 Tbsp honey

Mix all ingredients in a 2 quart casserole; cover and bake 45 minutes at 350 degrees. Serves 8 to 10.

GARBANZO MEDLEY

1/2 c. uncooked brown rice
1 (15 oz.) can garbanzo beans
1 green pepper, chopped
2 onions, sliced
1 eggplant, chopped

3 (15 oz.) cans tomatoes
4 stalks celery, topped
2 carrots, diced
3 Tbsp Italian seasoning
Pepper to taste

Combine all ingredients in pot and brine to a boil. Cover and simmer until rice is tender, about 1 hour. Makes 6 cups.

KIDNEY BEANS

1 1/2 tsp Erewhon Miso per c. of
beans, preferably barley miso
Spring water

1 strip Erewhon Kombu,
6 to 8 inches long
1 c. kidney beans

Wash and soak the beans for 6 to 8 hours. Put the kombu in the bottom of a heavy pot. Set the beans on top of the kombu and add water to just cover the beans. Bring to a boil. Reduce the heat to medium-low and cover. Simmer until the beans are about 80 percent done, or about 1 hour. Add cold water following the basic shocking method as needed. When the beans are 80% done, add the pureed miso. (Barley miso is best to use with this dish.) Just add the miso on top of the beans and do not mix in. The miso will filter down into the beans as they continue to cook. Continue to cook until the beans are soft and creamy, another 20 to 30 minutes. Transfer to a serving bowl and serve.

Variation: Pressure cook the beans for 45 minutes. Then add the pureed miso and cook, not under pressure, about 20 to 30 minutes longer.

MUNG DALE

* 1 c. mung beans
7 c. water
1 c. chopped tomatoes
1 med. zucchini, peeled and chopped
   in 1 inch cubes
1/2 Tbsp minced ginger
1 1/2 Tbsp cumin seeds
1 Tbsp black mustard seeds

1 green chili, minced
1/4 tsp hing
1 1/2 tsp turmeric
1 Tbsp salt
Fresh coriander leaves for
   garnish
Pam spray

*Mung beans are split yellow mung beans which can be purchased at all Indian grocery stores. If they are not available to you, you may use green split peas or yellow split peas with this same recipe.

In 1 gallon saucepan, spray with Pam. Add turmeric, hing, and beans. Fry for 30 seconds on medium heat. Add vegetables and fry for 1 more minute. Add water, salt, fresh chili, and diced ginger. Bring to a boil over high heat, then cover, lower heat, and let Dal simmer for 1 hour or until the beans have dissolved into a thick soup. Set aside.

In small skillet, spray with Pam. When hot, add cumin seeds and black mustard seeds. When the seeds start to crackle, pour the mixture into the pot of Dal. Garnish with fresh coriander leaves or parsley. Serve hot. Serves 6.

PINTO BEANS

4 to 5 c. dry pinto beans
Water to cover beans

1 to 2 Tbsp vinegar

In a large pot, combine above ingredients and boil for 5 minutes. Drain the water and refill with fresh water and more vinegar. Let beans soak on stove for about 1 hour (no heat). After beans have soaked and expanded, drain beans again and refill with fresh water.

Add to beans:

1 onion, chopped
1 clove garlic, minced
2 Tbsp onion powder

1 Tbsp garlic powder
1/4 c. chili salsa
1 chunk fresh ginger

Cook beans, adding water when needed, for about 4 to 5 hours.

SAUTEED BEAN SPROUTS - Fast Weight Loss

6 c. bean sprouts   1 c. chopped green onions
3 carrots, shredded   6 tsp water

Put water in a non-stick skillet and heat. Gently stir in carrots and onions; cook, stirring, until carrots are tender but not soft. Mix in bean sprouts and cook, uncovered, over high heat, stirring until bean sprouts are hot. Serves 5 to 6.

BROCCOLI IN CURRY SAUCE - Fast Weight Loss

1 bunch fresh broccoli,   1/8 tsp dry mustard
  sliced lengthwise   2 tsp unsweetened apple juice
1 c. chicken broth, defatted   1 Tbsp cornstarch
1/3 tsp curry powder

Cook broccoli until tender. Bring broth to a boil and add cornstarch (dissolve in small amount of water before adding to broth); stir constantly until mixture thickens and clears. Add remaining ingredients and cook for 1 minute; pour over broccoli and serve. Serves 4.

CABBAGE PLATE - Fast Weight Loss

3 c. coarsely chopped cabbage   1/2 c. apple juice (unsweetened)
2 c. sliced carrots   2 tsp lemon pepper
1 c. chopped celery   (or Instead of Salt)
1/4 c. hot water

Combine vegetables. Add apple juice, lemon pepper, and water. Cook in covered pot until just tender, 10 to 15 minutes. Makes 8 servings.

CABBAGE ROLLS

1 med. head cabbage   1 1/2 c. brown rice, cooked
1/2 c. chopped onion   1 c. tomato sauce
1/2 c. chopped celery   1/4 tsp sage
1/4 c. water   1/4 tsp garlic powder
1/2 c. chopped green bell pepper

Steam cabbage until leaves can be removed. Simmer vegetables in water until nearly tender. Mix cooked rice, seasonings and vegetables. Place 1/2 cup mix in cabbage leaf and roll. Place in baking dish with tomato sauce and water mixed; pour over rolls. Bake at 350 degrees for 45 minutes, covered until last few minutes. Serves 4.

HERBED CABBAGE - Fast Weight Loss

1 med. onion, thinly sliced	1/2 tsp oregano, crushed
1 c. cabbage, shredded	1/2 tsp dill weed
1 c. carrots, shredded	1 tsp water

In a non-stick skillet, sauté onion in water for 5 minutes. Stir in cabbage and carrots. Cover and cook over medium heat 8 minutes more. Stir in oregano and dill weed. Serves 4.

SPICED RED CABBAGE - Fast Weight Loss

3 1/2 c. shredded red cabbage	1/8 tsp ground nutmeg
1/4 c. cider vinegar	2 tart apples, peeled, cored,
1/2 c. water	and diced
1/4 tsp ground cinnamon	1/4 Tbsp sugar
1/4 tsp ground allspice	

In a saucepan, combine with all other ingredients, except apples. Cover and cook over moderate heat for 15 minutes, tossing several times so the cabbage will cook evenly. Add apples, then cover and cook 5 minutes longer. Add sugar. When dish is done, all water should have cooked away. Serves 6.

STUFFED CABBAGE

12 lg. cabbage leaves, prepared
    for stuffing

FILLING:

2 c. cooked brown rice	1/4 tsp cayenne
3/4 c. mushrooms	1/4 c. almonds, sliced
2 egg whites	2 green onions, chopped

SAUCE:

2 c. tomato juice	1 stalk celery, sliced
4 slices onion	1/2 c. green pepper strips

To prepare filling, mix rice, egg whites, and seasonings until evenly blended. Place a small mound of filling, about 3 tablespoons, on each cabbage leaf and roll into bundles.

To prepare sauce, combine broth, onion, celery, and green pepper in a 15 inch skillet. Bring to a boil. Place cabbage rolls in sauce, cover, and with heat very low simmer for 30 minutes. Spoon sauce over cabbage once or twice during cooking. Makes 12 rolls.

To prepare cabbage leaves for stuffing, boil in water until soft.

SWEET - SOUR CABBAGE ROLLS

1 lg. cabbage, cored

SAUCE:

2 onions chopped
1 (28 oz.) can tomatoes
1 (8 oz.) can tomato juice
1/2 c. lemon juice
1/2 c. raisins

1/4 c. frozen apple juice
  concentrate
1 Tbsp soy sauce
1/4 tsp cayenne pepper

FILLING:

1/2 c. cooked brown rice
1 Tbsp soy sauce
1 Tbsp ground coriander
1 tsp dill weed
1/4 tsp fennel seed, ground in
  blender
1 1/2 c. chopped onion

2 c. peeled potatoes, diced
  med. fine
1 1/2 c. chopped celery
1/2 c. chopped green bell
  pepper
2 egg whites, fork beaten

Set the cabbage, cored side down, in a steamer over boiling water covered, for about 10 minutes or until leaves are soft. Let cool and separate leaves. Prepare sauce by sautéing the onions in 1/2 cup boiling water in a large skillet. Cook, stirring frequently, until the water has evaporated and the onions are slightly browned. Stir in the other ingredients; bring to a boil, reduce heat, and simmer (covered) for about 10 minutes.

Prepare filling by spreading rice in a baking pan and place in a 400 degree oven for about 10 minutes to toast, stirring occasionally so the rice brown evenly. Bring 2 1/2 cups water to a boil in a saucepan. Stir in soy sauce, spices, and rice. Return to a boil then reduce heat to low, cover tightly, and cook for 40 to 45 minutes. Keep covered for an additional 10 minutes to allow rice to fluff from steam. Combine the rice, potatoes vegetables, and egg whites, mixing well. Fill the rolls and bake in a covered dish for an hour and 15 minutes at 350 degrees. Makes 12 rolls.

INDIAN - STYLE CARROTS - Fast Weight Loss

4 med. sized carrots
1 c. chicken stock (homemade or
   canned no salt added)
3 Tbsp apple juice
1 tsp Butter Buds

1/2 tsp cumin
1/2 tsp mint
Dash of cayenne pepper
Dash of cinnamon

Peel or scrape carrots. Cut in medium sized rounds (1/4 inch). Heat chicken stock in saucepan to boil. Add carrots; reduce heat to light boil. Cook until about 3/4 of the stock is boiled away. Add sweetener and spices. Cook, stirring occasionally, until carrots begin to glaze. Remove from heat; serve hot or cold.

CARROT SOUFFLE FOR ONE - Fast Weight Loss

1 (4 oz.) jar pureed carrots(use
   Gerber's brand or other baby
   food without salt or sugar added)

1/4 c. minced onion or shallots
1/2 c. thinly sliced mushrooms
1 egg white

SUGGESTED SPICES:
1/4 tsp sage
1/4 tsp nutmeg

1 Tbsp parsley

Sauté onions (or shallots) with spices in chicken stock. Sauté mushrooms separately and place them in the bottom of a soufflé or oven-proof dish. Mix carrot puree into sautéed onion and spices. Whip egg white into soft peaks and fold in the carrot mixture. Pile this mixture on top of the mushrooms. Bake for 20 minutes or until lightly browned on top at 350 degrees. Garnish with parsley. Note: Mushrooms may be mixed in with the carrot mixture, if preferred.

SWEET CARROTS

1 (4 oz.) can frozen apple or orange
   juice concentrate
2 oz. water

8 lg. carrots, sliced
1/2 tsp cinnamon

Place juice and water in a medium saucepan. Heat slowly until defrosted. Add carrots and cinnamon. Cook on medium heat until tender, about 10 to 15 minutes. Serves 8.

Main Dishes: Casseroles, Stews, Veggies, Etc.   323

CAULIFLOWER CURRY

1 head cauliflower, cut into
   1 inch pieces
2 onions, chopped fine
1/2 c. lentils

1/2 tsp chili powder
1 tsp curry powder
Juice of 1 lemon

Sauté onion in small amount of water 5 minutes. Add cauliflower, lentils, and spices. Add cup of water and cook until cauliflower is tender on low flame. Add lemon juice. Serves 4.

CORN BREAD STUFFING

3 c. crumbled cornbread
1 c. whole wheat bread crumbs
2 c. chicken broth, defatted
4 stalks celery, finely chopped

1 onion, chopped
2 egg whites
1/2 tsp poultry seasoning
Ground pepper to taste

Combine all ingredients in a large bowl and mix well. May be baked at 350 degrees for 40 minutes in a non-stick baking dish.

CORN - ON - THE - COB

4 ears of corn
Water

Butter Buds
Garlic powder

Remove the husks from corn and place husks in the bottom of a 4 quart pan. Add about 1 inch of water. Remove silky threads from cobs and rinse. Place cobs in pan. Cover tightly and steam for 15 minutes. Remove from pan and dip in Butter Buds and sprinkle with garlic powder. 4 servings.

DAL

1 c. lentils
2 Tbsp fresh grated ginger
1/4 tsp ground turmeric
1/4 tsp cayenne pepper
1/2 tsp cumin
2 Tbsp fresh cilantro

Pinch of cardamom
1 qt. chicken stock
   (homemade or canned,
    no salt added)
Lemon juice

Rinse the lentils and combine them in a medium sized saucepan with the stock. Bring the stock to a boil, then lower the heat and simmer for 1 hour. Add spices, continue to cook briefly and serve with fresh, whole wheat chapati.

DILLED GARDEN BEANS - Fast Weight Loss

2 beef bouillon cubes
1 c. water
2 Tbsp chopped onion
1/2 c. chopped green pepper

1/2 tsp dill seed
1 (20 oz.) pkg. frozen French
    cut green beans

In a saucepan, dissolve bouillon cubes in water over a medium heat. Add next 3 ingredients and cook several minutes. Add beans and cook, covered, 8 to 10 minutes until beans are just tender. Serves 6.

FANCY GREEN BEANS - Fast Weight Loss

1 (20 oz.) pkg. French cut green
1 c. sliced mushrooms beans

2 (5 oz.) cans water chestnuts,
    drained and sliced

Cook beans according to directions; add water chestnuts and cooked mushrooms. Season with pepper to taste.

LOUISIANA GREEN BEANS - Fast Weight Loss

1 lb. fresh green beans
2 c. tomatoes, diced
1/2 c. chopped celery

1/4 c. chopped green bell
    pepper
1/2 tsp onion powder

Cook beans until tender, then add remaining ingredients and cook over medium heat until cooked through, about 15 minutes. Serves 8.

GREEN BEANS ALMONDINE - Fast Weight Loss

3 c. fresh green beans, chopped
10 mushrooms
1 med. red onion
1 clove garlic

1 packet Butter Buds
1/2 c. hot water
2 Tbsp wine (white)

Dissolve Butter Buds in water and heat in skillet along with wine. Sauté onions and garlic until soft. Add green beans and mushrooms; simmer until soft.

GREEN BEANS OREGANO - Fast Weight Loss

1 (10 oz.) pkg. French cut green beans
1 tomato, diced
1/2 c. celery, diced
1/2 c. green bell pepper, diced

3 Tbsp onion, chopped
1/2 tsp dried oregano
1/3 c. water
Lemon wedges

Combine all ingredients in saucepan and bring to a boil. Reduce heat and simmer, covered, for 6 to 8 minutes or until beans are done. Garnish with lemon wedges. Serves 4.

SCANDINAVIAN GREEN BEANS - Fast Weight Loss

1 lb. fresh tender green beans
1 Tbsp low sodium vegetable
    seasoning
1 Tbsp low-sodium Dijon or
    champagne mustard

2 Tbsp fresh dill weed, minced
3 Tbsp rice milk
1 Tbsp red wine vinegar or
    apple cider vinegar

Prepare green beans; snap off stems and cut if needed. Steam in vegetable steamer until tender. Toss with seasonings and serve.

SPANISH GREEN BEANS - Fast Weight Loss

4 c. cooked green beans
1 onion, chopped

1/2 c. tomato puree
Pepper to taste

Brown onion in water until golden. Add rest of ingredients. Mix and heat through. Serves 6 to 8.

LIMA BEANS, PEARL ONIONS, & CARROTS

1/2 c. Butter Buds liquid
1 clove garlic, crushed
1 (16 oz.) bag frozen pearl onions

3 carrots, sliced
3 (10 oz.) bags frozen
    lima beans

Sauté garlic in Butter Buds. Add carrots and onions. Let simmer a few minutes. Add lima beans and simmer until all vegetables are tender.

BREADED EGGPLANT

1 green bell pepper, chopped	4 slices whole grain bread,
1 onion chopped	crumbled
2 Tbsp tomato paste	8 (1/4 inch thick) sliced
2 egg whites	eggplant
2 tsp oregano	2 tomatoes, sliced thin
2 tsp basil	

In blender, blend first 6 ingredients. Pour this mixture over bread crumbs in a large bowl. Mix thoroughly, then arrange eggplant slices on a non-stick cookie sheet (use non-stick spray). Top with bread mixture. Bake at 350 degrees for 30 minutes. Top with fresh tomato slices before serving. Serves 2.

DELGADO GADO

2 lg. potatoes boiled and sliced	1 c. cauliflower flowerettes
1 c. carrots, sliced into 1/4 inch pieces	1 c. sliced cabbage
1 c. fresh green beans, sliced into	1/4 lb. bean sprouts
1 inch pieces	1 cucumber, sliced

SAUCE:

3/4 c. pecans	1 tsp ground ginger
3/4 c. almonds	1/4 tsp ground cumin
1/4 c. chopped onion	1 1/2 c. coconut milk
4 garlic cloves, minced	3 Tbsp fresh lemon juice
2 tsp crushed red pepper	4 Tbsp soy sauce

Blanch beans, carrots, cabbage, and cauliflower separately in water for 3 minutes each. Drain vegetables and arrange on platter. Top with bean sprouts and surround with cucumber and potato slices. Serve from platter topping each plate with sauce.

To make sauce, place nuts in food processor and mix to paste. In a saucepan, add onion and garlic; sauté about 1 minute. Add coconut milk, peppers, ginger, cumin, lemon juice, and soy sauce; bring to a boll. Add nuts and cook until sauce is thickened, about 5 minutes.

TOMATO KALE

1 1/2 bunches kale (1 to 2 lbs.)
1 sm. onion
1 clove garlic
1 tsp cumin seeds or ground cumin

1/2 c. tomato paste
1 c. tomatoes, chopped
1/2 c. peas
Salt (if needed)

Wash kale; strip off stems and chop. You should have 12 cups, more or less. Steam until tender and drain.

Meantime, sauté onion (and garlic, if desired,) in non-stick pan with water as needed, adding cumin when onion is soft. Continue to cook a moment more until the cumin is fragrant. Add the tomato paste and tomatoes; stir to heat through. Add peas, cooking until tender, then add kale. If you have used canned tomatoes or frozen peas, you may not need to add more salt; check and adjust salt to taste. Makes about 4 cups.

Variation: Instead of peas, add a cup of cubed steamed potato or winter squash.

BLACKEYED PEAS - INDIAN STYLE

1 c. dried black eyed peas
1 sliced carrot
1/4 tsp turmeric
1/2 tsp shredded ginger (keep fresh
   ginger root in freezer until
   ready for use)
1 chopped onion

2 Tbsp coconut
1/4 tsp cumin
1 tsp S & B Sun Bird
   oriental curry powder
   (a combo of spices)
1 tsp honey or waffle syrup
3 c. water

Add all ingredients to boiling water and simmer until liquid is absorbed and peas are tender. Makes 4 servings.

BLACK - EYED PEAS SOUTHERN STYLE

1 c. black eyed peas
1 med. onion, chopped
2 cloves garlic, minced
1 green bell pepper, chopped
1 red bell pepper, chopped
2 c. (1 lg. can) whole tomatoes, chopped

3 Tbsp Butter Buds
1 Tbsp Worcestershire sauce
1 Tbsp chili powder
1/4 tsp ground cumin
Pepper to taste

Wash black-eyed peas; cover with water (4 cups) and soak overnight (or bring to boil - boil 3 minutes and let stand 1 hour). Drain and throw away soak water. Cover peas with fresh water and boil gently until tender. Drain. While peas are cooking, sauté onion, peppers, and garlic in Butter Buds for 5 minutes. Add tomatoes and seasonings; simmer 3/4 to 1 hour. Combine with black-eyed peas and reheat.

SPLIT PEA PUDDING

1 lb. green split peas	1 tsp dried spices or herbs
1 carrot, chopped fine	according to your taste as
1 onion, chopped fine	marjoram, thyme, mint,
1 celery stalk, chopped fine	dill, and/or parsley
2 egg whites	Pepper

Place peas, carrot, onion, and celery in a large pot. Cover with 8 cups water. Bring to a boil; cut back to a simmer and cook gently, covered, for 45 minutes. Preheat oven to 350 degrees.

Drain peas through a colander, reserving liquid for another soup if you wish. Puree peas and vegetables in a food processor, blender, or food mill and blend in egg whites. Add herbs or spices and pepper according to taste. This dish can be eaten hot or cold. Bake in 6 cup baking pan for 45 minutes. Serving size: 1/8 recipe. 77 calories, 3 grams fat, 0 cholesterol, 21 milligrams sodium.

BAKED POTATO - Fast Weight Loss

Microwave potato, covered by glass Pyrex bowl. A plain baked potato can be a delicious snack. As topping use chili salsa, barbecue sauce, ketchup (not sugar), or Butter Buds.

BAKED STUFFED POTATOES - Microwave

4 baking potatoes, scrubbed, pierced	1 pkg. Butter Buds, prepared
1/2 c. frozen peas	1/8 tsp white pepper
1/3 c. chopped green onions	

Place a paper towel in bottom of microwave oven. Arrange potatoes in a circle on paper towel. Microwave on full power 9 to 11 minutes or until potatoes give slightly when squeezed. Cool. Cut in 1/2 lengthwise. Scoop pulp from each potato half, leaving a 1/4 inch thick shell, into a medium bowl, set shells aside. Mash potato pulp. Stir in peas green onions, Butter Buds, and pepper. Spoon potato mixture into shells. Arrange stuffed potatoes on a plate. Microwave on full power 3 minutes. Sprinkle with paprika. 8 servings.

SCALLOPED POTATOES

5 potatoes, peeled and sliced
1 onion, chopped
1/4 tsp paprika
1/4 c. whole wheat flour

1/4 tsp pepper
1/4 tsp dill weed
1/2 c. ground nuts
1 c. water

Layer the potatoes and onions in a large casserole dish. Sprinkle with paprika, flour, pepper, and dill weed. Mix ground nuts an water together. Pour over potatoes and onions. Bake at 375 degrees, covered, for 1 hour.

MASHED POTATOES - Fast Weight Loss

4 med. potatoes, peeled and cut
   into lg. chunks
1 med. onion., chopped
2 cloves garlic, crushed

2 Tbsp parsley flakes
1/2 tsp basil
1/2 tsp thyme

Place potatoes, onions, garlic, and spices in a large saucepan. Add water to; cover. Bring to a boil. Cover and cook over medium heat until done, about 30 minutes. Drain and reserve the cooking liquid. Add 1 cup hot cooking liquid back to the pot. Beat the cooked vegetables with electric mixer until smooth. Serve with gravy or sauce. Serves 4.

NEW POTATOES AND BEANS

1 lb new potatoes, sliced
   1/4 inch slices
1/4 c. julienne green pepper
   (1 1/2 x 1/4inch strips)
1/4 c. julienne red pepper
   (1 1/2 x 1/4 inch strips)
1/4 c. chopped onion
2 Tbsp defatted chicken broth

1 lg. clove garlic, minced
1/4 tsp dried rosemary
   leaves, crushed
2 Tbsp snipped fresh parsley
1 (16 oz.) can Great Northern
   beans or kidney beans,
   rinsed and drained

In 2 quart casserole, combine all ingredients, except beans. Cover Microwave at high for 10 to 14 minutes or until potatoes are tender, stirring once. Add beans; mix well. Microwave at high for 1 1/2 to 2 minutes or until beans are hot. 8 servings. Per serving: 107 calories, 4 g protein, 19 g carbohydrates, 2 g fat, 4 mg. sodium, 3 g fiber.

How to Look Great & Feel Sexy

POTATO AND CABBAGE VEGETABLE - Fast Weight Loss

1 cabbage, sliced very thin	1 Tbsp coriander powder
3 lg. potatoes, cut in 1/2 inch cubes	1 tsp salt
1 sm. jalapeno chili, diced finely	1 sm. slice lemon
1 Tbsp black mustard seeds	Pam spray
1/4 tsp turmeric	

In pan, heat Pam spray, mustard seeds, chili, and turmeric. When mustard seeds start to crackle, add potatoes. Stir for 8 minutes on medium heat. Add cabbage and cook for 15 more minutes until cabbage and potatoes are both tender. Add salt and coriander powder. Sprinkle with lemon juice. Serve hot. Serves 4.

POTATOES IN MUSHROOM - TOMATO SAUCE

6 potatoes	1/2 c. celery chopped
1 1/2 c. defatted chicken stock	3 cloves garlic, minced
1 lg. onion, chopped	1 Tbsp soy sauce (low sodium)
1 c. mushrooms, chopped	1/4 tsp cayenne pepper
1/2 c. green bell pepper, chopped	1 (16 oz.) can tomatoes in juice

Place potatoes in pot of boiling water and cook for 25 minutes over moderate heat until partially done. Remove from pot and cool briefly; peel and halve lengthwise. Bring stock to a boil in a large skillet, then add onion, mushrooms, green pepper, celery, and garlic. Cook vegetables over moderate heat for 5 minutes, stirring occasionally. Add soy sauce and pepper. Cover and simmer for 5 minutes, stirring if needed. Stir in tomatoes. Bring the sauce to a boil, then lower heat. Place in pan and simmer for 15 minutes until potatoes are tender. Stir occasionally. Serves 6.

POTATO PANCAKES I - Fast Weight Loss

2 lbs. baking potatoes, peeled and cut	2 egg whites
1 inch pieces	Pepper to taste
1 c. minced onions	Applesauce
2 Tbsp whole wheat flour	

Finely chop potatoes in processor until pulpy. Do not puree. Transfer to large bowl. Mix in onions. Let stand until water forms at bottom of bowl, about 10 minutes. Drain potatoes and onions through fine sieve, pressing down to extract all liquid. Stir 2 tablespoons flour and egg whites into potato mixture. Season with pepper. Form into patties and place in non-stick skillet. Cook until potatoes are brown, 1 to 1 1/2 minutes. Turn and cook until the other side is brown. Serve with applesauce. 12 pancakes.

TWICE BAKED POTATOES - Fast Weight Loss

4 baking potatoes
2 egg whites
2 Tbsp prepared Butter Buds

1 Tbsp thyme
2 tbsp finely chopped onion

Bake potatoes 50 minutes at 400 degrees. Slice lengthwise in halves. Scoop out pulp into mixing bowl; beat potato pulp with remaining ingredients. Return mixture to potato shells; top with paprika and bake 15 minutes at 350 degrees. Serves 6 to 8.

POTATO PANCAKES II - Fast Weight Loss

3 lg. potatoes (such as Idaho)
1 med. onion, coarsely grated
2 egg whites
3 Tbsp matzo meal

1 tsp unsalted Dijon style
    mustard
1/4 tsp baking powder
1 Tbsp low sodium soy sauce

1. Peel and coarsely grate potatoes. Place them in a large bowl and cover completely with cold water. Refrigerate 12 hours.
2. Drain the potatoes, then press them in a kitchen towel to extract as much moisture as possible. Return them to the empty bowl and mix in grated onion.
3. In a small bowl, combine soy sauce, mustard, baking powder, and matzo meal. Slowly mix thoroughly into potato mixture. Beat egg whites until stiff and fold into potato mixture.
4. Heat a non-stick skillet, or a regular skillet coated with a nonstick cooking spray, over medium heat. (Pan is ready when a drop of water dances across its surface.) Drop potato mixture onto the skillet by the tablespoon. Cook until well browned and crisp on both sides. Serve hot. Makes 16 pancakes. Potato pancakes may be served with 1/4 cup unsweetened applesauce per serving.

GLAZED SWEET POTATOES

3 lbs. sweet potatoes cut crosswise   1 tsp Butter Buds
   into 1/2 inch slices, peeled   1/2 tsp cinnamon
1/3 c. orange juice concentrate, thawed

Preheat oven to 350 degrees. Arrange sweet potatoes in a single layer in 2 large, shallow baking dishes. Mix orange juice concentrate, Butter Buds, and cinnamon; pour over sweet potatoes. Cover dishes tightly with foil and bake until tender, about 30 minutes. Serves 8.

SWEET POTATO STUFFING

3 c. chopped onion   1 1/2 tsp dried marjoram
2 c. chopped celery   1/2 tsp sage
4 c. mashed sweet potato   1 tsp pepper
8 c. cubed whole wheat bread   1/2 c. rice or soy milk
2 tsp dried thyme   2 egg whites, beaten

Sauté onion and celery in small amount of water until onion is done. In a large bowl, mix next 6 ingredients together well. Add onion and celery; mix well. In a separate bowl, mix milk and egg whites. Beat lightly and pour over rest of ingredients. Toss together. Stuff a 12 pound turkey or 3 chickens. If not for stuffing, bake in a non-stick casserole dish at 350 degrees for 30 to 35 minutes. Serves 8.

ORANGE SWEET POTATOES

4 med. sweet potatoes or yams   2 Tbsp apple juice concentrate
1/2 tsp grated orange rind   1/4 tsp cinnamon
1/2 c. orange juice

Steam potatoes and peel. Mash all ingredients together. Bake in casserole dish, covered, for 25 minutes at 350 degrees.

RATATOUILLE I - Fast Weight Loss

1 eggplant, diced (peeled optional)
1 lg. yellow onion, diced
4 sm. yellow or green zucchini, sliced
1 bell pepper (red is best,
    green will do), diced
1 sm. peeled and sliced cucumber
1 can salt-free tomatoes or 4 fresh
    tomatoes, diced

1 c. red wine
1/4 c. tomato paste or
    Progresso crushed tomatoes
1 clove garlic, crushed
2 Tbsp sweet basil
Dash of hot red pepper to taste
1 Tbsp apple juice concentrate

This dish is simple to make and delicious served with a salad of Romaine and fresh crusty bread. Combine all ingredients in a large saucepan. Cook on low heat 30 to 45 minutes until all vegetables are tender. Stir occasionally. Serves 6.

RATATOUILLE II - Fast Weight Loss

1 med. eggplant
6 med. zucchini
2 green bell peppers
2 lg. onions, sliced
4 lg. tomatoes, cut into chunks

1 clove garlic, minced
1/2 c. minced parsley
1 tsp crushed oregano
1 tsp low-sodium soy sauce

1. Cut unpeeled eggplant into 1/2 inch cubes. Slice zucchini into 1/2 inch rounds. Remove seeds from green bell peppers and cut into 1/2 inch squares.
2. Combine all ingredients and mix thoroughly.
3. Place mixture in a 6 quart casserole with a cover. Bake at 350 degrees for 1 1/2 hours, covered, and 1/2 hour, uncovered. During the first hour, baste top occasionally with some of the liquid to ensure even flavoring.
4. Serve hot from oven, or cold. Cool to room temperature before refrigerating. Flavors are enhanced if chilled and then reheated before serving. Makes 8 servings. Each serving contains 75 calories, 8% fat, 33 mg sodium, 0 mg cholesterol.
    Variation: Place all ingredients in a 6 quart pot. Add 1/2 cup red wine, 1/2 cup tomato juice. Cook, covered, on top of stove for 35 minutes.

RATATOUILLE ESPECIAL

2 c. eggplant, diced
1 c. zucchini diced
1/2 c. green bell pepper, chopped
1 1/2 c. cooked mushrooms, chopped
1/2 c. onions, cut in chunks

4 c. cooked brown rice
2 c. water
2 Tbsp vegetable broth
   seasoning

In large pot combine water and remaining ingredients, except rice, and cook over medium heat for 30 minutes. Serve over hot cooked brown rice. Serves 4 to 6.

HERBED TOMATOES

6 tomatoes
1/2 tsp pepper
3 tsp dill weed

2 tsp grated sap sago cheese
(optional)

Arrange tomatoes in baking pan making a cross on top of each. Sprinkle insides with remaining ingredients. Place under broiler for 8 to 10 minutes. Do not overcook or tomatoes lose their shape. Serves 6.

STUFFED TOMATOES - BELL PEPPERS - Microwave

6 lg. firm, ripe tomatoes
1/2 c. green onion, chopped
1/4 c. celery, chopped
2 Tbsp Butter Buds
1/2 c. Seitan wheat meat, shredded
2/3 c. cooked brown rice

1 (4 oz.) can mushrooms,
   drained
1/4 tsp basil
1/8 tsp pepper
Dash of cayenne pepper

Cut 1/4 inch slice off top of each tomato. Scoop out pulps; drain and reserve. Place onion, celery, and Butter Buds in 1 quart casserole. Heat on full power 2 minutes or until onion and celery is tender. Add tomato pulp and remaining ingredients to onion and celery. Spoon mixture into tomatoes. Place in casserole dish. Cover with plastic wrap. Bake on full power for 3 minutes.

MARINATED VEGETABLES - Fast Weight Loss

1/4 c. vinegar
1 Tbsp lemon juice
1/2 tsp coriander seed, crushed
1 clove garlic, minced
1/2 tsp pepper

1 c. water
1/2 c. sliced zucchini
1/2 c. sliced yellow squash
1/2 c. chopped broccoli
1/2 c. green beans

Place first 6 ingredients in a pot and bring to a boil. Add vegetables and reduce heat. Simmer until vegetables are crisp-tender. Chill and serve cold. Serves 2 to 3.

VEGETABLE CURRY

1 med. onion, chopped
3 Tbsp whole wheat flour
1 c. chicken broth, defatted
1 1/2 tsp curry powder
1/2 c. water
1 c. broccoli flowerettes
1 c. cauliflower pieces
2 med. carrots, sliced

4 stalks celery, sliced
1 lg. zucchini, sliced
1 med. red or green pepper,
   chopped
1/2 c. frozen green peas
1 (8 oz.) can water chestnuts
1/2 c. raisins

Sauté onion in a little water until soft. Add flour, chicken broth, curry powder, and water. Bring to a boil and add broccoli, cauliflower, carrots, and celery. Cook until veggies start to get tender (broccoli will be bright green). Add zucchini and bell pepper. Cook for about 3 to 5 minutes. Add peas, water, chestnuts, and raisins. Heat another 3 minutes. Serve plain for weight loss or serve over brown rice.

SPICY ZUCCHINI - Fast Weight Loss

2 med. zucchini, thinly sliced
1 lg. carrot, coarsely grated
1 med. onion, chopped
2 stalks celery, chopped

1/2 med. green pepper, thinly
   sliced
2 med. tomatoes, sliced

SAUCE:

1 c. mild green chili salsa
1/4 tsp dried basil

1 clove garlic, crushed
2 tsp prepared mustard

Prepare vegetables as directed and layer in a casserole dish, all except for the tomatoes. Combine ingredients for the sauce and pour over the layered vegetables. Place sliced tomatoes over the top. Cover and bake at 325 degrees for 45 minutes. Remove cover and bake for 15 minutes longer. Serves 6 to 8.

How to Look Great & Feel Sexy

STUFFED ZUCCHINI

4 lg. zucchini	1 1/4 c. tomato juice
1 onion, chopped	1 tsp dried oregano
1 green pepper, chopped	2 slices whole wheat toast
3/4 c. chopped tomatoes	

Cut the zucchini in half lengthwise, then scoop out pulp. Save shells for stuffing. Dice scooped out zucchini, then place in non-stick skillet with next 4 ingredients and 1/3 cup tomato juice and oregano. Cook until vegetables are limp and fill the shells with cooked mixture and place on baking dish. Pour remaining juice around zucchini and sprinkle with crumbled toast. Bake at 350 degrees for 30 minutes. Serves 8.

ZUCCHINI BOATS - Microwave

2 med. zucchini, cut in half	1/4 tsp pepper
lengthwise	1/4 tsp basil
1/4 c. chopped green onions	1/2 c. smashed, cooked
1/2 c. chopped fresh tomatoes	garbanzo beans
1/8 tsp marjoram	

Hollow out inside of each zucchini half, leaving a 1/4 inch thick shell. Chop zucchini pulp. In a medium bowl, mix zucchini pulp, green onions, tomato, 1/4 cup of spices, and garbanzo beans. Fill zucchini halves with mixture. Place in a shallow dish. Cover tightly. Microwave on high for 5 minutes. 4 servings.

ZUCCHINI COLACHE - Fast Weight Loss

1 lb. zucchini, unpeeled and sliced	2 c. whole kernel corn
1 onion, sliced	1/8 tsp oregano
1/2 c. green bell pepper, diced	1/4 tsp basil
1/4 c. water	1/4 tsp marjoram
1 c. diced tomato	Freshly ground pepper to taste

Sauté zucchini, onion, and pepper in non-stick skillet (use non-stick spray) until vegetables are limp. Add water, tomato, and corn. Cover and cook squash until tender, adding more water if necessary. Add pepper to taste and other seasonings. Serves 6.

ZUCCHINI LOAF

3 c. shredded zucchini
1 c. cooked brown rice
1 c. oat bran
1 c. chopped walnuts
2 c. sliced, fresh mushrooms
4 green onions, sliced

1 tsp oregano
4 garlic cloves, minced
1/2 tsp thyme
1/2 tsp sage
Pepper
1/2 c. apple juice

Preheat oven to 375 degrees. Combine all the ingredients in a large bowl. Mix until well blended. Pour into a 9 x 5 inch loaf pan. Sprinkle top with remaining cheese. Bake for 50 minutes or until brown. 6 servings.

ZUCCHINI SQUARES

3 c. shredded zucchini
3/4 c. whole wheat flour
1 pkg. Butter Buds
2 tsp parsley
2 cloves garlic, minced

1/2 c. onion, chopped
1 tsp baking soda
6 egg whites
1 Tbsp low sodium soy sauce
Dash of Tabasco sauce

Preheat oven to 350 degrees. Mix soy sauce, Tabasco and egg whites. Beat until stiff peaks form. Mix dry ingredients; blend with egg white mixture. Pour into 13 x 9 x 2 inch pan sprayed with non-stick spray. Bake 25 to 30 minutes until golden brown. Makes 2 to 3 dozen squares.

ZUCCHINI - STUFFED TOMATOES - Fast Weight Loss

1 lb. zucchini, chopped
5 med. tomatoes
1 sm. onion, chopped
1 sm. green pepper, chopped
1 clove garlic, minced
1 tsp each oregano and basil

1/2 tsp vegetable seasoning
1/4 tsp pepper
1/2 c. egg whites
4 Tbsp grated Lite Line
    cheese(optional)

Cut out core of tomato. Set upside down to drain. Sauté onion and pepper in small amount of liquid until soft. Stir in zucchini, garlic and spices, and seasonings. Cook, stirring often for about 5 minutes. Stir in egg whites and 2 tablespoons of the cheese. Evenly spoon mixture into tomato shells; sprinkle with remaining cheese. Bake at 350 degrees for 15 minutes. Serves 6.

Soups & Salads

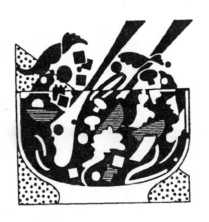 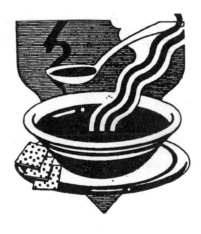

How to Look Great & Feel Sexy

AZTEC SOUP

Baked tortilla pieces
3 Tbsp Butter Buds
2/3 c. pine nuts
3/4 c. walnut halves
1 lg. red onion, chopped
2 cloves garlic, minced
12 c. chicken broth, defatted

4 c. diced, peeled butternut or
  acorn squash
2 pkgs. frozen corn
3/4 c. toasted, shelled
  pumpkin seeds
1 lg. avocado

Bake tortillas in oven at 400 degrees until crispy, about 10 minutes.
In a pan over medium heat, melt 1 tablespoon of the Butter Buds. Add pine nuts and walnuts; cook, stirring until golden. Remove nuts and set aside.
Melt the remaining 2 tablespoons Butter Buds in pan and cook onion and garlic until onion is golden. Place onion and garlic in a large pot; add chicken broth and squash and bring to a boil. Reduce heat, cover, and simmer until squash is tender. Add corn and cook for 5 more minutes. Sprinkle with pumpkin seeds just before serving. Peel and dice avocado. Place avocado, nuts, and tortilla pieces in bowl and pass as condiments at the table to add to the soup. Serves 19.

BARBECUE BEAN SOUP

1 1/4 c. dried legumes (use as many
  different kinds as possible)
1/4 tsp ginger
1 lg. onion, chopped
1/4 tsp lemon pepper
1 Tbsp barbecue sauce

1 sm. clove garlic, chopped
1 (16 oz.) can tomatoes
1/2 tsp chili powder
2 tsp ketchup
2 stalks celery, chopped
1/2 tsp crushed red pepper

Soak the beans overnight. The next day cook the beans for at least 12 hours to eliminate any gas problems. Add the ginger while they are cooking. Add the remaining ingredients and cook for 3 hours.

BEET BOSCHT - Fast Weight Loss

3 c. water
1/2 c. salt free tomato juice
1 med. onion, finely chopped
1/4 head cabbage, finely
  shredded(about 1 1/2 c.)

2 Tbsp fresh lemon juice
1 sm. beet, cooked, peeled,
  and julienned
1 Tbsp cider vinegar
2 Tbsp apple juice concentrate

In a large saucepan, combine 3 cups water, tomato juice, onion, and cabbage. Bring to a boil, reduce heat, and simmer (covered) about 15 minutes until vegetables are tender. Add remaining ingredients and mix thoroughly. Makes 4 servings. This soup freezes well.

BLACK BEAN SOUP

1 c. black beans
4 c. water
3 bay leaves
4 cloves

2 onions, chopped
2 cloves garlic
1/4 tsp dry mustard
1 1/2 tsp chili powder

Add all ingredients to boiling water and simmer until tender. Puree. Serves 4 to 5.

BLACK BEAN SOUP WITH CHILLED SPICED RICE

3 beef bouillon cubes
5 c. hot water
1/4 c. minced dried onion
1 med. green pepper, seeded and
   chopped (3/4 c.)
3 cloves garlic, minced or pressed
1 1/2 tsp ground cumin
1 1/2 tsp dried oregano

2 (15 oz.) can black beans
   drained (pinto or red
   beans can be substituted)
1 (4 oz.) can chopped
   green chilies
2 Tbsp cider vinegar
Chilled spiced rice

In a 3 quart saucepan, combine all ingredients. Stir, bring to a boil, cover, and simmer for 20 to 30 minutes. Ladle into bowls and top with a generous spoonful of chilled spiced rice.

Chilled Spiced Rice: (The rice is best when made the night before or at least 30 minutes before serving to allow flavors to blend.) Combine 1/2 cup finely chopped green onion, 1/2 teaspoon oregano, 1/4 cup each no oil Italian salad dressing and cider vinegar. Mix with 3 cups cooked brown or white rice. Chill thoroughly before serving. Nutrient values per serving: Yields: 6 (1 cup) servings. 113 calories, trace fat, 0 cholesterol, 22 gm carbohydrates, 940 gm sodium, 7 mg protein.

The distinctive contrast of temperatures and textures make this an especially enjoyable main dish. Serve it with a green salad topped with canned mandarin orange sections and creamy avocado slices with poppy seed dressing. Pass crusty, whole grain rolls to complete the meal.

BROCCOLI LEMON SOUP - Fast Weight Loss

1 c. broccoli, chopped	1 Tbsp sweet basil
2 c. clear chicken stock, defatted	1 clove garlic
2 egg whites	1 carrot, diced
1/4 c. lemon juice	1/4 c. diced onion
1/4 c. cooked brown rice or pastini (pasta)	1 Tbsp apple juice concentrate

In heavy bottomed saucepan, add all ingredients, except lemon and egg whites. Simmer 1/2 hour. Beat egg whites together with lemon juice. Add to soup. Makes 4 to 6 servings.

BETH'S BLACK KETTLE SOUP

1 c. dried black beans (available in specialty stores if not in your market)	2 tbsp fresh green cilantro or dried coriander, minced
3 c. salt free or vegetable broth, defatted	1 bay leaf, remove before serving
1 c. mild green chili salsa (check for sodium content)	Sprinkle of green scallion onions, chopped as garnish
2 cloves minced garlic	1 Tbsp Bakon seasoning or liquid smoke
1/2 c. dry red wine or sherry	

This soup makes itself. To shorten cooking time, soak beans in bowl of water overnight. Discard water before using beans. Place all ingredients, except scallions, in heavy bottomed saucepan or soup kettle (if you have an iron pot, it's best to use). Simmer 2 1/2 hours or until beans are plump and tender. Place in bowl and sprinkle with scallions. Serve more salsa and cilantro on the side. Add a salad for a simple,. complete, and satisfying meal. Makes 8 to 10 servings. Freeze leftovers for an easy meal later.

This Black Bean soup is a savory dish popular in Latin American and Cuba. While it is simmering on the back of your stove, it will fill your home with a seductive, mouth-watering aroma.

CABBAGE - VEGETABLE SOUP - Fast Weight Loss

1/2 head cabbage, chopped
3 lg. red potatoes, cubed
4 carrots, sliced
1 (15 oz.) can kidney beans, rinsed
   and drained
1 (15 oz.) can tomato sauce

3 c. water
1 1/4 c. chicken broth, defatted
2 tsp chili powder
1 1/2 tsp cumin
Juice from 1/2 of lemon
1/4 c. tomato paste

Combine all ingredients together in large saucepan and simmer on stove, covered, for about 2 hours.

CARROT AND PARSNIP SOUP - Fast Weight Loss

1 1/2 qts. water
1 lg. onion, chopped
2 bay leaves
1/2 tsp thyme

2 stalks celery and leaves,
   chopped very fine
1 lg. parsnip, grated
2 to 3 lg. carrots, grated

Simmer onion in 1/4 cup water for 5 minutes. Add remaining water, bay leaves, pepper, and thyme. Bring to a boil slowly. Add vegetables to the stock and simmer gently for 1 hour. Puree 2 cups of this soup for a creamier texture. Garnish with carrot curls or chopped parsley. Serves 4.

CAULIFLOWER SOUP - Fast Weight Loss

5 c. water
1 head cauliflower, chopped
   into sm. pieces
1 c. corn

1 sm. zucchini, chopped
1 1/2 c. cooked barley
1 1/2 Tbsp vegetable broth
   seasoning

In a medium saucepan, combine all ingredients in water and bring to a boil. Simmer for 20 minutes.

CHILI BEAN SOUP

1 onion, chopped fine
1 (28 oz.) can kidney beans
1 (28 oz.) can tomatoes

1 (6 oz.) can tomato paste
1 Tbsp chili powder
1/2 Tbsp ground cumin

Slowly sauté onion in small amount of water in a 2 quart saucepan. Put the tomatoes in a blender and blend for 30 seconds or until they have a lumpy consistency. Add the beans and tomatoes to the onion. Add tomato paste and mix well. Add chili powder and cumin; mix well, then bring the mixture to a boil. Reduce heat and simmer for 30 minutes. Soup is best when prepared a day ahead, refrigerated overnight, and reheated. Serves 4.

How to Look Great & Feel Sexy

CHINESE HOT AND SOUR SOUP

5 c. chicken stock, defatted
(low-sodium)
10 oz. broccoli or wheat meat
3 egg whites, lightly beaten
1/2 c. mushrooms, halved
1 carrot
1 bunch scallions
2 Tbsp dry sherry (optional)

2 stalks bok choy (use cabbage,
if not available)
1/4 c. (or to taste) hot
Szechuan chili paste,
or Sanj Szechuan Sauce
2 cloves garlic
1 tsp ground ginger

Heat stock; add pepper, garlic, and ginger. Slice vegetables, add to broth simmer for 10 minutes. With temperature just under boiling, drip egg whites, stirring lightly. Add vinegar and simmer for 5 more minutes.

For a variation, add bean sprouts or diced pepper instead of tofu. Serves 4.

LIMA LEEK SOUP

1 leek, white part only, finely chopped
2 c. cooked dried lima beans
1 c. chopped watercress

2 c. defatted chicken broth
2 Tbsp lemon juice (to taste)

Sauté leek in chicken broth or a little water. Add balance of chicken broth and lima beans. Cover and simmer 1/2 hour. Let the mixture cool to room temperature. Puree in a blender of food processor. Mix in lemon juice and pepper to taste.

CHINESE TOMATO - Fast Weight Loss

1 green chili, seeded, rinsed, and
finely chopped
1 c. salt-free tomato sauce
15 oz. can salt-free tomatoes
3 c. low sodium chicken stock, defatted
1 c. bok choy, cut into slices
2 celery stalks thinly sliced
1 med. onion, thinly sliced

2 garlic cloves, minced
1/2 c. chopped scallion
1/4 c. cooked brown rice
(optional)
1 Tbsp low sodium soy sauce
1/2 tsp curry powder
1 tsp chili powder
1 c. bean sprouts

In a medium saucepan, cook chili, tomato sauce, tomatoes, chicken stock, bok choy, celery, onion, and garlic over medium heat for 15 minutes. Add scallion, rice (if using), soy sauce, curry, and chili powders; mix thoroughly. Cook for 5 minutes. Add bean sprouts and cook for 1 minute more. Serve hot. Makes 6 servings.

CHICK - PEA SOUP

12 oz. chick peas (garbanzos)
6 c. water
3 or 4 med. parsnips (1/2 lb.), sliced
4 or 5 med. ribs celery (1/2 lb.), sliced
2 med. onions or leeks (1/2 lb.), chopped
1/4 tsp nutmeg

3 or 4 carrots (1/2 lb.), sliced
6 c. additional water
1/4 to 1/3 c. tamari (soy sauce)
2 Tbsp Vogue's Vege-Base or
    Mrs. Dash seasoning

Soak chick peas overnight. Next day add the vegetables and additional water. Simmer over low heat 1 1/2 hours or more until chick peas are tender. Remove about half the soup and whiz in blender or food processor a few seconds. Return to pot. Add seasonings. This recipe can easily be cut in half for a smaller group. Serves 10 to 12.

CIDER ZUCCHINI SOUP

3/4 c. apple cider
1/4 c. water
3 Tbsp sliced green onion
1/2 tsp grated ginger root
1/4 tsp dried basil

Dash of pepper
2 1/2 c. shredded zucchini
1/2 c. shredded carrots
1/8 tsp finely shredded
    orange peel

In a small saucepan, combine cider, water, and next 4 ingredients. Bring to the point of boiling; reduce heat, cover, and simmer 5 minutes. Add zucchini, carrots, and orange peel. Return to the point of boiling; reduce heat. Cover and simmer for 3 to 5 minutes more. Serves 1.

COLD AVOCADO BEAN SOUP

2 (10 1/2 oz.) cans chicken broth,
    chilled and defatted
1/2 c. kidney beans
1/2 c. green beans

Dill weed
Dash of lemon juice
2 ripe avocados, diced
1 oz. sherry

Put chilled broth into blender; add cubed chicken, diced avocados, sherry, and lemon juice. Blend well. Sprinkle with dill weed. Serves 4.

CURRIED CREAM OF BROCCOLI SOUP

1 pkg. Butter Buds
1 lg. (1 c.) onion, chopped
2 cloves garlic, chopped (2 tsp)
3/4 tsp curry powder or more to taste
1 c. soy "lite" milk or rice milk
Freshly ground black pepper, if
    desired, to taste
1 c. water

1 2/3 c. chicken broth (canned
    or homemade)
1 bunch broccoli (about 1 lb.),
    cut into flowerettes, stems
    cut into 1/2 inch slices
1 lg. potato, peeled and cut
    into 1/2 inch cubes

1. In a large saucepan, add Butter Buds and sauté the onion and garlic for a few minutes.
2. Add the curry, pepper, broth, and water to the pan and bring the soup to a boil.
3. Add the broccoli and potato. When mixture returns to a boil reduce the heat, cover the pan and simmer soup for about 20 minutes or until the vegetables are tender.
4. Puree the soup in batches in a blender or food processor. Return the puree to the pan, stir in the milk, and cook the soup over low heat until it is hot but do not boil it

You needn't worry about the calories in creamed soups when the "cream" is actually rice milk. Preparation Tip: This soup has enough flavor to permit omission of all added salt. It can be frozen before or after pureeing but preferably before the addition of the milk.

CURRIED ZUCCHINI SOUP - Fast Weight Loss

3 sm. zucchini, diced
2 lg. onions, sliced
2 to 3 tomatoes, sliced
1 qt. vegetable stock plus 3 Tbsp
1 tsp whole wheat flour
4 Tbsp water

1 tsp curry powder
1/8 tsp ginger
Dash of cayenne pepper
Basil
Garlic powder

Heat 3 tablespoons stock and sauté zucchini and onion until onion is soft. Add remaining stock and cook 20 minutes. Sauté tomatoes in stock and then add to the other vegetables and bring to a boil. Mix flour, water curry, ginger, and cayenne. When blended, add to soup. Simmer 6 minutes. Force the mixture through a strainer or spin in blender. Season to taste with basil and garlic powder. Serves 4.

CORN CHOWDER

3 c fresh or frozen corn kernels
2 c low sodium chicken stock, defatted
1 celery stalk, finely chopped
1 onion, finely chopped
1 carrot, peeled and finely chopped
1 potato, peeled and diced
4 Tbsp potato starch or salt-free
instant mashed potato flakes

1 red bell pepper, seeded and
finely chopped
4 garlic cloves, finely chopped
4 oz. canned green chilies,
rinsed and chopped
1/4 tsp white pepper
2 Tbsp natural rice vinegar

1. In a blender, puree 1 1/2 cups corn kernels and 1 cup chicken stock until smooth. Transfer to a large saucepan and add remaining corn and chicken stock, celery, onion, carrot, potato, pepper, and garlic. Bring to a boil; cover and simmer for 20 minutes.
2. Add chilies, vinegar, and pepper; simmer another 20 minutes.
3. Stir in the potato starch (or instant potato flakes) and cook for a few minutes until the soup is thickened. Makes 8 servings.

EGGPLANT BEAN SOUP

Soak overnight 1/2 cup each: Black eyed peas, pink beans, white beans, red beans, and black beans. Drain water of the next morning.

In a large pot on stove simmer beans in 6 cups water. Season with garlic and onion powder and Instead of Salt. About 6 hours later, add:

1 chopped onion
1 c. brown rice
1 spear fresh broccoli, sliced

1 sliced zucchini
1 fresh yellow crookneck squash
1/2 diced eggplant

Simmer another 45 minutes to cook and add fresh chopped parsley last. Ready to serve and enjoy anytime.

FRENCH ONION SOUP - Fast Weight Loss

2 lg. onions, thinly sliced lengthwise
4 c. low-sodium French onion stock

1/2 tsp low-sodium soy sauce
1/4 c. dry sherry

1. In a large skillet, cook onions over a very low heat, covered, until soft. Remove lid, increase heat to high, and brown onions (stirring constantly to avoid burning). When completely browned, reduce heat to low and add 1/4 cup stock and mix well.
2. Transfer onion mixture to a larger saucepan. Add remaining stock, soy sauce, and sherry; bring to a boil. Reduce heat and simmer, uncovered, for 30 minutes. Makes 4 servings.
Variation: French onion soup with croutons. Add 1/3 cup whole wheat bread croutons to each cup of soup.

FRENCH VEGETABLE SOUP - Fast Weight Loss

8 c. water
2 onions, coarsely chopped
2 potatoes, chopped coarsely
1 clove garlic, crushed
2 stalks celery, thickly sliced
1 carrot, thickly sliced
1/2 lb. mushrooms, sliced
4 zucchini, thickly sliced and cut in half
2 leeks, sliced or bunch green
   onions sliced

1 c. fresh or frozen peas
1 c. chopped cauliflower pieces
1 tsp thyme
1 tsp dill weed
1 tsp marjoram
1 tsp basil
Fresh, ground black pepper
2 c. chopped broccoli pieces
3 Tbsp low-sodium soy sauce
1 c. dry white wine

Place 8 cups water in a large soup pot. Add onions, potatoes, garlic, celery, and carrots. Bring to a boil; reduce heat, cover, and simmer for 15 minutes. Add remaining ingredients; cook an additional 30 minutes.

Sprinkle with finely chopped green onions before serving, if desired. Serves 8 to 10.

FLAVORFUL BEAN SOUP

2 c. cooked Great Northern beans
   (about 3/4 c. raw)
2 c. cooked kidney or red beans
   (about 3/4 c. raw)
1 med. onion, chopped
2 lg. celery stalks, chopped
1 med. potato, scrubbed and diced
4 med. tomatoes

1 tsp dried summer savory
1 tsp paprika
1/2 tsp coriander - cilantro
1/2 tsp ground cumin
Ground pepper to taste
3/4 c. string beans, cut into
   1 inch pieces
1/4 c. dry red wine

Soak the northern and kidney beans overnight and then cook them for several hours until tender. Place the onion, celery, potato, and string beans in a large pot with just enough water, including the liquid remaining from the cooked beans to cover. Bring to a boil, cover, and simmer until vegetables are just tender. Add the cooked beans and all the remaining ingredients, plus 2 more cups of water. Simmer covered, over low heat for 20 to 25 minutes. Taste to be sure that everything is done to your liking.

SPICY POTATO CABBAGE SOUP - Fast Weight Loss

6 c. defatted chicken broth
2 lg. potatoes, peeled and cubed
6 to 8 stalks celery, cut into
   1/2 inch slices
10 fresh mushrooms, sliced

1/2 c. kernel corn, drained
1/2 head cabbage, shredded
3 to 4 tsp Mrs. Dash Extra Spicy
3 to 4 tsp garlic powder

Combine all ingredients in a large pot. Cook on low to medium heat 15 to 25 minutes or until potatoes are tender. Seasoning can be adjusted to taste as it is very spicy.

GARLIC SOUP - Fast Weight Loss

1 1/2 qts. water
4 potatoes
1 carrot
2 stalks celery

1 onion
2 lg. bulbs garlic
1/2 tsp thyme
Dash of cayenne pepper

Bring water to a boil. Cut potatoes, celery, and onion into 1/2 inch pieces and place in boiling water. Break garlic bulbs and peel individual cloves. Place in soup together with spices. Cook over medium heat for 20 to 30 minutes. When soup is ready, it can be served in either of 2 ways: (1) Strain and serve as a clear broth or (2) Puree in blender and serve as a "cream of garlic" soup. Serves 6 to 8.

COLD TOMATO HERB SOUP - Fast Weight Loss

2 beef bouillon cubes
1 c. boiling water
3 c. tomato juice
1 sm. onion, grated
1 c. celery, chopped
1 green pepper, minced

1 clove garlic
3 Tbsp lemon juice
Dash of Tabasco sauce
2 Tbsp dried basil
1 cucumber diced
2 ripe tomatoes, peeled and diced

Dissolve the cubes in water. Cool slightly, then add the next 4 ingredients. Cut the garlic in half and stick a toothpick through both halves. Add to the mixture. Mix and refrigerate for several hours. Just before serving, remove the garlic and add remaining ingredients. Serve cold. Serves 6.

GAZPACHO SOUP I - Fast Weight Loss

2 1/2 c. chopped tomatoes
1 c. chopped zucchini
1 c. peeled and chopped cucumber
3/4 c. chopped celery
1/2 c. chopped green onion

1/4 c. chopped green pepper
4 c. tomato juice
1 c. canned green chili salsa
1/4 tsp Tabasco sauce

Puree 1/3 of the tomato, zucchini, and celery with some of the tomato juice. Mix in the rest of the ingredients. Chill. This Spanish soup, which should be served icy cold, is really a salad in the guise of a soup. Makes almost 2 quarts.

GAZPACHO II

2 lg. cucumbers, peeled and seeded
   (if hot house Belgium type, no
   need to seed)
4 to 5 ripe red Big Boy type
   tomatoes, peeled if you have the
   time (to peel, pierce skin and
   place in pan of boiling water 1
   minute or microwave until the
   skin easily slips off)
1/3 to 1/2 c. chopped green scallions
2 cloves garlic
1/3 c. red wine vinegar or herbed
   vinegar, such as tarragon,
   oregano or raspberry
1 c. chicken stock (salt-free)

1 c. low sodium V-8 juice
Few drops of Tabasco to
   your taste
3 Tbsp fresh basil or 1 Tbsp
   dried, minced lemon wedges
Whole wheat bread, rubbed
   with garlic, toasted until
   dry and crusty and cut into
   cubes for croutons (may use
   sourdough bread or check
   your market for an
   unseasoned crouton)
1 bell pepper, cut with seeds
   and pith discarded

This is another soup that makes itself in minutes, despite the long list of ingredients. Place all ingredients in a food processor, process with an on-off motion, until chunky and partially pureed. If using a blender, use same on-off motion, but process in smaller batches. Refrigerate 1 hour before serving. Add lemon, if desired. Serve with crouton garnish. Serves 8 to 10.

Gazpacho is a soup from Spain. There are as many recipes for this soup as there are cities and villages. Some are hot, some cold, some tomato based, and some with no tomatoes! One thing they all have in common is bread or croutons as garnish an ingredient often left out in Americanized versions. Gazpacho literally means "soaked bread !" This version is wonderful chilled and poured from a pitcher into chilled bowls on a hot summer day.

ITALIAN SOUP

1/2 lb. zucchini, sliced
1 (15 oz.) can garbanzo beans
1 tsp minced basil leaves
Pepper (if desired)
1 1/2 c. dry white wine

2 onions sliced
1 (16 oz.) can tomatoes, chopped
2 tsp minced garlic
1 bay leaf

Combine zucchini, onions, beans, tomatoes with liquid, wine, garlic, basil, and bay leaf in baking dish. Cover and bake at 400 degrees for 1 hour, stirring once after 30 minutes. Season to taste with pepper or other seasoning, if desired. This may also be cooked on top of stove.

HOT OR COLD TOMATO LEEK SOUP - Fast Weight Loss

2 lbs. ripe tomatoes
1/2 c. firmly packed parsley (fresh)
1 lg. leek
2 cloves garlic, minced
1 (6 oz.) can tomato paste
2 Tbsp dry red wine

1 Tbsp minced fresh dill
1 1/2 tsp paprika
1/2 tsp dried marjoram
1/4 tsp dried thyme
Ground pepper to taste

Cut 1 1/2 pounds of the tomatoes into quarters and place them in the blender. Add the parsley and process until well pureed. Dice the remaining tomatoes and set aside. Slice the white part of the leek into 1/4 inch slices. Chop the tender, light green parts of the leaves. Reserve 2 or 3 of the tough green leaves, wash them, cut in half, and discard the rest of the green leaves. Separate the leek slices into rings by poking them in the center. Wash carefully, removing all grit and put them in a large pot along with the reserved green leaves and garlic. Cover with 3 cups of water or vegetable stock; bring to a boil, then reduce heat and simmer for 5 minutes. Add the pureed and diced tomatoes and all remaining ingredients; continue to simmer on low heat for 20 to 25 minutes or until the leek rings are tender. Chill, or let stand for 30 minutes if you are serving this hot, then heat through before serving. Remove green leaves before serving. Serves 4 to 6.

LEEK SHIITAKE SOUP - Fast Weight Loss

5 shiitake mushrooms
2 lg. leeks
1 (7 inch) piece wakame
1 celery stalk with leaves, chopped
6 c. water

2 sm. carrots, sliced and
cut in half
2 scallions, chopped (optional)
Chopped wakame
1 Tbsp tamari

Pour a cup of boiling water over shiitake mushrooms. Let soak 20 minutes, remove mushrooms, and chop. Chop bottom ends off the leeks. Wash ends, boil 10 minutes for stock with 6 cups water and wakame. Remove and discard ends. Remove and chop wakame. Clean rest of leeks carefully, slice white and green parts, keeping separate.

Heat a non-stick pan or use Pam cooking spray and fry briefly the sliced white part of leeks and the chopped green leek tops.

Use a non-stick pan to sauté the celery and carrots for 3 minutes, then add scallions and shiitake mushrooms. Add to kettle with wakame and tamari. Simmer for 10 minutes. Taste and add a little more tamari, if desired. Top each bowl with whole wheat croutons and minced parsley. Yield: 6 servings. Per serving: 35 calories, 1 gm protein, 3 gm carbohydrates, and 2 gm fat.

KALE - POTATO SOUP

1 lg. onion
1 clove garlic
2 big potatoes
1 lg. bunch kale

5 c. hot water or stock
1/2 tsp salt to taste
Black pepper

An utterly satisfying soup. How many winter nights does this seem to be the only possible choice? A classic a favorite, a stand-by. With fresh young kale, it is, perhaps, even a world-class soup.

Sauté onion in butter and non-stick pan with water, cooking and stirring until clear and slightly golden. About halfway, add the garlic. When the onion is done, crush the garlic with a fork.

Add the potatoes and 2 cups of water. Simmer, covered, until potatoes start to soften around the edges. Meantime, wash the kale, remove stems, chop, and steam. (Don't try to cook it with the potatoes, the flavor will be too strong.)

When the potatoes are very well done, puree half of them with remaining water and the salt and pepper. Combine all and heat gently, correcting the consistency if necessary by adding hot water or milk. Makes about 6 cups and serves 4 if no extra water is added.

LEMON GRASS SOUP

5 c. thin coconut milk
3 c. broccoli, cut into bite sized pieces
3 Tbsp dried lemon grass
3 green onions, finely chopped

2 Tbsp coriander leaves, chopped
4 fresh Serrano chilies
Juice of 2 limes

To make coconut milk, boil a piece of coconut in 5 cups water, or if you cannot obtain fresh coconut, you may substitute shredded, packaged coconut (1 cup) and boil it in water. Strain off the coconut and the resulting liquid is coconut milk.

Lemon grass is available in oriental markets.

In a saucepan, bring the coconut milk to a boil. Add the broccoli pieces and lemon grass. Reduce heat and simmer until the broccoli is tender, about 15 minutes. Do not cover. When the broccoli is tender, add the green onions coriander leaves, and chilies. Bring the heat up just below boiling. Remove the pan from heat and stir m the lime juice. Serve. Makes 6 servings.

LENTIL SOUP

1 lb. lentils
1 onion, chopped
2 1/2 c. tomato sauce
2 lg. tomatoes, chopped
2 carrots, sliced
2 lg. red potatoes, diced

2 garlic cloves, minced
1/2 tsp black pepper
1 tsp basil
Dash of onion powder
Dash of cinnamon

Cook lentils in about 6 cups of water until tender, about 1/2 hour. Add rest of ingredients, simmer for an hour or two or until vegetables are tender.

LENTIL AND BROWN RICE SOUP

1/2 c. raw lentils, washed
1/3 c. raw brown rice
2 cloves garlic, minced
2 Tbsp soy sauce
1 bay leaf
1 sm. onion, thinly sliced
2 med. carrots, thinly sliced
1 lg. celery stalk, finely chopped
1 tsp paprika

Handful of celery flakes
1 (14 oz.) can imported plum
    tomatoes with liquid, chopped
1/2 c. tomato sauce or
    tomato juice
1 tsp dried basil
1/2 tsp dried marjoram
1/2 tsp dried thyme
1/4 c. dry red wine

Place the first 5 ingredients in a large pot and cover with 3 cups of water. Bring to a boil, cover, and simmer for 7 to 8 minutes over low heat. Add 2 additional cups of water along with all remaining ingredients. Cover and simmer over low heat for 25 to 30 minutes or until vegetables, rice, and lentils are done to your liking. Serves 6.

How to Look Great & Feel Sexy

LIMA BEAN CHOWDER

2 1/2 c. dried baby lima beans
8 c. water
2 onions, finely chopped
2 carrots, finely chopped
2 stalks celery, chopped
2 cloves garlic, pressed
1 c. rice, soy, or nut milk

1 Tbsp parsley flakes
2 tsp caraway seeds
1 tsp dill weed
1/4 tsp crushed red pepper
1 (10 oz.) pkg. frozen lima
beans, thawed

Place dried lima beans and water in a large pot. Bring to boil, boil 1 minute, remove from heat, cover, and let rest 1 hour. Return to heat; add onion, carrots, celery, garlic, and seasonings. Bring to boil, reduce heat, cover, and cook over medium-low heat for 1 hour. Add thawed lima beans and acceptable milk. Cook an additional 15 minutes. Serves 6 to 8.

MEDITERRANEAN BROCCOLI AND MUSHROOM SOUP
Fast Weight Loss

1 med. onion, chopped
1/2 c. raw barley
2 cloves garlic, minced
2 1/2 to 3 c. chopped broccoli
1/2 lb. chopped mushrooms
1 sm. turnip, peeled and chopped
1 (8 oz.) can imported plum tomatoes
(with liquid), chopped

3 Tbsp minced fresh parsley
1 tsp paprika
1 tsp dried marjoram
1/2 tsp basil
1/4 tsp dried rosemary
2 bay leaves
Freshly ground pepper to taste
1/4 c. dry red wine

Place first 4 ingredients in a large pot and cover with 2 cups water or vegetable stock. Bring to a boil, cover, and simmer over low heat for 10 minutes. Add the remaining ingredients to the pot along with an additional 2 1/2 cups of water or stock. Cover and simmer over low heat for about 35 minutes or until the vegetables and barley are tender. Ideally this soup should stand an hour before serving. Serves 6 to 8.

MINESTRONE SOUP

1 onion, chopped
1 clove garlic, minced
2 Tbsp chopped parsley
1/2 tsp thyme
1/2 tsp oregano
3 Tbsp tomato paste
1 lg. can (28 oz.) pureed tomatoes

3 stalks celery, chopped
2 carrots, diced
2 c. shredded cabbage
2 zucchini, diced
1 c. uncooked brown rice
3 c. cooked dried beans
1 1/2 qts. chicken broth, defatted

Put all ingredients, except rice and beans into soup pot. Bring to a boil; add rice, then simmer (covered) for 1 hour. Now add the beans. Stir, heat, and serve.

BASIC MISO SOUP - Fast Weight Loss

1 (3 inch) piece dried Erewhon
   Wakame
1 c. thinly sliced onions
1 1/3 to 1 1/2 Tbsp Erewhon Miso

1 qt. spring water
Chopped scallions, parsley,
   ginger or watercress for
   garnish

Rinse the wakame in cold water for 3 to 5 minutes and slice it into 1/2 inch pieces. Put wakame and onions in a pot and add the water. Bring to a boil, lower the heat and simmer for 10 to 20 minutes or until tender. Reduce the heat to very low but not boiling or bubbling. Put the miso in a bowl or suribachi. Add 1/4 cup of the broth from the pot and puree until miso is completely dissolved in the liquid. Add pureed miso to the soup. Simmer for 3 to 5 minutes and serve. Garnish with scallions, parsley, ginger, or watercress.

MUSHROOM SOUP - Fast Weight Loss

1 1/2 lbs. mushrooms, sliced
1 onion, thinly sliced
1 lg. clove garlic, crushed
2 bay leaves
1 1/2 tsp basil
2 tsp dill weed

1 tsp paprika
Fresh ground black pepper
1 c. chicken stock
3 to 4 Tbsp low-sodium soy sauce
4 c. water
3/4 c. white wine (or apple juice)

Combine all ingredients in large saucepan. Bring to a boil, reduce heat, cover, and simmer for about 30 minutes. Serves 6.

How to Look Great & Feel Sexy

MUSHROOM BARLEY, AND NAVY BEAN SOUP

1 c. dry navy or pea beans, soaked or
2 c. canned beans, drained and
   rinsed
1/2 c. pearled barley
2 tsp garlic powder
1 lb. mushrooms, sliced thin

1(8 oz.) can no salt added
   tomato sauce
2 qts. fat free chicken broth or
   water
Tabasco

Place all ingredients, except Tabasco, in a large 8 quart pot. Slowly bring to a boil and simmer, covered, for 2 hours, if you are using soaked dried beans, or for 1 hour if you are using canned beans. If the level of liquid goes down, replace it with water or the soup will end up being too thick. Season to taste with Tabasco. This soup keeps on improving with each reheating. Serving size: 1 cup, 126 calories, 1 gram fat, 0 cholesterol, 13 milligrams sodium.

NAVY BEAN SOUP

8 c. low-sodium chicken stock, defatted
1 1/4 c. dry navy beans
1 clove garlic, peeled and crushed
10 oz. pkg. frozen cut green beans
3/4 c. chopped celery
3/4 c. chopped onion
3/4 c. diced fresh tomato
2 bay leaves

1/2 c. peeled diced potato
1/4 c. sliced leek
1/4 tsp dried basil
1/4 tsp dried dill
1/4 tsp dried thyme
1/4 tsp garlic powder
1/4 tsp onion powder
1/4 tsp dry mustard

1. In a large pot, combine stock, beans, and bay leaf. Bring to a boil over medium-high heat, then reduce heat; cover pan and simmer for 1 hour or until beans are just tender.
2. Remove and discard bay leaves. Transfer 1/3 of the beans to a food processor or blender; add garlic and process until pureed. Return puree to pot.
3. Add green beans, celery, onion, tomato, potato, and leek; cover pot and simmer for about 40 minutes.
4. Stir in basil, dill, thyme, garlic, and onion powders and mustard. Simmer, covered, for another 10 minutes, adding more stock if soup is too thick. Makes 10 serv.

ONION LEEK SOUP - Fast Weight Loss

2 onions sliced into rings
2 leeks, sliced (white and light green)
12 green onions, sliced
1/4 c. minced shallots
2 cloves garlic, crushed
2 tsp grated fresh ginger root
1/16 tsp cayenne pepper

2 tsp whole wheat flour
Fresh ground pepper
Fresh chives, snipped
1/4 c. low-sodium soy sauce
2 tsp lemon juice
7 c. water
1 c. white wine or use water

Sauté onions in 1/2 cup water for 5 minutes. Add leeks, green onions, and shallots with another 1/2 cup water. Sauté a few minutes to soften. Add garlic, ginger, and cayenne. Stir a few times, then add flour and stir for a couple of minutes. Slowly mix in water, wine, and soy sauce. Bring to boil, reduce heat, cover, and simmer for 45 minutes.

Add lemon juice and several twists of ground pepper. Mix. Ladle into bowls and garnish with snipped chives. Serves 6 to 8.

ORIENTAL EGG DROP SOUP - Fast Weight Loss

1 oz. dried shiitake mushrooms
3 c. chicken broth
2 tsp soy sauce (low-sodium)
1/8 tsp ground ginger
2 Tbsp cornstarch

2 Tbsp water
2 egg whites
3 Tbsp thinly sliced green
   onions, including top
White pepper

Place mushrooms in a bowl, pour in warm water to cover and let soak for about 30 minutes. Then drain mushrooms.

In a 2 quart saucepan, combine chicken broth, soy sauce, ginger, and mushrooms. Stir together cornstarch and water; add to soup. Bring to a boil, cover high heat, stirring constantly. Drop egg whites into boiling soup. Remove from heat and continue stirring until egg separates into shreds. Sprinkle with onions and season to taste with pepper. Serve immediately. 5 servings.

QUICKIE CORN CHOWDER

1/2 c. water
2 c. frozen corn
1 1/2 c. rice milk
2 tsp dried onion flakes

1/4 tsp garlic powder
1/2 tsp chili salsa
2 tsp lemon juice

Bring water to a boil. Add corn and cook according to directions. Drain corn and put into blender with remaining ingredients. Blend about 10 seconds. Pour soup into saucepan and simmer on low about 2 to 3 minutes or until heated through. Stir constantly. Serves 2.

POTATO CELERY CHOWDER - Fast Weight Loss

1 lg. onion, coarsely chopped
4 stalks celery, sliced
1 green pepper, chopped
2 carrots, sliced
2 cloves garlic, crushed
1 (28 oz.) can chopped tomatoes in
    their juice

4 lg. potatoes, cubed
2 tsp low-sodium soy sauce
1 tsp basil
1/2 tsp paprika
1/4 tsp pepper
6 1/2 c. water

Place onion, celery, green pepper, carrots, and garlic in a large soup pot with 1/2 cup water. Sauté for 5 minutes until vegetables are crisp-tender. Add potatoes, soy sauce, basil, paprika, pepper, and remaining water. Bring to a boil, reduce heat, cover, and cook over medium low heat for 30 minutes. Add tomatoes, cover, and cook an additional 15 minutes. Serves 10.

RED PEPPER SOUP - Fast Weight Loss

1 sm. cauliflower, coarsely chopped
2 sm. red peppers, sliced
1 sm. can tomatoes, chopped
2 inch piece of cucumber, peeled
    and chopped

3 3/4 c. vegetable stock
Pinch of dry mustard
Bean sprouts to garnish
1 onion, chopped
Seasoning to taste

Combine all ingredients in a large saucepan and bring to a boil. Cover pan and simmer 15 to 20 minutes or until everything is cooked but still crisp. Soup can be pureed to make a smooth soup. Adjust seasoning and garnish with a sprinkling of bean sprouts. Serves 2.

SAVORY SOUP

1/2 c. uncooked lentils
1/3 c. uncooked brown rice
2 cloves garlic, minced
2 bay leaves
1 sm. onion, chopped
2 Tbsp soy sauce
2 med. carrots, sliced
1 celery stalk, chopped

4 lg. tomatoes, chopped
1 tsp paprika
1/2 tsp marjoram
1 tsp basil
1/2 tsp thyme
Ground pepper to taste
1/2 c. tomato juice
1/4 c. dry red wine

Place the first 6 ingredients in a large pot and cover with 3 cups of water. Bring to a boil, cover, and simmer over low heat for 7 to 8 minutes. Add 2 additional cups of water along with all the remaining ingredients. Cover and simmer over low heat for 25 to 30 minutes or until the vegetables, rice, and lentils are done to your liking. Makes 6 servings.

SPICY SOUP

6 c. water
1 1/2 c. Picante sauce
3 cloves garlic, crushed
2 onions, cut into wedges
5 carrots, sliced 1/2 inch thick
4 med. potatoes, cut into lg. chunks
1/2 c. long grain brown rice
1 green pepper, cut into 1/2 inch pieces

1 rib celery, cut into
   1/2 inch slices
1/2 sm. cabbage, shredded
2 c. corn kernels
2 tomatoes, cut into wedges
Fresh chopped coriander

Place 6 cups water in a large soup pot. Add Picante sauce (either mild, medium, or hot depending on your taste buds). Add garlic, onions carrots, potatoes and rice. Cook over medium heat for 30 minutes. Add green pepper, celery, cabbage, and corn. Cook 20 minutes longer. Add tomatoes and coriander (if desired); heat through. Serve in large bowls. Garnish with lemon wedges, if desired); Pass more hot Picante sauce to spoon on at the table. Serves 8.

SPINACH NOODLE SOUP

4 c. chicken broth, defatted
2 cloves garlic, crushed
10 oz. spinach, chopped

1 c. whole wheat pasta shells,
   cooked

Heat broth and add garlic. Stir in spinach and cover until cooked; add pasta and heat through. Serves 4.

SPINACH SPAGHETTI SOUP

2 oz. spinach spaghetti
1/2 onion, chopped
1/2 green bell pepper, chopped fine
1/2 head broccoli, chopped into
   1 inch pieces

1 c. cooked barley
1 c. garbanzo beans (canned)
3 Tbsp vegetable broth seasoning
1/4 c. spaghetti sauce
8 c. water

Bring water to a boil in a large pot and add first 6 ingredients. Let simmer for 20 minutes, then add remaining ingredients and cook 10 to 15 minutes longer. Serves 4.

SPLIT PEA CHOWDER

4 c. water
1 med. onion, sliced
1 potato, diced
1 c. dry split peas

1 med. carrot, grated
1/2 tsp sweet basil
1 c. brown rice, cooked or
   whole grain toast

Bring water to a boil and add next 3 ingredients. Cook until tender. Add grated carrot and basil. Serve over brown rice or whole wheat toast. Serves 2 to 4.

SPLIT PEA SOUP

5 c. chicken stock (salt-free)
1 c. split peas
1/2 c. diced celery
1 carrot, diced
1/4 c. diced onion
1/2 c. dry sherry (optional)
1 clove garlic

2 Tbsp vegetable seasoning
   (salt-free)
1 bay leaf
1 tsp Bakon seasoning or
   liquid smoke
1/4 tsp Tabasco sauce

In large pan, heat chicken stock. Add all ingredients, except sherry. Simmer, stirring occasionally, for 45 minutes, loosely covered. Add more liquid, if needed. Before serving, stir in sherry.

TARRAGON SOUP - Fast Weight Loss

6 c. water
3 leeks, white part only, cleaned and
   cut into lg. pieces
2 carrots, sliced
2 celery stalks, sliced
4 sm. potatoes, quartered

4 cloves garlic, peeled
1 bay leaf
6 whole peppercorns
Ground black pepper to taste
2 Tbsp tarragon, chopped (fresh)
1 onion, quartered

Combine all ingredients, except tarragon and pepper in a large pot and bring to a boil. Reduce heat and simmer, uncovered, for 30 minutes to an hour. Drain and discard vegetables. Return broth to pot. Heat broth and add pepper and tarragon. Serve at once. Serves 4 to 6.

THAI RICE SOUP

4 c. chicken broth
1 stalk broccoli
1 c. cooked rice
2 Tbsp fish sauce
1 Tbsp ginger, minced

1 Tbsp dried onion flakes
1 Tbsp cilantro, chopped
3 green onions, chopped
1 tsp dried red chili flakes

Heat chicken broth in a saucepan. Add the broccoli and bring to a boil. Reduce heat to simmer. Add the rice and cook for 2 minutes. Season with fish sauce. Sprinkle ginger, onion flakes, cilantro, onions, and chili flakes on soup. 4 servings.

TOFU AND SNOW PEA SOUP

4 c. defatted chicken broth
1 (4 oz.) cake tofu, cubed
1/2 c. mushrooms, sliced
1/2 c. minced green onions
1/2 c. chopped carrots

1 clove garlic, minced
1 tsp fresh ginger, grated
1 tsp soy sauce (low-sodium)
1 c. fresh snow peas

Place all ingredients, except snow peas, in a saucepan. Bring to a boil, lower heat and simmer, covered, for 20 minutes or until vegetables are tender. Add snow peas and cook briefly until just tender. Serves 4.

TOMATO BOUILLON - Fast Weight Loss

4 c. tomato juice
1/2 bay leaf
2 cloves garlic, minced
1/4 tsp oregano
1/4 tsp basil

1/4 tsp marjoram
1/4 tsp dill weed
2 Tbsp fresh chopped parsley
Freshly ground pepper to taste

Place all herbs, except parsley, in tomato juice and allow to stand for 1 hour to allow flavors to blend. Heat to boiling and remove from heat and strain. Garnish with parsley. Serves 4.

TOMATO - CORN CHOWDER SOUP

2 c. frozen Latino Mexicali Vegetable
Mix or corn kernels with kidney
  beans and red pepper
2 c. chicken stock
1/2 c. mild green chili salsa
1 c. diced tomatoes

2 tsp cumin
2 Tbsp minced fresh cilantro
  or coriander
1 tsp garlic powder
2 Tbsp salt free chili powder
1/8 c. cornstarch

Bring chicken stock to boil. Add all ingredients, except cornstarch and simmer 1/2 hour. In small cup dissolve cornstarch into water. Add to soup and stir until soup thickens slightly.

TOMATO - EGGPLANT SOUP

1 1/2 lb. eggplant, unpeeled and diced
1 lg. (28 oz.) can whole tomatoes
4 Tbsp sesame tahini
1 c. water

2 Tbsp Vogue's Vege-Base or
  Mrs. Dash Seasoning
2 Tbsp tamari (soy sauce)

Cook eggplant and tomatoes (chopped up a little) in water for about 20 minutes or until eggplant is done. Add tahini, tamari, and Vege-Base, if using. Puree in blender of food processor for a few seconds. If soup is too thick, add 1/4 to 1/2 cup additional water. Reheat and serve. Serves 6.

TOMATO - MUSHROOM SOUP - Fast Weight Loss

1/2 c. Butter Buds
3 celery stalks, chopped
1 leek (white part only), chopped
1/2 lb. mushrooms, chopped
5 c. peeled, seeded, and chopped
  tomatoes
3/4 c. dry vermouth

2 tsp tomato paste
1/4 tsp apple juice concentrate
1 bay leaf
1/4 tsp oregano
3 c. chicken broth
1 garlic clove, chopped
Pepper to taste

Sauté celery, leek, and garlic in Butter Buds until softened, about 8 minutes. Increase heat to high. Add chopped mushrooms and sauté until lightly browned, about 5 minutes. Add tomatoes, broth, vermouth, tomato paste, apple juice concentrate, oregano, and bay leaf. Season with pepper. Bring to a boil. Reduce heat., cover, and simmer until vegetables are tender (about 30 minutes). 6 servings.

TOMATO SOUP - Fast Weight Loss

3 c. canned tomatoes
2 c. water
1 sm. onion, chopped
1 stalk celery, chopped
1 sm. carrot, chopped

1/2 Tbsp parsley flakes
1 tsp basil
3/4 tsp oregano
1/8 tsp marjoram
Dash or 2 of Tabasco

Combine all ingredients in a soup pot. Bring to a boil. Cover and simmer over low heat for 30 to 45 minutes until vegetables are tender. Place in the blender and process until smooth for a delicious, familiar texture tomato soup. Serves 6.

TOMATO VEGETABLE SOUP - Fast Weight Loss

1 c. water
1 lg. onion, chopped
2 c. chopped cauliflower
1 c. chopped broccoli
1 c. chopped carrots
1 c. chopped celery
2 c. chopped spinach
2 (28 oz.), cans tomatoes, blended

Dash of ground ginger
2 Tbsp parsley
2 Tbsp low-sodium soy sauce
1/4 tsp each: Cumin, celery
   seed, basil, rosemary, curry
   powder, dill weed, paprika,
   cayenne pepper
Dash of black pepper

Place all ingredients in a large soup pot. Bring to a boil, reduce heat, cover, and cook over medium heat until vegetables are tender. Serves 5.

TOMATO VERMICELLI SOUP

1 (28 oz.) can tomatoes
1 onion, minced
4 garlic cloves (more to taste),
   minced or put through a press

Freshly ground pepper
1/2 tsp dried marjoram (more
   to taste)
1/2 c. vermicelli

Drain the tomatoes and retain the liquid. Return the liquid to the can and add enough water to fill the can. Put the tomatoes through the medium disk of a food mill into a bowl or puree and put through a sieve; set aside

Heat water in a heavy bottomed soup pot and sauté the onion with 2 cloves of the garlic until the onion is tender. Add the tomato puree and cook 10 minutes, stirring. Add the remaining garlic and the liquid from the tomatoes. Add salt and pepper to taste and the marjoram. Bring to a simmer and add the vermicelli. Cook until the pasta is al dente. Taste again; add more garlic if desired. Correct seasonings and serve, not too hot The soup will keep up to 3 days in the refrigerator and can also be frozen, in either case, add the vermicelli just before serving.

TORTILLA SOUP

8 corn tortillas
4 c. chicken stock or canned broth
2 lbs. fresh tomatoes, peeled or
   1 (28 oz.)can solid pack tomatoes
1 med. onion, chopped

2 cloves garlic, minced
1 c. fresh cilantro, coarsely
   chopped
Black pepper, red pepper, and
   lime juice to taste

Preheat oven to 350 degrees. Cut tortillas in half, then cut crosswise into strips 1/4 inch wide. Spread tortilla strips on a large ungreased cookie sheet. Heat in 350 degree oven for 10 to 20 minutes, tossing strips every 5 minutes. Remove strips from oven when they are crisp but not brown. Set aside.

Heat water in a large pot and add onion and garlic. Sauté over medium heat just until onion is transparent, about 5 minutes. Puree tomatoes in blender or food processor. Add puree and chicken broth to onions. Bring mixture to a boil. Reduce heat and simmer for 5 minutes. If soup is prepared in advance, stop at this point. Add fresh cilantro and adjust seasonings at time of serving. Season to taste with black and red pepper and lime juice.

Serve immediately, putting a handful of tortilla strips in each soup bowl. Ladle soup over chips. Serves 8.

VEGETABLE WHEAT MEAT SOUP

2 c. fresh green beans
2 Tbsp lemon juice
1 (2 lb.) can tomatoes
1 onion, chopped
6 carrots, peeled and chopped
3 stalks celery, chopped
4 c. chicken broth, defatted

1/2 head cabbage, shredded
6 oz. Seitan vegetarian wheat
   meat
1 c. brown rice, cooked
2 Tbsp fresh parsley
1/2 tsp pepper

Cut beans diagonally into thirds; toss with lemon juice and steam until tender. Combine next 5 ingredients with chicken broth in large pot; bring to a boil, reduce heat, and simmer 1 to 2 hours or until vegetables are tender. Add beans and cabbage; simmer 15 minutes. Add wheat meat and rice and heat through. Sprinkle with parsley. Serves 4 to 6.

VEGETABLE BEAN SOUP

2 c. kidney beans
3 qts. stewed tomatoes
6 qts. water

4 c. celery, chopped
3 lg. onions, peeled and chopped

Optional Ingredients - chose one or more:
12 c. cooked whole wheat noodles
2 lg. carrots, diced

4 sm. zucchini, diced
4 c. fresh corn

Soak beans overnight; drain off water. Add fresh water; bring water to a boil and simmer for 1 1/2 hours. Add remaining ingredients; simmer for 1 hour more and adjust seasoning to taste. Serves 25 to 30.

VEGGIE HARVEST SOUP - Fast Weight Loss

10 c. water
4 white potatoes, cubed and peeled
1 sm. cabbage, shredded
4 stalks celery, chopped
1 sm. cauliflower, cored and cut
    into 1 inch flowerettes
1 lg. onion, finely chopped
4 carrots, chopped

3 med. zucchini, sliced
2 c. banana squash, cubed
2 cloves garlic, minced
2 cubes vegetable bouillon
1/2 tsp thyme
1/2 tsp basil
Pepper to taste
2 Tbsp fresh lemon juice

In a large soup kettle, bring water to a boil and add all ingredients except lemon juice. Return to boil and simmer for 30 minutes, stirring frequently to break up squash. Stir in lemon juice when ready to serve. Serves 8 to 10.

WILD RICE SOUP

12 1/2 c. water
2 onions, sliced
4 stalks celery, sliced
3 carrots,. sliced
1 c. sliced green onions
2 oz. chopped pimento
2 Tbsp dill weed
2 bay leaves
Fresh ground pepper (several twists)

1/2 tsp ground cumin
1/4 tsp garlic powder
1/8 tsp horseradish powder
1/2 tsp poultry seasoning
1/2 tsp turmeric
3 Tbsp low-sodium soy sauce
1 lb. fresh mushrooms, sliced
3/4 c. wild rice
1/2 c. brown rice

Sauté onions, celery, carrots, green onions and pimento in 1/2 cup water for 5 minutes. Stir in spices and mix well. Add remaining water, the soy sauce, and both kinds of rice. Bring to a boil, reduce heat, cover and simmer for 1 hour. Add sliced mushrooms; cook an additional 10 minutes. Serve hot. Serves 8 to 10.

WINTER VEGETABLE SOUP

1/2 c. each: black-eyed peas, red
  beans, pink beans, white beans
6 c. fresh water
1 c. chopped celery
1 chopped onion

2 spears broccoli, sliced
1 (14 1/2 oz.) can S & W
  Ready cut peeled tomatoes
2 sliced carrots

Soak beans overnight. Drain off water; rinse next morning. Simmer in a large pot beans and water; sprinkle with favorite spices. Simmer, covered, over lowest heat for 6 hours. Add remaining ingredients. Simmer 1 more hour. Serve with hot whole grain bread. Serves 10.

VEGETABLE BROTH - Fast Weight Loss

6 c. water
2 med. onions, peeled and chopped
4 lg. carrots, peeled and chopped

6 to 8 celery stalks, chopped
1 bunch fresh dill or parsley
Pepper to taste

Bring water to a boil; add onions and carrots. Add celery leaves and stalks to pot; simmer 45 minutes. Drain, then add dill and parsley. Serves 4.

ALFALFA SPROUT SALAD - Fast Weight Loss

3 stalks celery, diagonally sliced
1 cucumber, peeled and sliced
6 shallots, cut diagonally
1 Tbsp chives
1 red apple, cored, and cut into strips

2 tomatoes, chopped
1 c. alfalfa sprouts
1 Tbsp parsley
10 button mushrooms,
  thinly sliced

Combine all ingredients and squeeze lemon juice over them. Toss lightly and serve in lettuce cups or on a bed of shredded lettuce. Serves 2.

ARTICHOKE PASTA SALAD

4 oz. Vegeroni
1 (6 oz.) jar marinated artichoke hearts
1/2 c. pitted olives
1/4 lb. mushrooms, sliced

1 c. cherry tomatoes, halved
1 Tbsp parsley, chopped
1/2 tsp dry basil leaves
Pepper

Cook Vegeroni according to directions. Turn into a large bowl. Add artichokes, mushrooms, tomatoes, olives, parsley, and basil; toss gently. Cover and refrigerate for 4 hours. Season with pepper. 6 servings.

THREE BEAN SALAD

1/2 c. fresh string beans, steamed
lightly and cut into bite sized pieces
1 c. cooked garbanzo beans (salt-free)

Red Bermuda onion, a few thin
slices (or dice)
1 c. cooked kidney beans
(salt-free)

MARINADE:
1 clove garlic, crushed and minced
1/4 c. fresh orange juice
1/4 c. red wine vinegar

2 tsp dill weed, dried or
1 Tbsp fresh, minced
1 tsp low sodium Dijon mustard

Combine all ingredients in a small bowl. Refrigerate and marinate several hours, or overnight, before serving.

BROCCO- BEAN SALAD

1 bunch broccoli
1 can red kidney beans, rinsed
3 Tbsp Mrs. Pickford's (no oil)
vinaigrette dressing

Dash of Mrs. Dash
Dash of salad herbs
4 green onions, chopped

Steam broccoli (cut up) for 8 minutes; cool slightly. Combine all ingredients and refrigerate 1/2 hour (or more) before serving.

BROCCOLI AND ONION SALAD - Fast Weight Loss

2 lbs broccoli, cut into 1 inch pieces
1 sm. red onion, sliced
2 Tbsp lemon juice
1/2 c. no oil Italian dressing

1/4 tsp dry mustard
1/2 tsp dried tarragon leaves
Ground pepper to taste

Steam broccoli for 1 minute. Cool and toss with onion. Mix together rest of ingredients and pour over broccoli and onion. Marinate in refrigerator for 6 to 8 hours. Serves 4 to 6.

BROWN RICE DELIGHT

2 c. cold cooked brown rice
1 1/2 c. corn kernels
1 c. celery, sliced

1 c. grated carrot
2 onions, chopped

Combine all ingredients and toss with a dressing of your choice. Serves 2.

How to Look Great & Feel Sexy

BULGUR WHEAT AND CHICK PEA SALAD

1/2 c. uncooked bulgur wheat
1/2 c. sliced green onion
1 c. boiling water
1/4 c. fresh lemon juice

1 c. cooked chick peas, drained
1/2 c. chopped parsley
1/2 c. chopped carrots
1 c. sliced mushrooms

Put bulgur in a large heat-proof bowl. Pour boiling water over the bulgur; mix to moisten evenly. Allow to stand for 1 hour, bulgur will expand. Pour lemon juice over the bulgur and mix with a fork. Place mixture in a bowl with a snug cover. Layer each vegetable on top of the mixture in this order: Green onions, mushrooms, chick peas parsley, and carrots. Cover and refrigerate. Toss before serving. Garnish with tomato wedges. Serves 4 to 6.

CABBAGE SALAD WITH DILL - Fast Weight Loss

1/4 head cabbage, cut into thin strips
1 sm. cucumber, peeled and sliced
1 Tbsp white wine vinegar

2 Tbsp lemon juice
2 Tbsp chopped dill
Black pepper to taste

Mix cabbage, cucumber, and onions in large bowl. Stir in vinegar and lemon juice; sprinkle in dill and black pepper. Cover with plastic wrap and chill for several hours. Serves 2.

CARROT SALAD

1/4 c. walnut pieces
1 Tbsp shredded coconut
2 c. grated carrot
1/2 c. orange juice
Zest and juice of 1/2 lemon

1 apple, cored and grated
1/2 c. currants
Mrs. Dash or Instead of Salt
1 1/2 tsp grated fresh ginger

Toast walnut pieces and coconut in a low 300 degree oven. The walnuts will take about 10 minutes and the coconut 5. Chill. Combine grated carrots, apple, lemon zest, orange, and lemon juices, currants, Instead of Salt, and ginger. Add walnuts and coconut and serve. Makes 3 cups to serve 4.

CARROT AND FRUIT SALAD

3 med. carrots
2/3 c. dates, finely chopped
3/4 c. seedless grapes
1 lg. dessert apple

1 bunch watercress
1/3 c. roasted sunflower seeds
1 to 2 Tbsp lemon juice

Grate carrots, then mix dates with grapes. Coarsely chop the apple and stir into the other ingredients. Add lemon juice at once and toss lightly. Make a nest of the watercress and spoon the carrot mixture into the center. Sprinkle with the sunflower seeds. Serve at once. Serves 2 to 3.

CUCUMBER MARINADE - Fast Weight Loss

5 cucumbers thinly sliced
1 onion, thinly sliced
1 c. red wine vinegar

1 to 2 Tbsp honey
3 tsp dill weed
Black pepper (optional)

Place vinegar and honey in a saucepan and heat until warm. Place cucumbers, onion, dill weed, and optional pepper into a large container. Pour heated vinegar mixture over the cucumbers and onions; mix well. Cover and refrigerate at least 2 hours. Tastes even better if eaten the following day. Serves 6 to 8.

CAULIFLOWER WITH HERB VINEGAR - Fast Weight Loss

Flowers of 1/2 head cauliflower
1 slice lemon

1/4 c. mint, chopped
2 c. herb or tarragon vinegar

Lightly steam cauliflower in boiling water with slice of lemon. Remove from boiling water and plunge into icy water. Lightly towel dry. Sprinkle with 1/4 cup mint and toss in herb vinegar. Chill for at least 2 to 4 hours, tossing cauliflower through vinegar frequently. Drain and serve. Serves 2.

How to Look Great & Feel Sexy

CAULIFLOWER MARINADE SALAD - Fast Weight Loss

Break a head of cauliflower into small pieces and drop into a kettle of boiling water with:

The juice of 1/2 lemon (to keep the white color)

1/2 tsp sea salt

Cook a few minutes; drain and cool. Combine in a salad bowl:

Drained cauliflower
4 green onions, chopped
2 carrots, cut in matchsticks

1 red or green pepper, cut in matchsticks
1/2 c. celery, sliced thinly

Toss to moisten with 1/4 cup Lemon Vinaigrette Dressing (no oil). Per serving: 89 calories, 3 gm protein, 8 gm carbohydrates, 1 gm fat. Yield: 6 servings.

CHICK PEA AND PASTA SALAD

2 c. whole wheat pasta shells
1 (16 oz.) can chick peas, drained and rinsed
3 tomatoes, chopped fine
1/2 bunch fresh broccoli, chopped into 1 inch pieces

1 c. NO OIL Italian dressing (Cook's choice or Kraft)
1/2 tsp fresh ground black pepper
1 tsp dried oregano
1/2 tsp garlic powder

Mix pasta, chick peas, and vegetables together. Mix remaining ingredients in small bowl, then pour over pasta and toss gently. Chill for 3 to 4 hours before serving. Serves 6 to 8.

CHINESE SALAD

2 (2 oz.) firm tofu or wheat meat (for a vegetarian alternative)
1/4 yellow onion, sliced thin
1/2 c. bok choy or napa cabbage, shredded
1 lg. carrot, sliced in thin matchsticks

1/2 red pepper, sliced in thin strips
2 c. fresh bean sprouts
Sesame seeds, water chestnuts, or cashews (as garnish)

DRESSING:

1/3 c. rice vinegar
1/3 c. pineapple juice
1 Tbsp Chinese parsley (cilantro)

1/4 tsp powdered ginger or
freshly grated onion

Cut tofu or wheat meat into bite sized pieces; stir fry or boil until tender. Prepare vegetables; toss in bowl with tofu or wheat meat and dressing. Marinate 1/2 hour before serving. Makes 4 servings.

CHINESE HOT SALAD - Fast Weight Loss

1 onion, sliced
1 Tbsp grated fresh ginger
3 cloves garlic, pressed
2Tbsp low-sodium tamari
2 stalks celery, thickly sliced
1 green pepper, cut into strips

2 c. bean sprouts
1 c. Chinese pea pods
1/2 cucumber, peeled and cut
into strips
6 lettuce leaves, coarsely chopped
1 Tbsp lemon juice

In a wok or large pan, sauté onion, ginger, and garlic in 2 tablespoons water for 1 minute. Add 1 tablespoon tamari and next 4 ingredients. Cook over medium heat, stirring for 6 minutes. Add the remaining tamari, cucumber, and lettuce. Continue to cook 3 minutes longer. Sprinkle with lemon juice. Mix well. Serve hot. Serves 6.

COLESLAW

2 c. shredded green cabbage
2 c. shredded red cabbage
1/2 c. diced carrot
1/2 c. diced celery
1/2 c. diced green pepper
1/2 c. chopped apple
1/2 c. diced, peeled cucumber
1/4 c. finely chopped green onions

1/4 tsp caraway seeds
1/4 tsp celery seed
1/4 c. chopped parsley
3 Tbsp cider vinegar
1 Tbsp Dijon mustard
1/2 tsp low-sodium soy sauce
1 tsp honey
1 Tbsp lemon juice

Mix vegetables together in a large bowl. Mix vinegar, mustard, soy sauce, and honey together. Pour over vegetables. Sprinkle seeds on top. Toss to mix well. Chill for about 2 hours to blend flavors. Serves 6. *Helpful Hints: If you have a food processor, this can be prepared quite quickly.*

CRUNCHY PEA SALAD

2 c. fresh peas, steamed and chilled
1 (7 oz.) can water chestnuts, drained
   and sliced
4 stalks celery, thinly sliced
1 c. shredded carrots
4 green onions, thinly sliced
2 Tbsp tomato juice

2 Tbsp red wine vinegar
1 Tbsp low-sodium soy sauce
1 tsp Dijon mustard
1 clove garlic, minced
1 tsp paprika
1 tsp frozen apple juice
   concentrate

Combine first 5 ingredients. To make marinade, mix the remaining ingredients and beat well: Pour over salad; blend well. Cover and chill for about an hour. Drain excess marinade before serving. Serves 8.

CRUNCHY BEST SLAW- Fast Weight Loss

3 med. beets, peeled and grated
1 med. carrot, grated
1/3 jicama, diced
1/2 tsp Dijon mustard

2 Tbsp orange juice
2 Tbsp lemon juice
Peel of 1 orange, finely grated

In a salad bowl, combine beets and grated carrot. And in another bowl, stir together orange peel, mustard, and juices. Dress slaw and chill briefly before serving. Serves 4.

FINOCCHIO SALAD

1 1/2 c. raw whole wheat macaroni
1/2 c. sliced Florence fennel*
1/4 c. chopped Italian parsley
1/4 c. diced bell pepper
1 c. sliced raw mushrooms
2 Tbsp chopped chives

1/3 c. sliced black olives
2 to 3 Tbsp lemon juice
2 Tbsp no oil Italian dressing
1/2 tsp Instead of Salt
Freshly ground black pepper

A mouth-watering pasta salad. Cook macaroni until tender in salted, boiling water. Cool and combine with fennel, parsley, bell pepper, mushrooms, chives and olives. Mix 2 tablespoons lemon juice, salt, and pepper. Toss salad in dressing; taste and add remaining tablespoon of lemon juice, if desired. Makes 5 1/2 cups.

*No fennel in sight? Substitute raw celery or blanched green beans or crisp-tender broccoli.

GARDEN SALAD - Fast Weight Loss

2 heads leaf lettuce
1/2 head shredded cabbage
6 Swiss chard leaves, chopped
3 Chinese cabbage leaves, shredded
1 head cauliflower, broken into
   flowerettes
3 stalks broccoli, chopped

1 zucchini, diced
5 lg. spinach leaves, chopped
3 carrots, diced
1 red pepper, diced
4 scallion tops, diced
1 beet, diced or grated

Tear lettuce into bite size pieces and cut greens. Combine all ingredients in a large bowl, adding no oil Italian dressing (see Dressings). Toss, chill, and serve. Serves 10.

GREEN SALAD - Fast Weight Loss

1 c. torn Romaine lettuce
1 c. torn red leaf lettuce
1 c. torn spinach leaves
1 c. chopped watercress
1/4 c. chopped parsley

1 tsp toasted sesame seeds
4 red bell pepper rings
1/2 c. alfalfa sprouts
1/3 c. grated raw beets

Toss together first 8 ingredients. Divide into 4 salad bowls and top with red pepper rings. Fill rings sprouts and top with beets. Serves 4.

GARDEN VEGETABLE SALAD - Fast Weight Loss

1 stalk broccoli (about 1 1/2 c.)
2 to 3 button mushrooms
Vinaigrette dressing or Italian
   no oil dressing
1 carrot

Wedge of cabbage (purple
   or green)
Thin slice of onion, minced
1 red pepper, sliced

Bring saucepan of water to boil. While broccoli is still whole, dip the flower head in the boiling water, briefly, about 20 seconds. Slice the pepper. Cut the broccoli into bite sized bits. Peel or scrape the carrot, slice thinly. Cut mushroom caps in half. Cut cabbage into bite sized wedges. Mince onion. Place in salad bowl and serve with vinaigrette dressing. Serves 4. *The success of this salad depends on FRESH ingredients!*

KIDNEY BEAN SALAD

2 c. kidney beans (canned)
1 red onion, sliced
3 stalks celery, diced
2 c. whole kernel corn (canned)

1 c. carrots, diced
1 c. parsley chopped
1 head red leaf lettuce, torn

Combine all ingredients. Chill and toss with no oil dressing of choice.

MACARONI SALAD

2 c. whole wheat macaroni
4 hard cooked egg whites, chopped
2 Tbsp green onions, chopped fine
2 Tbsp minced dill pickle
2 c. canned baby green peas

1/4 c. chopped pimento
4 Tbsp vinegar
2 tsp mustard
3 tsp vegetable broth seasoning

Cook macaroni according to package directions. Drain and rinse in cold water. Add remaining ingredients in order given, tossing with vinegar, mustard, and seasoning. Serve on bed of lettuce. Serves 4.

MEDITERRANEAN RICE SALAD

1 1/2 c. brown rice
3 c. chicken broth
3 Tbsp lemon juice
Dash of cinnamon
Sprinkling of cilantro
Pepper to taste

1 Tbsp Butter Buds (dry)
3/4 c. chopped pistachio nuts
1/2 c. raisins
1/2 c. sliced mushrooms
1/4 c. finely chopped mint leaves

Combine lemon juice, cinnamon, cilantro, and pepper; set aside. In medium saucepan with a lid, cover rice with chicken broth; add Butter Buds. Bring to a boil, then cover and simmer over low heat for 40 minutes. While hot, toss rice with dressing. Add remaining ingredients. Serves 6.

MEDITERRANEAN SALAD

1 lg. firm red tomato
1 cucumber
1 sm. red Bermuda onion

3/4 c. garbanzo beans (or sm. can), well rinsed

MARINADE:

1 Tbsp fresh oregano or 1/2 Tbsp dried
1 Tbsp apple juice concentrate
1/2 c. red wine vinegar

1 Tbsp fresh sweet basil or 1/2 Tbsp dried
1 clove garlic, crushed

Cut tomato into wedges. Peel cucumber; slice in half lengthwise. Scoop out seeds and cut into slices. Slice onion. Place vegetables into a small bowl. Add garbanzos. Press garlic and add vinegar, herbs, and sweetener. Allow to marinate at least 1 hour, refrigerated, before serving. Serves 3 to 4.

MUSHROOM AND WALNUT SALAD

4 c. bite size pieces of Romaine and butter lettuce
10 cherry tomatoes, halved
1/2 lb. mushrooms, sliced
2/3 c. walnut pieces
2 green onion (tops included), sliced

2 tsp Dijon mustard
1/8 tsp pepper
1/8 tsp paprika
2 tsp dry basil leaves
5 tsp white wine vinegar

In a salad bowl, combine basil, pepper, paprika, mustard, and vinegar. Beat with a fork until blended. Mix in mushrooms and green onions. Let stand at room temperature for at least 30 minutes. Add walnut pieces, lettuce, and cherry tomatoes; toss lightly. Serves 4.

NUTTY RICE SALAD

Have ready:
2 c. cooked brown rice

1/2 c. cooked wheat berries

Bring a quart of water to boiling, drop in:
1 c. green string beans, slivered

1 carrot, cut in matchsticks

Boil for 1 1/2 minutes, drain, and run cold water over to set color. Combine with cooked grains and add:
1/4 c. parsley, minced
1/4 c. chopped toasted walnuts

1/4 c. green onions, chopped

Serve on a bed of greens with Poppy Seed Dressing. Yield: 6 servings. Per serving: 112 calories, 3 gm protein, 18 gm carbohydrates, 3 gm fat.

ORANGE ALMOND SPINACH SALAD

1 bunch spinach   3 oranges, peeled and chopped
1/2 c. sliced almonds

DRESSING:

1/2 c. orange juice   1/2 tsp black pepper
1/4 c. red wine vinegar

Toss all ingredients together and chill for 1/2 hour.

ORANGE COLESLAW - Fast Weight Loss

1/2 head cabbage   1/2 c. red pepper, thinly sliced
2 oranges, peeled and segmented   1/2 tsp grated lemon rind
1/2 c. green pepper, thinly sliced   2 tsp lemon or orange rind

Combine all ingredients and let stand for 1 hour. Toss lightly and chill for 2 hours before serving. Serves 2.

DRESSING:

2 Tbsp orange juice   1 Tbsp vinegar
2 Tbsp lemon juice   Black pepper to taste

Combine all ingredients well and toss over cole slaw before serving. Serves 2.

POLYNESIAN FRUIT SALAD

1 lg. pineapple   1 c. strawberries, sliced
1 c. peeled, seeded, diced papaya   1/2 c. canned lychees
1 mango peeled, pitted, and diced   1/2 c. shredded coconut
1 banana, sliced

Halve pineapple lengthwise through crown. Cut out fruit, leaving a 1/4 inch shell. Remove core; dice fruit and place in large bowl. To pineapple, add other ingredients. Mix lightly. Spoon fruit into pineapple shells. Sprinkle with coconut. 4 servings.

RAISIN SALAD

6 shredded raw carrots
1 c. raisins
Section, 3 oranges

1 can crushed pineapple in its
own juice

Mix together in large bowl. Include pineapple juice and squeeze the juice from the orange after sectioning. Refrigerate and serve cold. No mayonnaise or salad dressing necessary.

POTATO SALAD - Fast Weight Loss

3 cooked potatoes, peeled and diced
1 celery stalk, chopped
1/2 onion, peeled and chopped
1 red bell pepper, seeded and chopped
1 tsp celery seed
1 tsp garlic powder

1/4 tsp dried dill
1 tsp mustard powder
2 tsp fresh lemon juice
1 Tbsp apple juice concentrate
1/2 c. red wine vinegar

1. In a medium bowl, combine potatoes, celery, onion, and pepper. Mix thoroughly.
2. In a small bowl, combine remaining ingredients. Pour over vegetables and mix thoroughly. Chill well before serving. Makes 8 servings.

QUICK ARTICHOKE PASTA SALAD

4 oz. (1 c.) whole wheat macaroni
1 (6 oz.) jar marinated artichoke
    hearts (water packed)
1/4 lb. mushrooms, quartered

1 Tbsp parsley, chopped
1/2 tsp dry basil leaves
1 c. cherry tomatoes, halved
Pepper to taste

Cook macaroni according to package directions. Drain, rinse with cold water, and drain again. Place into large bowl. Add artichokes and their liquid, mushrooms, tomatoes, parsley, and basil; toss gently. Cover and refrigerate for at least 4 hours. Before serving, season with pepper to taste. Serves 6.

RICE SALAD

1 1/2 c. cooked brown rice
1 lg. celery stalk, thinly sliced
1/4 c. raisins
1/4 of an onion, chopped

2 Tbsp mango chutney
5 Tbsp Italian no oil dressing
1 Tbsp curry

Combine rice, celery, raisins, onion, and chutney. Add curry and dressing; toss to blend. Chill before serving.

SPINACH PASTA SALAD

8 oz. spinach pasta Rotelle
1 c. frozen corn
1/2 c. frozen green beans
1 jar pimentos
1 can water pack artichoke hearts

1/4 c. toasted sesame seeds
Fresh, chopped parsley
Garlic powder to taste
No oil Italian dressing

Boil water; add Rotelle pasta and cook 11 to 12 minutes. Drain and rinse with cold water. Defrost and lightly cook corn and green beans. Drain and cool. Add remaining ingredients, draining can of artichoke hearts. Refrigerate and serve chilled.

SCANDINAVIAN HOT POTATO SALAD - Fast Weight Loss

4 med. sized new potatoes
1/2 c. chopped red onion

1/2 c. chopped celery

DRESSING:

1/3 c. cider or balsamic vinegar
2 Tbsp apple juice concentrate
1 Tbsp Veg-It seasoning
1 Tbsp low-sodium Dijon mustard

1 Tbsp fresh dill weed or 1 tsp
   dried dill weed
1 Tbsp "Bakon" seasoning or
   dash liquid smoke

Boil or steam new potatoes until tender, 15 to 20 minutes. Slice thin and place in bowl along with chopped onion and celery. In saucepan, heat together and briefly boil the dressing ingredients. Pour dressing over contents of bowl; gently stir. Cover and serve warm.

SNOW PEA AND RICE SALAD

4 c. brown rice, cold (cooked)   1/4 c. chopped parsley
1 c. fresh snow peas, coarsely cut   1/4 c. red bell pepper
1/2 c. chopped green onions

DRESSING:
1/4 c. orange juice   1 Tbsp pectin
2 Tbsp rice vinegar   2 tsp low-sodium soy sauce

Combine the rice and vegetables, then mix well. In a separate container, mix the dressing ingredients thoroughly. Pour dressing over vegetables, mixing well. Serve chilled. Serves 4 to 6.

SPINACH SALAD WITH RASPBERRY VINAIGRETTE

2 bunches fresh spinach   Cucumber, thinly sliced
Few slivers of red onion   2 hard boiled eggs (no yolk), sliced
Sesame seeds, slivered almonds or   1 peeled, sliced orange
  toasted pine nuts (as garnish)

VINAIGRETTE:
1/4 c. raspberry vinegar (Silver   1 Tbsp garlic, crushed and pressed
  Palate or other brand)

Combine all vinaigrette ingredients in shaker jar; shake and let blend. Cut off spinach leaves at stem, float in large tub of water to clean. Dry in salad spinner or towel; tear and place in salad bowl and add remaining ingredients. Toss with dressing and serve with garnish.

For a variation, warm salad dressing in small saucepan and serve warm on salad. Makes 4 to 5 servings.

SPROUT SALAD - Fast Weight Loss

SALAD:

2 c. mixed sprouts (lentils, pea, azuki, etc.)
3 to 4 green onions, sliced
1 stalk celery, sliced

2.2 oz. jar chopped pimentos
1 c. sliced mushrooms
3 to 4 Tbsp chopped fresh coriander or parsley

DRESSING:

2 tsp Dijon mustard
1 Tbsp water
2 Tbsp white wine vinegar

1 tsp Worcestershire sauce
1 Tbsp low-sodium soy sauce
1/4 tsp black pepper

Mix salad ingredients in a large bowl. Place the mustard and the water in a small bowl and mix well. Add remaining ingredients and mix, then pour over the sprout salad. Toss to coat. Refrigerate before serving.

STEAMED VEGETABLE SALAD - Fast Weight Loss

1 c. zucchini, sliced
1 c. carrots, sliced
1 1/2 c. broccoli flowerettes
3 med. tomatoes
1 red pepper

Pinch of mint
3 Tbsp salad dressing (no oil Italian or vinaigrette)
Juice of 1/4 to 1/2 lemon

Steam the carrots 5 minutes or until tender. Steam the broccoli and zucchini 2 to 3 minutes. Let the vegetables cool. Cut the tomatoes in wedges and the red pepper in narrow strips. Combine all the vegetables and toss with the dressing, lemon, and mint.

SUMI SALAD

Shred 1 head cabbage. Lightly brown 1/4 cup slivered almonds and 1/4 cup sesame seeds. Chop 8 green onions. Crunch up 2 packages Ramen noodles (uncooked without flavor packet). Add snow peas. Combine above ingredients. Add dressing and toss.

DRESSING:

2 Tbsp rice vinegar
Juice of 1 lemon
1/4 tsp salt
Pepper

1 tsp Dijon mustard
1 clove garlic, minced
2 green onions, finely chopped

Mix well and toss with salad.

STIR FRY SALAD

8 c. torn fresh spinach
2 c. wheat meat
1/2 c. water
1/2 c. tarragon vinegar
1/4 c. sliced green onion
4 tsp cornstarch
1/2 tsp dry mustard

1/4 tsp pepper
1 clove garlic, minced
1 c. sliced carrots
2 c. sliced cauliflower flowerettes
1/2 c. sliced celery
1 c. cherry tomatoes, halved
Non-stick spray coating

Place torn spinach in a large salad bowl;. set aside. Cut wheat meat (or chicken) into bite size pieces. For sauce, combine water, vinegar, onion, cornstarch, mustard, pepper, and garlic. Set aside.

Spray a wok or large skillet with non-stick spray. Preheat over a medium high heat. Stir fry carrots and cauliflower for about 5 minutes or until crisp-tender. Spray skillet or wok again and add half the wheat meat to the wok and stir fry for 3 to 4 minutes. Return all the wheat meat to the wok. Push the wheat meat from the center of the wok. Stir sauce, then add to the center of wok or skillet.

Cook and stir 2 minutes more. Return vegetables to wok. Add celery and tomatoes. Stir ingredients together to coat with sauce. Pour the wheat meat mixture over spinach in bowl. Toss lightly to coat. Serve immediately. Serves 6.

SUMMER SHREDDED SALAD

1 c. bulgur wheat
4 firm, fresh zucchini
2 lg. carrots
1 sm. yellow onion
Juice of 3 lemons or 1/3 c. (no salt, no oil) Italian dressing
2 Tbsp fresh mint leaves or 1 Tbsp dried
1 ripe red tomato

1/4 c. fresh parsley
1 sm. red bell pepper
1 bunch (about 1/4 c.) green scallion(spring onion)
1 1/2 c. hot chicken stock - (salt free, of course)
Dash of hot cayenne pepper

Bring 2 cups of water to a boil and add bulgur; cook for 40 minutes until soft. Place bulgur in small bowl. Cover with hot chicken stock and toss. Allow to sit 15 minutes. Mix in all ingredients. Add seasonings; toss again. Garnish with tomato wedges. This is best made ahead and refrigerated a few hours before serving. Serve in pita bread or Romaine lettuce leaves. Serves 4.

How to Look Great & Feel Sexy

SWEET POTATO - BANANA SALAD

4 baked sweet potatoes, peeled
    and cut in chunks
4 bananas sliced

1/2 c. raisins
2 apples, chopped
1/2 tsp nutmeg

Mix the first 4 ingredients together. Sprinkle the nutmeg over the top. Serves 4 to 6.

SUMMER FRUIT SALAD - Fast Weight Loss

1/4 watermelon
1/2 cantaloupe
1/2 honeydew melon
1 lb. seedless grapes

1 pt. strawberries
1 pt. raspberries
1 pt. cherries
1 pt. blueberries

Remove rind from melons. Slice melons into wedges. Stem grapes. Hull strawberries. Pile strawberries in the center of a large basket or tray; surround with melon wedges, raspberries, and cherries. Garnish with grapes and blueberries. Serves 8 to 10.

TABOULI

1 c. bulgur
8 scallions, chopped
1/4 c. finely chopped parsley
1/4 c. chopped fresh mint

3 ripe tomatoes, chopped
1/4 c. lemon juice
1/4 tsp black pepper

Bring 2 cups of water to a boil; add bulgur. Cook for 45 minutes. Place bulgur in a bowl with water to cover. Allow to soak 15 minutes, then drain and squeeze dry. Mix all ingredients and serve on lettuce leaves or with crackers.

TOMANGO (TOMATO - MANGO) SALAD - Fast Weight Loss

4 lg. mangos, peeled and chopped
Juice from 1/2 lemon

2 tsp basil
5 med. tomatoes, chopped

Combine mangos, lemon juice, and basil. Let chill in refrigerator for about 1/2 hour. Stir in tomatoes and chill until serving time.

CUCUMBER DRESSING

3 lg. cucumbers, peeled and cut
4 Tbsp apple juice concentrate (frozen)
4 Tbsp orange juice concentrate
  (frozen)
8 Tbsp lemon juice
1 tsp dill weed
2 cloves garlic, minced
1 tsp onion powder

Blend all ingredients in blender until very smooth. Serves 2 to 4.

DRESSING - Fast Weight Loss

1/2 c. tomato juice
2 tsp onion, finely chopped
Dash of oregano or dry mustard
1 tsp parsley
1 Tbsp lemon juice

Combine all ingredients in a jar with tight fitting lid. Shake well and refrigerate. Yield: 3/4 cup.

FRENCH DRESSING I

1/2 c. water
2 Tbsp orange juice
3 Tbsp concentrated apple juice
4 Tbsp lemon juice
1 1/2 Tbsp tomato puree
1/4 tsp dill weed
1 tsp onion powder
1 tsp garlic powder
1/2 tsp paprika
1 1/2 tsp cornstarch

Mix all ingredients, except cornstarch. Mix cornstarch with 1/2 tablespoon water and add to mix. Bring to a boil and chill. Serves 2.

FRENCH SALAD DRESSING II

2 c. V-8 juice
2 c. vinegar
1 c. tomato sauce
1/2 c. lemon juice
3 1/2 Tbsp apple juice concentrate
1/4 c. tomato paste
1/4 green pepper
1 tsp celery seed
1 tsp dill weed
1/2 tsp paprika
1/4 tsp cayenne pepper
1 Tbsp arrowroot
1 onion

Combine all ingredients in a saucepan. Heat to a boil and simmer 5 minutes. Cool. Chill thoroughly before serving.

FRUITY DRESSING

1 cucumber, peeled and seeded	1 Tbsp lemon rind, grated
2 cloves garlic	1 Tbsp orange rind , grated
1 c. orange juice	2 Tbsp chopped fresh herbs
1/2 c. lemon vinegar	(parsley, basil, chives, thyme)

Combine all ingredients, except lemon and orange rind and fresh herbs. Blend in a food processor for 1 minute. Add other ingredients but do not blend. Shake well and store in sealed jars in refrigerator. Yield: About 2 cups.

GARLIC DRESSING - Fast Weight Loss

1 c. vinegar	2 to 3 cloves garlic
1/2 c. water	1/2 cucumber, peeled and seeded
Juice of 1 lemon	Black pepper to taste

Combine all ingredients in food processor and blend for 1 minute. Place in sealed jars and store in refrigerator. Yield: About 2 cups.

HERBED SALAD DRESSING I - Fast Weight Loss

1 Tbsp powdered fruit pectin	1/8 tsp pepper
1 tsp apple juice concentrate	1/4 c. water
1/8 tsp dry mustard	1 Tbsp vinegar
1/8 tsp dried basil, crushed	1 sm. clove garlic, minced
1/8 tsp paprika	

Combine the pectin, apple juice concentrate, mustard, basil, paprika, and pepper. Stir in water, vinegar, and garlic. Cover and chill for 1 hour.

HERB DRESSING II

1 c. herb vinegar	1/2 cucumber, peeled and seeded
1 c apple juice	2 Tbsp mixed herbs (parsley,
Juice of 1 lemon	chives, thyme, dill)

Combine the first 4 ingredients in a food processor and blend for 1 minute. Add herbs but do not blend. Place in sealed jars and store in refrigerator. Yield: About 2 cups.

ITALIAN NO OIL DRESSING - Fast Weight Loss

1/4 c. lemon juice
1/4 c. cider vinegar
1/4 c. apple juice
1/2 tsp oregano
1/2 tsp dry mustard

1/2 tsp onion powder
1/2 tsp garlic powder
1/2 tsp paprika
1/8 tsp thyme
1/8 tsp rosemary

Combine all ingredients in blender and blend well. Refrigerate overnight or longer to allow flavors to mix. Yield: 3/4 cup.

SPICY DRESSING - Fast Weight Loss

1 1/2 c. unsweetened apple juice
1 c. cider vinegar
4 1/2 tsp garlic powder
4 1/2 tsp cornstarch
3 tsp crushed oregano

1 tsp onion powder
1 1/2 tsp mustard powder
1 1/2 tsp paprika
1/2 tsp black pepper

Combine all ingredients in saucepan and bring to a boil. Cook, stirring until thickened. Chill, covered, until ready to use. Shake well before using. Yield: About 2 1/2 cups.

SWEET SOUR VINAIGRETTE DRESSING

3/4 c. water
1/4 c. frozen apple juice concentrate
3 Tbsp rice vinegar
1 Tbsp cider vinegar
1 Tbsp lemon juice
2 tsp soy sauce
2 cloves garlic, crushed
1 Tbsp pectin

1 1/2 tsp arrow root
1 tsp oregano
1 tsp onion powder
1/2 tsp each garlic powder,
    savory, paprika, and dry
    mustard
Dash cayenne pepper

In a small saucepan, combine all ingredients and stir to blend well. Bring to a boil, then reduce heat and simmer, stirring constantly, until thickened (about 4 to 5 minutes). Serve chilled or warmed. Yield: 1 1/2 cups.

TOFU - GARLIC SALAD DRESSING

3/4 c. V-8 juice
2/3 c. lemon juice
2 Tbsp tamari, Quick-Sip, or soy sauce
3/4 c. water
1 lb. tofu

1 tsp garlic powder or 2 to 3
  garlic buds
1 c. sesame seeds
1/4 of an onion

Blend together the preceding ingredients:
This dressing is also very good served over baked potatoes, steamed veggies, and grains such as brown rice and millet.

TOMATO SALAD DRESSING - Fast Weight Loss

1 c. tomato juice
1 1/2 Tbsp frozen apple juice
  concentrate
1 1/2 Tbsp lemon juice
1 Tbsp chopped celery leaves

1 Tbsp chopped parsley
2 tsp garlic powder
1/4 tsp basil
1/4 tsp oregano

Place all ingredients in a blender and blend at high speed. Chill before serving.

TOMATO JUICE DRESSING - Fast Weight Loss

1 c. tomato juice
1/4 c. tarragon vinegar
1 c. grated onion

1/2 tsp dry mustard
1 clove garlic, minced
2 tsp parsley

Combine all ingredients in blender and mix well. Chill in refrigerator. Before serving, shake well. Yield: 2 cups.

How to Look Great & Feel Sexy

REFERENCES

1. Anderson, James W., M.D. *Diabetes - A practical new guide to healthy living.* New York, New York: Arco Publishing, Inc., 1981.
2. Bailey, Covert. *The Fit-or-Fat Target Diet.* Boston, Massachusetts: Houghton Mifflin Company, 1984.
3. Bennett, Cleaves M., M.D. *In 12 weeks you can control your high blood pressure without drugs.* Garden City, New York: Doubleday & Company, Inc., 1984.
4. Bronfen, Nan. *Nutrition for a Better Life.* Santa Barbara, California: Capra Press, 1980.
5. Burkitt, Denis, M.D., F.R.C.S., F.R.S. *Eat right - to stay healthy and enjoy life more.* New York, New York: Arco Publishing, 1979.
6. Dunne, Lavon J. *Nutrition Almanac.* New York, New York: McGraw Hill Publishing Company, 1990.
7. Guyton, Arthur C., M.D. *Textbook of Medical Physiology.* Philadelphia, Pennsylvania: W.B. Sanders Company, 1976.
8. Klaper, Michael, M.D. *Pregnancy, Children and the Vegan Diet.* Umatilla, Florida: Gentle World Inc., 1987.
9. Langley, Gill, M.A., Ph.D. *Vegan Nutrition.* Oxford, England: The Vegan Society Ltd., 1988.
10. Leonard, Jon N., and J.L. Hofer and Nathan Pritikin. *Live Longer Now.*
11. McDougall, John A., M.D. *McDougall's Medicine.* Piscataway, New Jersey: New Century Publishers, Inc., 1985.
12. McDougall, John A., M.D., and Mary A. McDougall. *The McDougall Plan.* Piscataway, New Jersey: New Century Publishers, Inc., 1983.
13. Pritikin, Nathan. *The Pritikin Permanent Weight Loss Manual.* New York, New York: Grosset and Dunlap, 1981.
14. Pritikin, Nathan. *The Pritikin Program for Diet and Exerclse.* New York, New York: Grosset and Dunlap, 1979.
15. Robbins, John. *Diet for a New America.* Walpole, New Hampshire: Stillpoint Publishing, 1987.
16. Sattilaro, Anthony J., M.D. *Recalled for Life.* New York, New York: Avon Books, 1982.
17. Swank, Roy Haver, M.D., and Barbara Brewer Dugan. The Multiple Sclerosis Diet Book. New York, New York: Doubleday 1977
18. Webb, Densie, Ph.D., R.D. The Complete "Lite" Foods Calorie, Fat Cholesterol and Sodium Counter, New York, New York: Bantam Books, 1990
19. Whitaker, Julian M., M.D. *Reversing Diabetes.* New York, New York: Warner Books, Inc., 1987
20. Whitaker, Julian., M., M.D. *Reversing Heart Disease.* New York, New York: Warner Books, Inc., 1985

How to Look Great & Feel Sexy

INDEX

BROWN RICE MUSHROOM RING, 315
BROWN RICE PUDDING, 231
BROWN RICE WITH ZUCCHINI, 315
BUCKWHEAT PANCAKES, 197
BULGUR WHEAT AND CHICK PEA
  SALAD, 371
BURGER BUNS, 209
BURRITOS, 257

C

CABBAGE - VEGETABLE SOUP, 346
CABBAGE PLATE, 322
CABBAGE ROLLS, 322
CABBAGE SALAD WITH DILL, 371
CAROB BROWNIES, 214
CARROT - APPLE JUICE, 183
CARROT AND FRUIT SALAD, 372
CARROT AND PARSNIP SOUP, 346
CARROT BREAD, 205
CARROT CAKE, 216
CARROT CASSEROLE, 302
CARROT SALAD, 275, 371
CARROT SOUFFLE FOR ONE, 325
CAULIFLOWER CURRY, 326
CAULIFLOWER MARINADE SALAD,
  373
CAULIFLOWER SOUP, 346
CAULIFLOWER WITH HERB VINEGAR,
  372
CHAROSES, 232
CHERRY COBBLER, 228
CHERRY SOUP, 242
CHICK - PEA SOUP, 348
CHICK PEA AND PASTA SALAD, 373
CHILES RELLENOS, 261
CHILI BEAN SOUP, 346
CHILI BEAN STUFFED PEPPERS, 260
CHILI BEANS I, 259
CHILI BEANS II, 259
CHILI PIE, 260
CHILI RANCH STYLE, 259
CHILI SAUCE DIP, 173
CHINESE BROCCOLI, CAULIFLOWER,
  & ALMONDS, 271
CHINESE EGGPLANT, 272
CHINESE FRIED RICE WITHOUT OIL,
  282
CHINESE FRUIT SALAD, 275
CHINESE HOT AND SOUR SOUP, 347
CHINESE HOT SALAD, 374
CHINESE NOODLES, 278
CHINESE SALAD, 373
CHINESE SALAD - RAW, 276
CHINESE SPICY VEGETABLES, 272
CHINESE TOMATO, 347

CHOCOLATE BANANA BROWNIES, 220
CHOCOLATE BANANA ICE CREAM, 234
CHOP SUEY, 284
CHOW MEIN I, 285
CHOW MEIN II, 285
CIDER ZUCCHINI SOUP, 348
CINNAMON PRUNE STICKS, 201
COFFEE CAKE, 217
COFFEE CAKE TOPPING, 217
COLD AVOCADO BEAN SOUP, 348
COLD NOODLE SALAD, 276
COLD TOMATO HERB SOUP, 352
COLESLAW, 374
CORN - ON - THE - COB, 326
CORN AND BROWN RICE STIR - FRY,
  315
CORN BREAD STUFFING, 326
CORN CHOWDER, 350
CORN TORTILLAS, 258
CORN ZUCCHINI CASSEROLE, 302
CORNMEAL HOT CEREAL, 195
CRANBERRY DELIGHT, 181
CRANBERRY GLOG, 182
CRANBERRY SAUCE, 173
CRANBERRY TEA PUNCH, 182
CRANBERRY SPRITZER, 182
CREOLE CASSEROLE, 303
CREPES, 192
CRUMB TOPPED FRUIT PIE, 222
CRUNCHY BEST SLAW, 375
CRUNCHY CARROT CAKE, 216
CRUNCHY PEA SALAD, 375
CRUNCHY RICE AND PEAS, 315
CUCUMBER DRESSING, 386
CUCUMBER MARINADE, 372
CUCUMBER ONION DIP, 174
CUCUMBER SALAD, 276
CURRIED CREAM OF BROCCOLI SOUP,
  349
CURRIED LENTILS AND BROWN RICE,
  316
CURRIED ZUCCHINI SOUP, 349

D

DAL, 326
DATE CAKE, 219
DATE FROSTING, 220
DATE NUT BREAD PUDDING, 231
DELGADO GADO, 329
DELICIOUS CORNBREAD, 207
DILLED GARDEN BEANS, 327

How to Look Great & Feel Sexy

How to Look Great, Feel Younger, Stronger and Sexier in 90 days*

"How to Look Great & Feel Sexy!" Only $31.95
Did you know that there are eight natural hormones in our bodies that control everything from our energy levels and libido to how fast we age? In fact, many of the complaints associated with aging such as decreased vitality and sex drive, increased body fat, and slower mental processing can be alleviated just by restoring these hormones to youthful levels!

Read this book by Dr. Nick Delgado, sought after speaker, talk show host, presenter of over 3,500 seminars, and an expert on aging and nutrition. He'll reveal how these hormones are helping thousands discover the secret of "The Fountain of Youth" - often within 90 days! And his simple techniques guarantee even the busiest people can get immediate results.
The book "How to Look Great & Feel Sexy!" explains:
- Amazing facts about diet programs to avoid like the Zone, Slim Fast, Weight Watchers, and Phen Fen.
- Ways to reduce the risk of heart attacks and strokes and improve the immune system in only 9 days.
- How testosterone and DHEA renew strength, reduce body fat, and improve sexual potency past age 40.
- How to determine the levels of each of these hormones in your own body.
- Where to find the best natural hormones rather than prescribed synthetics.
- How to improve mental acuity in 30 days with a combination of hormones, diet, and exercise.

Dr. Delgado, former director of the Nathan Pritikin program, conducts programs for Tony Robbins at Mastery University. This book, "How to Look Great & Feel Sexy!" discusses the latest on nutrition, exercise, vitamins, minerals, and hormones. You will learn techniques for achieving optimal mental attitude to achieve maximum health! Enjoy 600 tasty recipes, including Italian, Chinese, Mexican, Thai, and American cuisine's. 400 pages.

"Mastering the Powers of Your Inner Health" Only $19.95
This book gives you the secrets of how to live life to the fullest, beginning with practical information on nutrition for infants and the nursing or pregnant mother. You will find out the best drug free ways to build up muscle and reduce body fat. "Mastering the Powers of Your Inner Health" shows you how to enhance the immune system and overcome allergy symptoms. Discover how to establish health as a priority within your values and goals.

"Reverse Aging" Series 12 Cassette Tapes. Only $129
You will hear the essence of the best interviews conducted by Dr. Nick Delgado on his television program. Discussions cover slowing the aging process with nutrition, natural hormones, herb's, exercise, stress reduction and smoking cessation. Tapes on humor, happiness, fitness and discipline for busy people, how to preserve the earth's resources, senile brain damage from meat, male sexual impotency, and the reversal of atherosclerosis. Also learn relief for neck and back pain, improving circulation, skin rejuvenation, oxygen therapy, cosmetic procedures, supplements, homeopathy and allergies.

"Look and Feel Great" 8 audio tapes. Only $89.95
These tapes explain how to establish new winning habits, helping you to lose unwanted body fat and gain lean muscle tissue. This program will bring you high-energy living. Discover how to reduce cholesterol, triglycerides and achieve ideal body weight. Shop at the supermarket and order healthfully dinning out at almost any restaurant. Learn the cause and prevention of heart disease, diabetes, arthritis, cancer, osteoporosis, hypertension, hearing loss, digestive problems, ulcers, hernia, gallstones and varicose veins.

CD-ROM "Live Long & Love It!" $29.95
Dr. Delgado's plan provides an entertaining and informative multi-media experience. A dynamite addition toward personalizing your health & fitness plan. PC Minimum Requirements: 486/25Mhz w/10MB available on hard drive, 4MB RAM, SVGA, CD-ROM, Sound Card, Mouse, Windows™ 3.1, DOS 5.0 or higher and MPC Level 1 complaint.

"Wellness" video $23.95
Nick's dynamic video tape of his most popular nutrition presentation will stimulate and motivate you to stay on the health track. Filled with information that you can see and use now.

"Good Safe Sex" video and audio. Only $69
You'll appreciate the candor of this helpful discussion on sex. The audio: Sex is the Sizzle in Relationships. The video: Tasteful discussion of love-making techniques that will improve your sexual intimacy and transcend your relationship.

Special $229: "Reverse Aging" 12 audio tapes + "Look & Feel Great" 8 audio tapes and "Wellness" video.

* Money Back Guarantee - Study this program for 90 days, keep a wellness record of your body fat, cholesterol lipid level, exercise, supplements and 24 hour food recall once a week. If this program helps you to improve your health beyond your present level you will have met the Delgado challenge. If not satisfied, just send in a record of your tests and wellness diary and a refund minus shipping and handling costs will be returned without question.

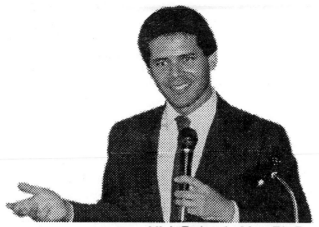

Nick Delgado Ms., Ph.D.
HEALTHY STUDIOS ®

25422 Trabuco Road, #105-141
Lake Forest, California 92630

<u>Inquiries; Orders **800-631-0232**</u>

Change the Course of Your Life Experience with the Best Health that You Can Attain.

Qty	Description	Unit Price	Total
	Special 20 Audio Tapes, 1 Wellness Video	$229.00	
	Reverse Aging Series - 12 Audio Tapes	$129.00	
	Delgado Diet and Exercise Plan - 8 audios	$89.95	
	Sex Series - 1 video, 1 audio tape	$69.00	
	"How to Look Great; & Feel Sexy"	$31.95	
	Nick's book titled "Fatigue to Vitality"	$22.95	
	"Mastering the Powers of Your Inner Health" Book	$19.95	
	Wellness - video	$23.95	
	Diet and Exercise Plan - CD ROM	$29.95	

USE THIS HANDY ORDER FORM

Postage & Handling			
Order Total	Postage	SubTotal	
Up to $35...............................$5		Postage and Handling	
Over $35...............................$9		Add 8% State Tax	
		TOTAL ENCLOSED	
Canada and Europe........Add $18			
Australia and Asia.........Add $35			

Allow 4 weeks for delivery.
_____*PAL video tapes add $10 per video*

Mail To: **Nick Delgado, Ms. Ph.D.**
Healthy Studios
25422 Trabuco Rd., #105-141
Lake Forest, CA 92630

FAX Orders **714-951-7013**
For Credit Card Orders Call
800-631-0232
(Leave detailed message of order, credit card #& expiration date.)

Today's Date:_____

Send to:

Name _____

Address _____

City/St/Zip _____

Daytime Phone_____

MasterCard _____ Visa _____ AmEx_____

CC# _____ Exp. Date_____

Signature _____